PREGNANCY SERIES I

PREGNANCY SERIES I

ALL YOU NEED TO KNOW ABOUT ANTENATAL CARE

AUTHORS:

DR. M. ABBEY

FELLOW FETAL MEDICINE FOUNDATION FMF LONDON,
MRCOG, PHD O&G, DMAS, VRACH/MBBS.

PROF. C. I. AKANI

MBBS IBADAN, FWACS, FICS.
PROVOST COLLEGE OF HEALTH SCIENCES,
UNIVERSITY OF PORT HARCOURT, RIVERS STATE, NIGERIA.

To order additional copies of this book, contact:
Xlibris
0-800-056-3182
www.xlibrispublishing.co.uk
Orders@xlibrispublishing.co.uk
517227

CONTENTS

List of Abbreviation

AC—Abdominal circumference
ACE—Angiotensin-converting enzyme
ACT—Artemisinin-based combination therapy
A&E unit—Accident and Emergency unit
AFP—Alpha-fetoprotein
AFV—Amniotic fluid volume
AIDS—Acquired immunodeficiency syndrome
APH—Antepartum haemorrhage aPL—ntiphospholipid antibodies
ART—Antiretroviral treatment
BMI—Body mass index
BP—Blood pressure
BV—Bacterial vaginosis
CBT—Cognitive behavioural therapy
C-CBT—Computer-based cognitive behavioural therapy
CEFM—Continuous electronic foetal monitoring
CMV—Cytomegalovirus
CRL—Crown-rump length
CTG—Cardiotocogram
CTPA—Computed tomography pulmonary angiogram
CVS—Chorionic villus sampling
DC—Dichorionic
DCDA—Dichorionic diamniotic
DNA—Deoxyribonucleic acid
DR—Detection rates
DVT—Deep venous thrombosis
EDD—Expected date of delivery
EFM—Electronic foetal monitoring
EFW—Expected foetal weight
EPAU—Early pregnancy assessment unit
FGR—Foetal growth restriction
FHR—Foetal heart rate
FPR—False positive rate
FMF—Foetal Medicine Foundation
FSH—Follicle-stimulating hormone
FVS—Foetal varicella syndrome
GA—Gestational age
GAD—Generalised anxiety disorder
GBS infection—Group B Streptococcus infection
GDM—Gestational diabetes mellitus
G6PD—Glucose-6-phosphate dihydrogenase deficiency

GP—General practitioner
GTT—Glucose tolerant test
HAART—Highly active antiretroviral therapy
HbA1C—Glycosylated haemoglobin
HBGM—Home blood glucose monitoring
HBV—Hepatitis B virus
HC—Head circumference
HCG—Human chorionic gonadotrophin
HIP—High blood pressure in pregnancy
HG—Hyperemesis gravidarum
HIV—Human immunodeficiency virus
HSV—Herpes simplex virus
IDDM—Insulin-dependent diabetes mellitus
INR—International normalised ratio
IOL—Induction of labour
IPT—Interpersonal therapy
ITN—Insecticide-treated nets
IVF—In vitro fertilisation
LBW—Low birth weight
LFD baby—Large-for-date baby
LFTs—Liver function tests
LGA—Large for gestational age
LH—Luteinising hormone
LMWH—Low-molecular-weight heparin
LMWH—Low-molecular-weight heparin
MC—Monochorionic
MCA—Middle cerebral artery
MCDA—Monochorionic diamniotic
MCMA—Monochorionic monoamniotic
MSU—Mid-stream urine
MMR—Measles, mumps, and rubella
NB—Nasal bone
NHS—National Health Service
NICE—National Institute of Clinical Excellence
NT—Nuchal translucency
NVP—Nausea and vomiting in pregnancy
OGTT—Oral glucose tolerance test
OC—Obstetric cholestasis
PAPP-A Pregnancy-associated plasma protein-A
PCP—Polycystic carinii parasitical infection
PCOD—Polycystic ovarian disease
PE—Pre-eclampsia

PIH—Pregnancy-induced hypertension

PP—Presenting part

PPROM—Preterm pre-labour rupture of the membranes

PPH—Post-partum haemorrhage

PRN—pro re nata (as the situation demands)

PTD—Preterm delivery

PTE—Pulmonary thromboembolism

PUL—Pregnancy of unknown location

RCOG—Royal College of Obstetricians and Gynaecologists

RBG—Random blood glucose

RFM—Reduced foetal movements

RM—Recurrent miscarriage

SCD—Sickle-cell disease

SFH—Symphysis-fundal height

SGA—Small for gestational age

SMP—Statutory Maternity Pay

SP—Sulphadoxine-pyrimethamine

STI—Sexually transmitted infection

T21—Trisomy 21 (Down's syndrome)

T13—Trisomy 13 (Patau's syndrome)

T18—Trisomy 18 (Edwards' syndrome)

TOP—Termination of pregnancy

TORCH—Toxoplasmosis, rubella, cytomegalovirus, herpes

TTTS—Twin-to-twin transfusion syndrome uE3—Unconjugated oestriol

UCLH—University College London Hospital

VBAC—Vaginal birth after Caesarean

WHO—World Health Organisation

VTE—Venous thromboembolism

V/Q—Ventilation/perfusion

VZIG—Varicella-zoster Immunoglobulin

Prepregnancy Care—Before You Get Pregnant

DEFINITION

Prepregnancy (preconception) health care is care given to you before pregnancy to manage conditions and behaviours which could be a risk to you or your future baby. So if you are planning to become pregnant, make an appointment with your doctor, who will offer you the care in the clinic. It is advised that your partner attends the clinic with you; your chances of getting pregnant will increase if he is in good health, too.

PREPREGNANCY-TO-PREGNANCY INTERVAL

This is the interval from the time that you start trying for a baby to the date that you actually become pregnant; it should be at least 3 months. You should start observing the following recommendations even sooner: quit smoking, reach healthy weight, and adjust your medications.

REPRODUCTIVE LIFE PLAN

This is a plan about 'when' and under what conditions you want to become pregnant. It also includes how to achieve those goals. Here are some examples:

- You may decide not to be pregnant until you have finished your university. You may, therefore, abstain from heterosexual sex or use a contraceptive.
- You may decide to have children when your relationship feels secure and you have saved enough money.
- You may decide to have two children and space your pregnancies by at least 2 years.

REVIEW OF YOUR PAST OBSTETRIC, GYNAECOLOGICAL AND MEDICAL HISTORY

Your doctor will ask you about the following:

- Past pregnancies and their outcome
  - Deliveries: year, age of the pregnancy (gestational age, GA) at delivery, mode of delivery, complications at delivery, and baby's weight.
  - Pregnancy complications: pre-eclampsia (PE), preterm labour, and so on.
  - Miscarriages: GA when they occurred, number, and year.
  - Past terminations: gestational age when termination of pregnancy took place, number, and year.
  - History of twins in your family.
- Past gynaecological history including menstrual and sexual problems, smear test, contraceptives, previous gynaecological problems, for example infertility, polycystic ovarian disease (PCOD), fibroid, history of gynaecological operations, and so on.

The purpose of asking you these questions is to identify possible obstetric risk that may be associated with your previous history and then prevent them from happening in your next pregnancy.

PROMOTING HEALTHY BEHAVIOURS

HEALTHY EATING AND TAKING SUPPLEMENTS INCLUDING FOLIC ACID

Please see page xxx.

WEIGHT—OVERWEIGHT AND UNDERWEIGHT

If you are obese or overweight, you may have difficulty conceiving. If overweight, try to lose some weight before becoming pregnant, but not during pregnancy. Drastic dieting in the months during pregnancy could deprive your baby of essential foods. Women who are overweight have a greater risk of pregnancy complications (page 319). You can get rid of your excess weight by

- eating healthy foods.
- doing exercise.
- joining a slimming class.
- getting support from a friend or your partner.
- getting help from your doctor and a dietician.

If you are underweight (Body Mass Index, BMI, less than 18.5), you may have high risk of miscarriage and giving birth to a low-birth-weight (LBW) baby. Therefore, if you are slightly underweight, you can gain a few pounds to prepare for pregnancy.

LIFESTYLE MODIFICATION

SMOKING

If you smoke, you are strongly advised to stop before getting pregnant. Tobacco smoke contains poisonous chemicals which will pass into baby's blood and cause problems (pages 150-156). If you find it difficult to stop smoking, then seek advice and help from your practice nurse or your doctor. The prepregnancy period is often a good time to persuade your partner to give up smoking, too.

ALCOHOL

Ideally, it is necessary to stop drinking when you are planning for pregnancy because of the ill effects alcohol can have on you and your baby during pregnancy (page 156-159). If you find it difficult to cut down on or stop drinking alcohol, then seek help from your doctor.

PREVENTION OF INFECTIONS

Some infections can harm you and/or your baby during pregnancy. It is therefore important that measures are put in place to safeguard you from those infections. Infections that are sexually transmitted infections (STIs) include the following:

- HIV (human immunodeficiency virus) infection
- Hepatitis B and C
- Syphilis
- Chlamydia
- Others

HIV INFECTION

If you are HIV positive, you can pass the virus on to your baby during pregnancy, at birth, or when breastfeeding. The infection can cause harm to you and your baby (pages 298-306) during pregnancy. Your doctor will offer you HIV testing, even if you have no symptoms. If you are positive, your pregnancy will be planned accordingly.

HEPATITIS B

You should confirm with your doctor about your hepatitis B status. If you have had it in the past, your care will be planned accordingly (pages 277-279). If you are not immune, then you should be given a jab against it. It is always a good practice not to be pregnant 3 months after the jab.

SYPHILIS

You will be offered test for syphilis when you book for antenatal care. You may also choose to be tested for the infection when you are trying for baby. If your test is positive, you will be treated accordingly before trying for baby.

CHLAMYDIA

Chlamydia infection causes infertility, ectopic pregnancy, or miscarriage or may infect the baby at birth. If you think there is a chance that you or your partner might have been infected, both of you should seek investigation and treatment, if necessary, before you become pregnant.

NON-SEXUALLY TRANSMITTED INFECTIONS THAT CAN BE PREVENTED BY GIVING JABS (IMMUNISATION.)

RUBELLA OR GERMAN MEASLES (PAGES 289-293), MUMP, MEASLES.

Confirm with your doctor that you are protected (immunisation) against these infections; you may need to have a blood test for that. If you are not protected, then you should be given the measles, mumps, and rubella (MMR) jab. You will need to wait for 3 months after the injection before trying for a baby. If you find out during pregnancy that you are not immune against, you should be offered an MMR immunisation immediately after your baby is born.

CHICKENPOX

If you have had chickenpox in the past, you will not have it again in the future, that is you are immune against it. If you are not sure about your status, then a blood test may be done to confirm it. If you are not immune, then you should be offered varicella-zoster vaccine. Chickenpox during pregnancy can affect you and your baby adversely (pages 279-285). The vaccination cannot be given during pregnancy, and you should avoid getting pregnant for 3 months after the injection.

OTHER INFECTIONS THAT CAN BE PREVENTED BY GIVING YOU JABS.
Women in their reproductive years should also have immunisations as a routine part of preventive care against the following infections:.

- Tetanus-diphtheria booster (every 10 years)
- Human papillomavirus (the vaccine is given once between the ages of 9 and 26)
- Influenza vaccine—especially if you live in the region of the world where there are cold seasons (autumn, winter, spring)

ASSESSMENT FOR GENETIC DISEASE

SICKLE-CELL DISEASE AND THALASSAEMIA
These are blood diseases. Some people are carriers of the genes for these diseases but do not actually have the disease itself. If the mother has any of the diseases or two carriers have a baby, then there is a risk that the baby will be born with the disease. If screening for these conditions was not performed before marriage, it should be carried out before trying for a baby. Your doctor will discuss this further with you.

CYSTIC FIBROSIS
In Europe, testing for cystic fibrosis is offered, but not universally. It is a lifelong illness (usually diagnosed in the first few years of life), which causes problems with digestion and breathing. The risk is higher if both you and your partner have Caucasian ancestry. A blood test before pregnancy or in early pregnancy can tell if you or your partner carry the gene that causes the disease and, thereby, indirectly assess the chance of your unborn baby having it.

PRE-EXISTING HEALTH PROBLEMS
Women who have medical problems may need special care when preparing to get pregnant and also during pregnancy. Therefore, you should see your doctor when preparing for pregnancy if you have any medical problems, especially those outlined below.

• Diabetes	• High blood pressure (BP)
• Epilepsy	• Obesity
• Certain infections, for example HIV	• Diseases of different organs and systems of the body
• Eating disorders	• Mental health issues (such as depression), and so on

DOMESTIC VIOLENCE

If you are a victim of domestic violence, you are even more likely to be abused during pregnancy. So inform your doctor, nurse, or social worker when it happens. In the developed countries, you can be helped to get in touch with support services for abused women, such as crisis hotlines, domestic violence programmes, legal aid services, or counselling.

STREET DRUGS

If you take street drugs by mouth or you inject them, you are strongly advised to stop before getting pregnant. Drugs such as cannabis, heroin, crack cocaine, amphetamines, and so on, are likely to affect fertility adversely, cause miscarriage, increase the risk of premature or low birth weight babies, and may cause damage to the developing baby. The safest course of action, therefore, is to avoid using any of these drugs before and during pregnancy. If you cannot come off drugs easily, see your doctor for help.

YOUR MEDICATION

If either you or your partner is taking medication for an illness or long-term condition, ask your general practitioner (GP) or consultant whether it might affect the pregnancy. If there is a risk to the pregnancy, you might want to ask whether the medication could be changed, reduced, or even stopped. On the other hand, you may need to balance the risks to your pregnancy with the risks to your health without the medication. Some of these medications are as follows:

- Drugs used for the treatment of high BP or epilepsy.
- Isotretinoin—used for treatment of cystic acne. It is associated with increased risk of miscarriage and developmental defect.
- Streptomycin—causes hearing loss in the baby.
- Tetracycline—causes underdevelopment of the teeth. It is also absorbed into bone.

Generally, when trying for a baby or during pregnancy, it is advised to consult your doctor before taking any drug.

ENVIRONMENTAL ISSUES, HOME AND WORKPLACE HAZARDS

HEAT HAZWARD

Research has shown that high heat from a fever, hot bath, or hot tub during the first 3 months of pregnancy may cause birth defects. You may not know that you are pregnant during the first 4 weeks, so it is better to avoid heat when trying for a baby and also during pregnancy.

HARMFUL SUBSTANCES

Some substances found at home or work can make it harder for you to become pregnant or can harm your foetus, for example heavy metals like lead, copper, and mercury; radiation, acids, anaesthetic gases, and carbon disulphide. Talk with your doctor about your workplace and home environments to find out if there are any dangers.

You should be sure that your job does not pose a risk to you or your baby. Some risks can be avoided, for example, by changing your working conditions or hours of work. If a risk cannot be avoided, your employer should offer you suitable alternative work with similar terms and conditions to your present job. If this is not possible, you should be suspended on full pay. This is what is obtainable in developed countries.

METHYLMERCURY AND LEAD

Some fish contain high levels of methylmercury, which can harm an unborn child's developing nervous system. These fishes are swordfish, tilefish, king mackerel, and shark. So if you're thinking about becoming pregnant, you should be aware of these risks and take steps to prevent exposure to mercury. Lead is used in industries that deal with lead smelting, paint manufacture, printing, ceramics, and pottery glazing, and so on. It can adversely affect the development of your baby's brain, so avoid it.

HUSBAND OR PARTNER AND PREPREGNANCY CARE

It takes two to be pregnant. The physical health of a couple in the 3 months before conception will influence the quality of both the sperm and the egg which will eventually join to produce a baby. Sperm are produced constantly and take 12 weeks to become mature. A bad diet, smoking, drinking, taking illicit drugs, and unhealthy working conditions can affect immature sperm adversely and therefore stop you getting pregnant.

It is, therefore, worth ensuring that you and your partner are both in good health before conceiving. Your partner can improve his own reproductive health by observing everything that has been suggested for you, as outlined above.

Your partner's fertility can be affected by exposure to chemicals used in photography, solvents, heavy metals such as lead and mercury, and some pesticides. They can damage sperm. If your partner works with chemicals or other toxins, he needs to be careful so that he does not expose you to them. For example, if he uses fertilisers or pesticides in agricultural jobs, he should change out of dirty work clothes before coming near to you. He should handle and wash soiled clothes separately.

SOURCES

- The UK NHS Pregnancy Book. Your complete guide to: a healthy pregnancy, labour and childbirth, 2009.
- Prepregnancy counselling. American College of Obstetricians and Gynecologists. ISSN 1074-8601. January 2007.
- Department of health and human resources. Centre for Disease Control and Prevention. Preconception Care Questions and Answers. April 2006.
- Preparing for another pregnancy. A brief guide to pre-pregnancy care after miscarriage. The Miscarriage Association, 2000, revised 2005, 2007.
- Antenatal Care: Routine Care for the Healthy Pregnant Woman. NICE Clinical Guideline, March 2008.

The Reproductive System

THE MALE REPRODUCTIVE SYSTEM

The system gives men the ability to fertilise an egg and produce a baby. It is made up of the following organs as illustrated in figure1:

- Testes
- Scrotum
- Penis
- Several tubules (epididymis, vas or ductus deferens, ejaculatory duct, urethra)
- Accessory sex glands (prostate gland, seminal vesicles, and Cowper's or bulbourethral glands)

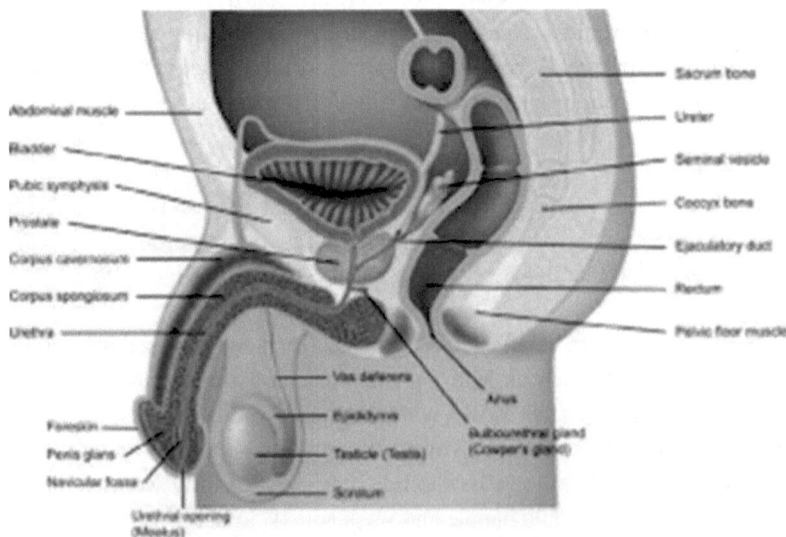

Figure 1. Male reproductive organ

Scrotum: This is a fleshy sac of skin between the upper thighs. The major function of the scrotum is to keep the testes cooler than the body temperature in order to enhance sperm production. The scrotum brings the testes closer to the heat of the body in the pelvic region when the ambient temperature is cold and takes the testes away from the body when it is warm.

Testes and the tubules: The testes are located in the scrotum. The hormone testosterone, which is produced in the testes, stimulates the production of immature sperm cells; these cells are then stored in the epididymis where they complete their maturation. The epididymis is an approximately 2-inch long tube and coiled at the top and to the back of each testis. The left and right epididymides continue into the left and right vas deferens. These tubules enter into the prostate where each joins with the tubule from the seminal vesicles of its side to form the ejaculatory duct, which then empties into the urethra.

The urethra: This is the last part of the urinary tract that runs down the length of the penis from the bladder, through the prostate gland, to an opening at the tip of the penis. It is both a passage for urine and for the ejaculation of semen, which contains sperm and seminal vesicle fluids.

The penis: It contains the urethra and is made up of three main parts - the root, body, and the glans. The root is the part which is attached to the lower abdomen. The body is made up of a spongy tissue, which swells when blood enters into it and becomes hard and erect. The glans is the slightly larger area which is located towards the end of the penis and contains the opening of the urethra.

FUNCTIONS OF THE MALE REPRODUCTIVE SYSTEM
- The male reproductive cell called sperm fertilises the female reproductive cell called the ovum.
- It helps men to develop the characteristics associated with being male, namely pubic hair, enlargement of the penis, and deepening of the voice.

SPERM PATHWAY AND THE PROCESS OF EJACULATION AND FERTILISATION

When orgasm occurs, the muscles around the reproductive organs contract and sperm is forcefully expelled from the epididymis into the vas deferens, the ejaculatory duct, the urethra, and then the vagina at the speed of about 70 mph. This process is called ejaculation and is not consciously controlled. The accessory glands release seminal fluid into the urethra where it mixes with sperm when it reaches there to form semen. The semen and urine do not mix because when the sperm reaches the urethra, the opening that drains urine from the bladder into the urethra closes up. From the vagina, semen makes its way up through the cervix, the uterus, and then the fallopian tube, where it meets the egg, if ovulation has already taken place. Fertilisation then takes place.

THE FEMALE REPRODUCTIVE SYSTEM

INTRODUCTION
The female reproductive system is divided into two parts:
- External sex organs
- Internal sex organs

THE EXTERNAL SEX ORGANS (VULVA)
They are as illustrated in figure 2 and include the following:
- Mons pubis
- Labia majora (outer lips of the vulva)
- Labia minora (inner lips of the vulva)
- Clitoris
- Opening of the urethra (meatus)
- Vaginal vestibule
- Vestibular bulbs
- Vestibular glands

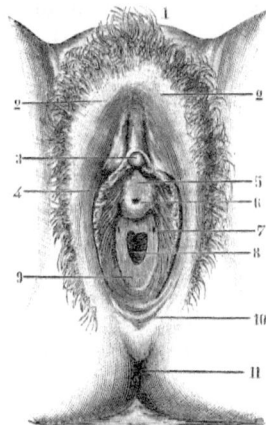

Figure 2—Front to rear view of the vulva

MONS PUBIS
This is fatty tissue covering the pubic bone. It protects the pubic bone and vulva from the impact of sexual intercourse. After puberty, it is covered with pubic hair, usually in a triangular shape.

THE LIPS OF THE VULVA

The two outer lips (labia majora) wrap around the vulva from the mons pubis to the perineum. They are usually covered with hair and contain numerous sweat and oil glands. The two inner lips of the vulva (labia minora) lie within the labia majora fold and protect the vagina, urethra, and clitoris. There is no hair on them, but there are oil glands. Both the labia majora and minora are quite sensitive to touch and pressure.

CLITORIS

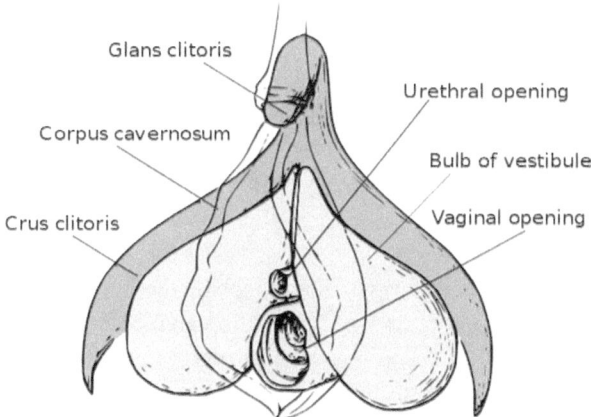

Figure 3. Clitoris (from the free encyclopaedia Wikipedia)

It lies between the top of the labia minora. Only the tip or glans of the clitoris is seen, but the organ itself is long and branches into two forks called the crura, which extend downwards along the rim of the vaginal opening towards the perineum (figure 3).

During sexual excitement, the clitoris erects and extends, and the hood (spongy tissue formed by the two labia minora at the top of the clitoris) retracts, making the clitoral glans more accessible. The size of the glans varies between women. In some, it is very small, while in others, it is large.

OPENING OF THE URETHRA

The urethra is the urinary pipe that takes urine from the bladder to outside the body and is 1.5 inches long. Its opening lies just below the clitoris. It is not a sex organ. Because the urethra is so close to the anus, women should always wipe themselves from front to back to avoid infecting the vagina and urethra with bacteria.

HYMEN

The hymen is a thin fold of membrane that separates the entrance into the vagina from the urethral opening. Contrary to traditional belief, an intact hymen is a poor indicator of virginity because a normal hymen does not always completely block the vaginal opening. A woman can actually have the first sexual encounter with the hymen still present after the act.

Furthermore, the blood that is sometimes, but not always, observed after first penetration can be due to the tearing of the hymen or it can also be from injury to nearby tissues. Masturbation and tampon insertion can, but are generally not forceful enough to, cause penetrating trauma to the hymen.

PERINEUM

The perineum is the short stretch of skin starting at the bottom of the vulva and extending to the anus. This area forms the floor of the pelvis. In some women, the perineum may tear or may be cut during childbirth to enhance delivery.

INTERNAL SEX ORGANS

The organs are as illustrated in figure 4 and include the following:

- Vagina
- Cervix
- Uterus
- Fallopian tube
- Ovaries

VAGINA

The vagina is a canal that leads from the cervix down to the vulva, where it opens out between the legs. It is situated between the urinary bladder and the rectum and is about 8 cm (3 inches) long. The muscular walls are lined with mucous, which keeps it protected and moist. The vagina is very elastic, so it can easily stretch around a man's penis during sex or around a baby during labour. The sperm that survive the acidic condition of the vagina continue on through the cervix and uterus to the fallopian tubes, where fertilisation may occur.

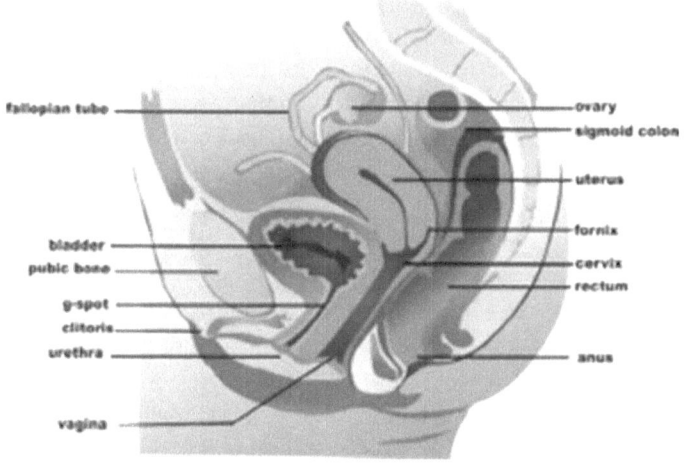

Figure 4. Cross-sectional diagram of the female reproductive organs

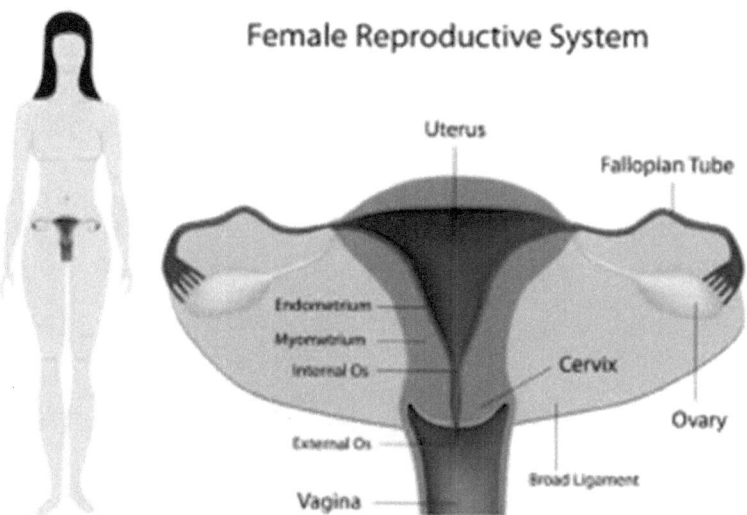

Figure 5. Projection of the female reproductive organs on the body.

CERVIX

The cervix is the neck of the womb; it joins with the top end of the vagina. It is conical in shape and protrudes through the upper anterior vaginal wall into the vaginal space. Approximately half its length is visible to the naked eye, the remainder lies above the vagina beyond view. During labour it retracts and opens and is taken up completely(effaced)

23

UTERUS

The uterus or womb is the major female reproductive organ. It contains three suspensory ligaments that help stabilize its position and limits its range of movement. It is a pear-shaped muscular organ that accepts a fertilized egg which becomes implanted into its lining the endometrium. It houses the baby during pregnancy, contacts, retracts, opens up and expels the baby during labour and childbirth.

FALLOPIAN TUBES

These are narrow tubes that are attached to the either side of the upper part of the uterus. At the other end of each fallopian tube is a fringed area that looks like a funnel. This fringed area, called the infundibulum, lies close to the ovary but is not attached. Within each tube is a tiny passageway through which the egg passes.

OVARIES

The ovaries are small, oval-shaped glands that are located on either side of the uterus. They produce eggs (ova) and the female sex hormones; the latter are released into the blood.

THE PELVIS

The pelvis is the bony structure through which baby passes during childbirth.

HIP JOINT
OSTEOARTHRITIS

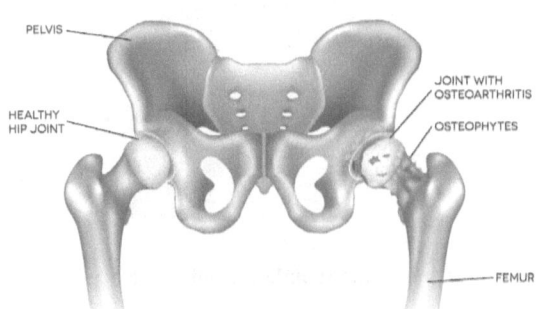

Figure 6. The bony pelvis

SOURCES

- American Social Health Association; www.ashastd.org
- Human Anatomy by Kent M. Van De Graaff, 2002. ISBN-10: 0072907932 | ISBN-13: 9780072907933

- Human female reproductive system. Wikipedia
- RCOG Pregnancy Book, 2008.
- Valerie C. Scanlon and Tina Sanders, Essentials of anatomy and physiology, by Web MD, http://www.webmd.com
- Wikibook: Sexual Health.
- www.patient.co.uk

The Menstrual Cycle and Getting Pregnant

INTRODUCTION

The menstrual cycle is defined as the duration from the first day of your menstruation, that is day 1 of bleeding, to day 1 of your next menstruation, and it normally lasts for about 28 days, but it can be less or more.

In this chapter, we will discuss what happens during your menstrual cycle, including the period in a month when you are likely to be pregnant. We will also explain the natural process of getting pregnant, signs and symptoms of pregnancy, and your reaction to it.

THE FIRST PHASE OF THE MENSTRUAL CYCLE
(FIRST 14 DAYS OF A 28-DAY CYCLE)

The first phase of the cycle involves development of the egg in your ovary and ovulation. The sequence of events that take place during this first phase is as following:

- Menstruation for about 5-7 days, starting from day 1 of the cycle.
- Development of about 20 small immature follicles in the ovaries from the last few days of menstruation. This continues throughout the cycle. A follicle is a female reproductive unit and is made up of a group of cells including the egg.
- Two hormones are produced in the brain by the pituitary gland, and they are discharged into the bloodstream; one of them called follicle-stimulating hormone (FSH) encourages the maturation of the follicles while luteinising hormone is very important during ovulation.
- The follicles start to release increasing amounts of hormone called oestrogen as they grow. The more the oestrogen produced, the less the amount of the hormone FSH released in the brain; this process is called 'a negative feedback'. This helps to prevent too many follicles growing at the same time. Eventually, one follicle outgrows the rest and becomes the mature follicle.
- Ovulation.

OVULATION

This is the process by which the egg from a mature follicle is released into the pelvis. It normally occurs each month and usually takes place around the fourteenth day of a 28-day cycle. Occasionally, more than one egg is released, usually within 24 hours of the first egg.

Around the time that ovulation is to occur, the follicles produce very high levels of oestrogen. In contrast to the negative feedback as stated above, these high levels of oestrogen encourage the brain to release more FSH into the bloodstream, and this is called 'a positive feedback'. At this point, another hormone that is produced in the brain called luteinising hormone (LH) encourages the follicle to burst through the outer layer of the ovary and release the egg—ovulation has taken place. The egg is then swept into the pelvic cavity (open space in the pelvis). The 'fingers' at the end of the fallopian tube then help to direct the egg down into it.

During this first phase of the menstrual cycle, the oestrogen that is produced stimulates the repair of the lining of the uterus, which was destroyed by menstruation. Furthermore, the mucus in the cervix, which was originally thick before menstruation, becomes thin under the influence of oestrogen so that sperm can easily swim through it.

SIGNS OF OVULATION
- Thinning of the mucus in the cervix.
- Temperature change: Temperature should be checked first thing in the morning before you get out of bed. In the first phase of the cycle, a normal temperature will be around 97.0-98.0 Fahrenheit (36-36.7oC.) On the day of ovulation, the temperature spikes down, usually into the 96.0-97.0 Fahrenheit range (35.6-36, oC.) and then the next morning, it will spike up to normal of around 98.6 Fahrenheit (37oC.) and stay in that range until menstruation begins.

THE SECOND PHASE OF THE MENSTRUAL CYCLE
(SECOND 14 DAYS OF A 28-DAY CYCLE)
What happens in the second phase of the cycle depends on whether the egg is fertilised or not.

THE EGG IS NOT FERTILISED
What is left of the mature follicle after the egg is released develops into another group of cells called the 'corpus luteum'(yellow body), which produces the hormones progesterone and oestrogen. Progesterone supports secretion in the womb. The yellow body can live only for a further 2 weeks after ovulation. As it begins to breakdown, it secretes less of its hormones.

The decrease in progesterone secretion caused by the breakdown of the yellow body stimulates the release of chemicals that eventually bring about shedding of the lining of the womb, which appears as the menstrual blood flow.

The low levels of oestrogen and progesterone that are produced by the yellow body can no longer control the levels of the two hormones FSH and LH, which are produced in the brain - no more negative feedback. So the secretion of the two hormones increases, and new follicles with their eggs begin to develop in the ovaries. This is the start of a new menstrual cycle, which begins with menstrual bleeding.

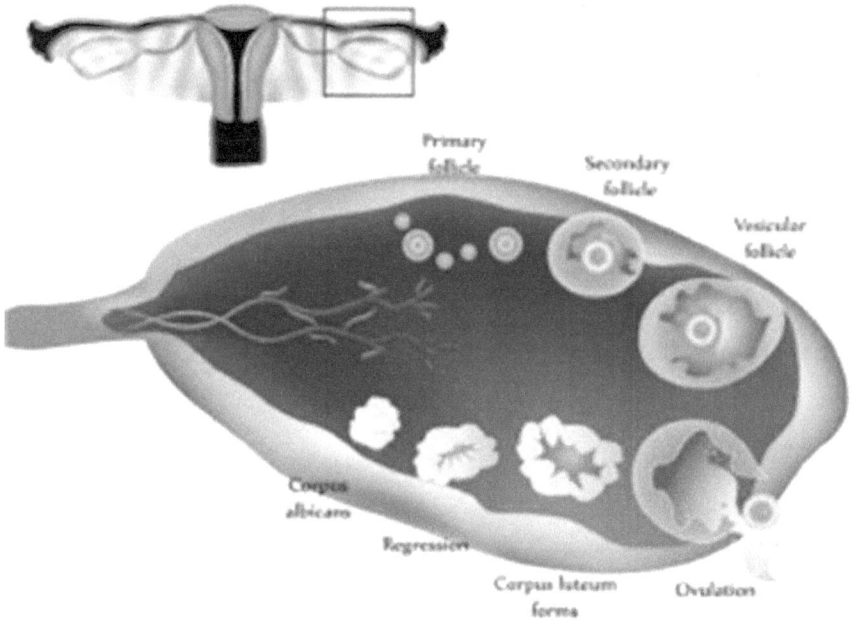

Figure 7. Development of follicles in the ovary

Menstruation forms a normal part of a natural cyclic process occurring in healthy women. The onset of menstruation, known as menarche, occurs at an average age of 12 years but is normal anywhere between 8 and 16. Factors such as hereditary, diet, and overall health can accelerate or delay the onset of menarche.

The Egg is Fertilised
If fertilisation has taken place in the tube, you will be pregnant.

Sex Determination
During fertilisation, both the egg and the sperm each containing 23 chromosomes merge together to form a future baby called the zygote, which contains 46 chromosomes. Chromosomes are tiny thread-like structures that carry our DNA (deoxyribonucleic acid) in which our genes are located. They are present in all the cells of our body. Genes determine the characteristics that we inherit from our parents, for example hair and eye colour, nose, blood group, height, and build.

The sex chromosomes are paired, XX in a woman and XY in a man. At fertilisation, the future baby (zygote) acquires one chromosome from each parent. If the egg, which always contains the X chromosome, is fertilised by a sperm containing an X chromosome, the baby will be a girl (XX). If the sperm contains a Y chromosome, the baby will be a boy (XY).

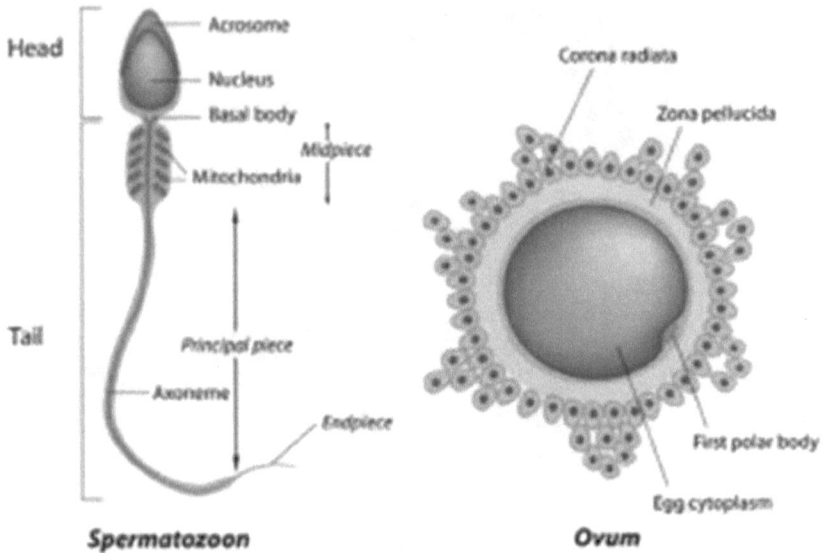

Figure 8. The male and the female eggs

TIMING OF A FERTILE WINDOW IN A MENSTRUAL CYCLE

The general belief is that pregnancy is likely to occur if you have sex around the time of your ovulation. If we assume that ovulation takes place at the middle of your menstrual cycle, then in a 28-day cycle, ovulation should take place on the fourteenth day. However, most women ovulate between 12 and 14 days before their next period, that is day 14 to day 16 of the menstrual cycle. An egg lives for about 12-24 hours after it is released from the ovary. Pregnancy can only happen if the sperm meets the egg during this window that the egg lives.

The good thing is that sperm can live for up to 7 days inside a woman's body. So if you have had sex within 7 days of ovulation, the sperm will have had time to travel up the fallopian tubes to 'wait' for the egg to be released. So the most fertile window for you to be pregnant is from 2 days before to 2 days after ovulation. If you have sex during this window, there is high chance you will be pregnant. This is illustrated below.

12, 13, 14, 15, 16 days in the cycle.

The most likely period to get pregnant in a cycle that lasts 28 days.

N/T
- *Day 14: This is the middle of a 28-day menstrual cycle.*
- *Days 14-16: These are the days when ovulation is likely to occur.*
- *Day 1 of your menstrual cycle: This is the first day of bleeding.*
- *Your menstrual cycle may be longer or shorter than 28 days.*

However, recent research has shown that using the above policy to plan for pregnancy may put unnecessary pressure on you and your partner. It is, therefore, generally advised that you have sex about 2-3 days in a week.

FINDING OUT ABOUT YOUR PREGNANCY

There are various symptoms that can indicate you might be pregnant. You may notice one or more of these symptoms. It is also perfectly possible to be pregnant without noticing any of the 'classic' signs of pregnancy listed below.

Missed period: This is the earliest and most reliable sign if you have a regular monthly cycle. Though it is possible to have a little light bleeding or spotting around the time you expected your period, even if you're pregnant.

Tiredness: You may feel unusually tired in the first few weeks of pregnancy. This is probably due to rising levels of the hormone progesterone.

Sickness: You may feel sick, or even be sick. This is commonly known as 'morning sickness', and it starts between the second and eighth week of pregnancy, but it can happen at any time of the day.

Passing urine more often: About 6-8 weeks after conception, you may find that you have to get up in the night to go to the loo. Some pregnant women also find that they 'leak' a bit when they cough, laugh, or sneeze.

Changes in your breasts: You may notice your breasts getting larger, feeling tender, or tingling in the early weeks of pregnancy. In addition, the veins on your breasts may show up more and your nipples may get darker.

Constipation: This may be due to the hormone progesterone which is produced during pregnancy.

Increased vaginal discharge: An increased vaginal discharge without any soreness or irritation may also occur.

Strange taste in your mouth: Many women describe the taste as metallic.

Changing tastes in food: You may find you go off certain things like tea, coffee, or fatty food. Some women also feel cravings for types of food they don't usually like.

Mood swings and stress: You may feel rapid changes in mood in the early stages of pregnancy and even start to cry sometimes, without knowing why. This is probably because of the changes in hormone levels taking place in your body.

PREGNANCY TESTS

You can do a pregnancy test from the first day of your missed period. If you have regular periods, you'll probably know when this is. Some very sensitive tests can be used even before you miss a period. If you're not sure when your next period is due, you can do a pregnancy test 21 days (3 weeks) after you last had unprotected sex. Urine collected at any time of the day in a clean soap-free, well-rinsed container can be used for the test.

WHERE TO DO THE TEST?

Pregnancy test can be performed at your primary health centre, at your doctor or midwife unit, at a pharmacy or chemist. You can buy the kits and do the test yourself in private.

WHAT'S BEING TESTED?

Pregnancy tests check for the presence of the pregnancy hormone, human chorionic gonadotrophin (HCG) in your urine. After you conceive, your body begins to produce HCG.

RESULTS OF THE TEST

A positive test result is almost certainly correct. If you do a pregnancy test on the first day of your missed period and it's positive, it's probably about 2 weeks since you conceived. You can use the pregnancy due date calculator to work out when your baby is due. A negative result is less reliable. If you still think you're pregnant after a negative result, wait a week and try again or see your GP or midwife.

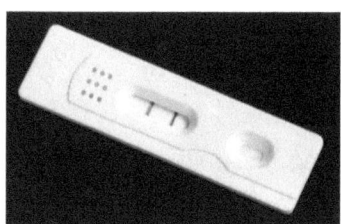 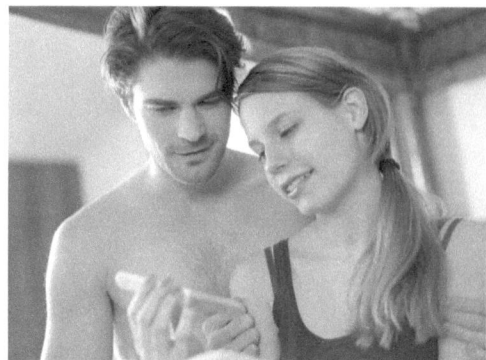

Figure 9. A positive pregnancy test

MEDICATIONS AND PREGNANCY TEST
Some medications can affect test results, including
- promethazine used to treat conditions such as allergies
- sleeping tablets (hypnotics)
- diuretics (medicines that increase production of urine) used to treat conditions such as heart failure
- anticonvulsants (medicines that prevent seizures or fits) used to treat conditions such as epilepsy
- medicines used for infertility
- others

If you are taking any medication, the patient information leaflet that comes with it will tell you whether it affects test results or not; talk to your doctor or midwife if concerned.

REACTION ON FINDING OUT THAT YOU ARE PREGNANT AND IMMEDIATE SUPPORT
You may feel happy and excited, or shocked, confused, and upset. Everybody is different; don't worry if you're not feeling as happy as you expected. Some of this may be caused by changes in your hormone levels, which can make you feel more emotional. Even if you feel anxious and uncertain now, your feelings may change. Talk to your midwife or doctor.

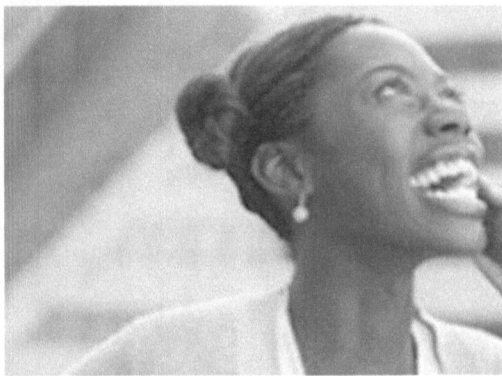

Figure 10. Happy after a positive pregnancy test

Men may also have mixed feelings when they find out their partner is pregnant. Your partner may find it hard to talk about these feelings because he doesn't want to upset you. Both of you should encourage each other to talk about your feelings and any worries or concerns you may have.

TELLING PEOPLE THAT YOU'RE PREGNANT

You may decide to tell your family and friends about your pregnancy or wait until you have confirmed that you want to keep the pregnancy. You may decide to wait until your first scan before you tell people. Members of your family and friends may have mixed feelings or react in unexpected ways to your news. Do not worry yourself; discuss this with your midwife or doctor.

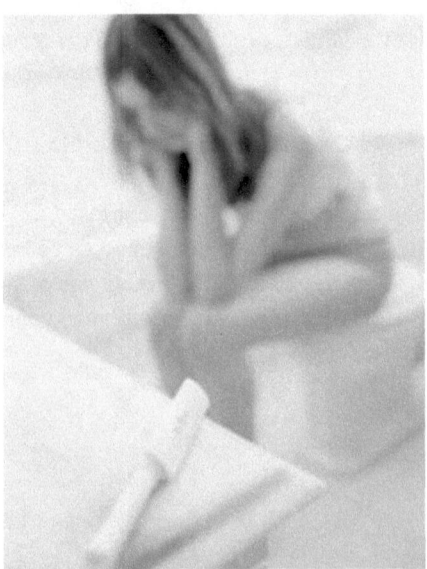

Figure 11. Positive pregnancy test and worried

HELP FOR YOUNG MOTHERS

If you are a young mum or teenager who is pregnant, there is a wide range of services to support you during pregnancy and after you have had your baby. Your midwife or health visitor can give you details of local services. Unfortunately, if you live in the Sub-Saharan Africa, such support services are not available; even if they are, they are not free. This is because governments of countries that belong to Sub-Saharan Africa do not have social security schemes for their citizens.

IF YOU ARE ON YOUR OWN

Sorting out problems, whether personal or medical, is often difficult when you are by yourself. It is better to find someone with whom you can share your feelings and who can offer you support than let things get you down.

CARRYING ON WITH YOUR EDUCATION

Becoming a mother doesn't have to mean the end of your education. If you are still of compulsory school age, your school should not exclude you on grounds of pregnancy or health and safety issues connected with your pregnancy. However, they may talk to you about making alternative arrangements for your education. You will be allowed up to 18 calendar weeks off school before and after the birth. After your return to education, you can receive help with childcare costs through the Care to Learn scheme. This is what is obtainable in the UK.

SOMEWHERE TO LIVE

Many young mothers want to carry on living with their own family until they are ready to move on. In the developed countries, if you are unable to live with your family, your local authority may be able to help you with housing.

CALCULATING YOUR DUE DATE

Your practitioner calculates your due date (and your baby's GA) starting from the first day of your last menstrual period. Pregnancy lasts about 38 weeks from fertilisation, but since it's often difficult to pinpoint exactly when egg and sperm merged, doctors and midwives simply count 40 weeks of pregnancy, beginning with the onset of your last period. That's why you're already considered to be 2 weeks into your pregnancy when fertilisation occurs.

REFERENCES
- Your NHS Guide to Having a Baby. Your pregnancy guide: pregnancy care planner, NHS Choice, UK, 2011.
- ACOG Committee Opinion No. 349, November 2006: Menstruation in girls and adolescents: using the menstrual cycle as a vital sign. Obstet Gynecol. 2006 Nov; 108(5): 1323-8.

- RCOG Pregnancy Book, 2008.
- www.clearblue.com/pregnant/pregnancy-symptoms

Early Pregnancy Assessment Unit and Early Pregnancy Problem

In developed countries, most early pregnancy problems are managed through a specialised unit called 'Early Pregnancy Assessment Unit' (EPAU) and/or 'Accident and Emergency (A&E) Unit', for example in the UK.

This unit is dedicated to early pregnancy problems. The following happens in the unit:
- Diagnosis and treatment of women with signs and symptoms of early pregnancy complications.
- Support and counselling for women who experience early pregnancy loss.
- Research into early pregnancy problems with particular emphasis on the use of ultrasound and other minimal invasive procedures.

INDICATIONS FOR IMMEDIATE ASSESSMENT IN THE EPAU

You should go to the EPAU or the A&E immediately if any of the following is applicable to you:
- Bleeding or lower abdominal pain with a positive pregnancy test and you are less than 16 weeks pregnant. This is because miscarriages and a life-threatening condition—ectopic pregnancy present with those symptoms
- Acute onset of severe lower abdominal pain
- You are in the first 13 weeks of your pregnancy and you have any of the risk factors for ectopic pregnancy (page 40).
- Pelvic inflammatory disease unresponsive to antibiotic treatment.
- Severe vomiting (hyperemesis gravidarum, HG).

INDICATIONS FOR ROUTINE ASSESSMENT IN THE EPAU

Your GP will refer you to the EPAU for the following reasons:
- Recurrent miscarriage (RM)—reassurance scans
- Dating of pregnancy

MISCARRIAGES

DEFINITION

Miscarriage is the spontaneous loss of a pregnancy at any stage up to the age of viability, which is the twenty fourth week. A loss after this time is called a stillbirth. Early miscarriage is when a woman loses her pregnancy in the first 3 months.

PREVALENCE

It is the most common complication of pregnancy occurring in 10-15 out of every 100 pregnancies and mostly before 13 weeks. Most miscarriages occur as a 'one-off' (sporadic) event and the vast majority of women who miscarry go on to have a successful pregnancy next time.

CAUSES OF MISCARRIAGE

Much is still unknown about why early miscarriages occur. The most common cause of miscarriages before 14 weeks is chromosomal problem. This is usually an isolated genetic mistake and rarely occurs again. In order to grow and develop normally, a baby needs a precise number of chromosomes which are normally 23 pairs. If there are too few or too many chromosomes, the pregnancy may end in a miscarriage.

Less common causes of miscarriage, especially late miscarriages, are as follows:
- Abnormalities of the womb
- Imbalance of hormone in your blood
- Weakness of the neck of the womb (cervix)
- Certain blood clotting problems
- Infections like listeria and rubella
- Problems in the placenta
- Obesity

Other risk factors for miscarriage are as follows:
- Age at pregnancy—Please see page 37 under RMs.
- Health problems—for example, poorly controlled diabetes.
- Lifestyle factors—smoking, heavy drinking, and drug abuse.
- Drinking more than 200 mg caffeine per day.

Miscarriage is not caused by lifting, working, constipation, straining at the toilet, stress, worry, sex, eating spicy foods, or doing normal exercise.

PRESENTATION

There are different types of miscarriage which are determined by their clinical presentation, condition of the cervix on vaginal examination, and ultrasound findings but all the types present with bleeding. There may be abdominal pain and symptoms of anaemia, e.g. feeling dizzy or faint, headache, etc.

MANAGEMENT

As stated above, you should go to the A&E or EPAU if you have the symptoms. Doctors will assess you and plan your treatment accordingly. We have not discussed this topic further in this book.

REFERENCES

- The management of early pregnancy loss, Royal College of Obstetricians and Gynaecologists (2006)
- Mark Deutchman, Amy Tanner Tubay. First trimester bleeding. American Family Physician. June 2009. 1; 79(11): 985-992.
- Bleeding during pregnancy. Frequently asked questions. American college of obstetricians and gynecologists. Copyright Aug. 2011
- Early miscarriage: information for you. Royal College of Obstetricians and Gynaecologists (RCOG) January 2008.
- Royal College of Obstetricians and Gynaecologists (RCOG). Information about recovering from surgical management of a miscarriage.
- Information leaflet. Miscarriage. www.patient.co.uk
- EPAU protocol, 2009, King's College Hospital, London.

RECURRENT MISCARRIAGE RM

DEFINITION

This is the loss of three or more consecutive pregnancies. Around 1 in every 100 pregnant women has RMs. For some women, there must be a specific reason for their losses. For others, their repeated miscarriages may be due to chance alone. As the number of miscarriages increases, the risk of chromosome abnormalities decreases and the risk of underlying maternal cause increases. In developed countries, ideally, couples are seen together by a gynaecologist with special interest in RM, and where available, in a RM clinic.

INVESTIGATIONS FOR RECURRENT PREGNANCY LOSS

We have tackled this question, taken into consideration, possible causes of the problem.

Your age. This will be ascertained because the older you become, the more the decline in both the number and the quality of the remaining eggs in your ovaries and therefore, the greater your risk of having a miscarriage. It is particularly so if you are 35 years of age or more and your partner is 40 years of age or more.

Maternal age	Miscarriage risk (%)
16-20	15
21-25	11
26-30	12
31-35	17
36-40	30
41-45	60

Table 1. Maternal age and the risk of miscarriage

Assessment of body mass index BMI. This is necessary because recent research has shown that obesity increases the risk of both sporadic miscarriage and RM.

Investigation for polycystic ovarian disease PCOD: PCOD can predispose to recurrent miscarriages. Blood will be taken from you to test for the hormones that are associated with PCOD and pelvic ultrasound will be performed to confirm that the ovaries have small cysts in them.

Testing for conditions that cause sticky blood. Certain conditions cause sticky blood in the arteries of the placenta with resultant RM, preeclampsia, FGR, preterm labour, in other arteries with resultant adverse effects and in veins to cause blood clots in them. They are called thrombophyllia; they are either acquired (Antiphospholipid aPL antibodies) or inherited.

1. **Antiphospholipid antibodies.** Antibodies are substances that are produced in our blood to fight off infections. Some people produce antibodies that react against their own tissues; this is known as an autoimmune response and it is what happens to women who have aPL antibodies. Blood is normally taken for the antibodies when you are not pregnant. Two positive tests, at least 12 weeks apart, are necessary to confirm the diagnosis.
2. **Tests for inherited conditions that cause sticky blood (inherited thrombophilias).** They can cause second-trimester miscarriages. Your blood should be screened for these conditions.

Couple's blood to be tested for rearrangement of chromosomes. In approximately 2-5 out of 100 couples with RM, one of the partners has abnormal chromosomal rearrangement. Although such abnormalities may cause no problem for you or your partner, they may result in a pregnancy that is at increased risk of miscarriage.

Analysis of the chromosomal and/or genetic content of retained products of conception after a miscarriage. Chromosomal abnormalities is the most common cause of single miscarriages. However, the more miscarriages that you have, the less likely that chromosomal abnormality is responsible.

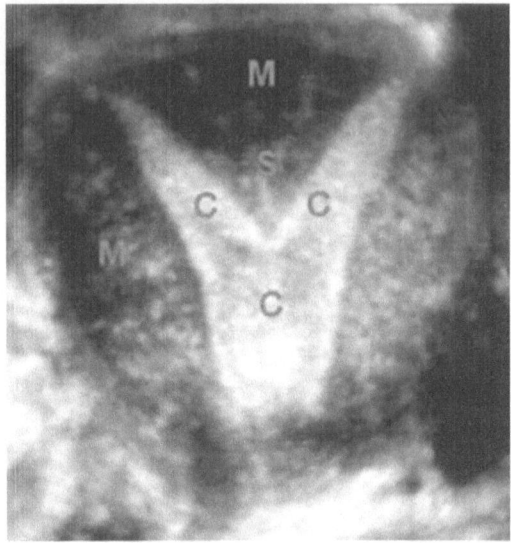

Figure 13. Ultrasound picture of an abnormal womb

Vaginal swab test. A vaginal swab will be taken and tested for a group of bugs called bacteria vaginosis BV which has been associated with second-trimester miscarriages and preterm delivery (PTD).

3D ultrasound of the pelvis. This is used to rule out abnormalities of the womb (figure 13) which can predispose to RM. Other investigations that can be offered for suspected abnormalities of the womb are
- Hysteroscopy (looking inside the womb through the vagina with a telescope)
- Laparoscopy (assessing the outside of the womb through the tummy by a keyhole surgery)

PECULIARITIES OF MANAGEMENT OF RM IN A LOW-INCOME SETTING, FOR EXAMPLE SUB-SAHARAN AFRICA

The information that is outlined above is what is obtainable in a developed country, for example the UK. The peculiarities of management of RM in developing countries are as follows:
- A dedicated RM clinic is unlikely to be found.
- Screening for inherited and acquired thrombophilias is unlikely to be available. Therefore, treatment of these important causes of RM is unlikely to be offered.

- Screening of pregnancy products for genetic abnormality is unlikely to be offered and so is parental screening for abnormal chromosomal rearrangement. Therefore, genetic counselling services will not be offered.
- A well-organised ultrasound service is unlikely to be available, so checking for PCOD or uterine abnormality and counselling in that respect may not be offered.
- Management of suspected cervical weakness may be completely different from the service offered in the developed countries.

So you should discuss with your doctor to find out about the available services wherever you live. If certain service is indicated, you should ask your doctor to refer you to places where it is offered.

Sources

- Repeated miscarriages. Frequently asked questions. ACOG. 2013
- The Management of Recurrent Miscarriage. RCOG Green-top Guideline, May 2003.
- Evaluation and management of recurrent pregnancy loss. Opinion of American Society for Reproductive Medicine. Fertil. Steril. 2012; 98:1101-11
- RCOG Green-top Guideline No. 17. Recurrent miscarriage, investigation and treatment of couples, 2011.
- RCOG patient's information. Couples with recurrent miscarriage. August 2004.
- Information leaflet. Recurrent miscarriage. www.patient.co.uk.
- Nybo Andersen AM, et al. Maternal age and foetal loss: population based register linkage study. BMJ. 2000;320:1708.

Ectopic Pregnancy

Definition and Location of Ectopic Pregnancy

An ectopic pregnancy is a pregnancy in which the foetus grows outside the womb(Figure 15). In the UK, 1 out of 90 women get ectopic pregnancy. The corresponding figure for developing countries, especially Sub-Saharan African countries, should be higher, may be twice or thrice as much. The sites where ectopic pregnancy occurs are as follows:

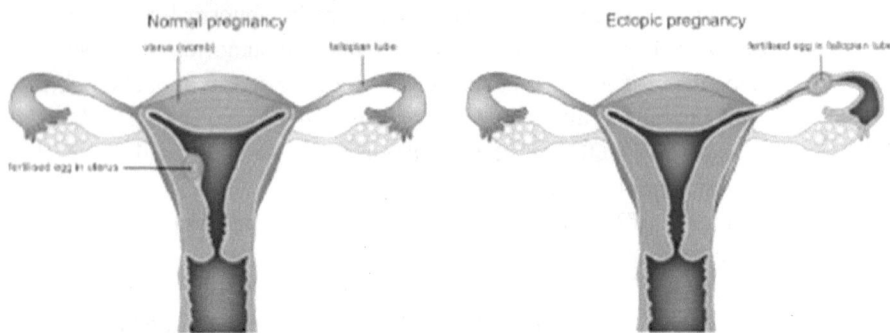

Figure 15. Ectopic pregnancy

- Fallopian tube, which is the main site of occurrence—tubal pregnancy
- Rare sites of occurrence include
    - ovaries—ovarian pregnancy
    - cervix—cervical pregnancy
    - abdomen—abdominal pregnancy
    - heterotopic pregnancy—ectopic pregnancy associated with pregnancy in the womb

Risk Factors for Ectopic Pregnancy

Ectopic pregnancy can occur in any sexually active woman. The 'at-risk' groups are as follows:

- Previous ectopic pregnancy: The more ectopic pregnancies you have had in the past, the more the chance that you will have an ectopic pregnancy again.
- Damaged fallopian tube: Ectopic pregnancy can be caused by a fertilised egg getting stuck in a damaged fallopian tube. The tube can be damaged due to the following factors:
    - pelvic infection
    - previous sterilization; if pregnancy occurs, about 1 in 20 will be ectopic
    - any other previous surgery to the fallopian tube or nearby structures
    - pelvic endometriosis (a condition that affects the uterus and the pelvis in general)
- Usage of coil for contraception; high chance of ectopic if pregnancy occurs.
- Usage of the progesterone-only contraceptive pill (mini-pill).
- Assisted conception treatments.
- Age above 40.
- Smoking.

If you are in any of the above groups, see a doctor as soon as you think you may be pregnant.

THE NATURAL HISTORY OF A TUBAL ECTOPIC PREGNANCY

A pregnancy cannot survive in the fallopian tube and sadly cannot lead to the birth of a baby. So if the pregnancy is not identified early and treated, as it gets bigger, the following can happen:

- The pregnancy often dies after a few days. About half of ectopic pregnancies probably end like this. You may have no symptoms, and you may never know that you were pregnant. Sometimes, there is slight pain and some vaginal bleeding like a miscarriage. Nothing further needs to be done if this occurs.
- The pregnancy may grow for a while in the narrow fallopian tube. This can stretch the tube and cause symptoms. This is when an ectopic pregnancy is commonly diagnosed.
- The pregnancy can run out of space to grow in the fallopian tube and therefore burst it, causing severe pain and internal bleeding. This is a potentially life-threatening situation and therefore a medical emergency.
- The pregnancy can detach itself from the wall of the fallopian tube and move out of it not to the womb but to the opposite end of the tube and then the abdomen. This will send blood into the abdomen and cause pain.
- Rarely, the pregnancy may burst through the fallopian tube into the abdomen without causing much pain and bleeding; it will then grow as abdominal pregnancy with its consequences (not discussed in this book).

PRESENTATION

Symptoms typically develop around the sixth week of pregnancy but may develop at any time between the fourth and the tenth week. They include one or more of the following:

- Pain in the lower abdomen: This may develop suddenly for no apparent reason or may come on gradually over several days. It may be on one side only. It can be severe.

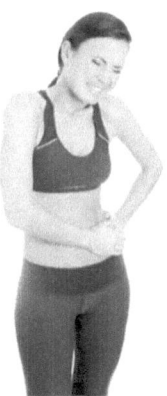

Figure 16. Presenting with pain in ectopic pregnancy

- Vaginal bleeding often occurs, but not always.
- Shoulder tip pain may develop. This is due to some blood leaking into the abdomen and irritating the diaphragm (the muscle used for breathing). This pain is there all the time and may be worse when you are lying down. It is not helped by movement and may not be relieved by painkillers.
- Other symptoms such as diarrhoea, feeling faint, or pain on passing faeces (stools) may occur.

MANAGEMENT

If you have any of the outlined symptoms and you have had sex for at least within the last 3-4 weeks (even if you have used contraception and have not had a positive pregnancy test), you might be pregnant. You should, therefore, get medical help immediately in A&E unit or EPAU. In the hospital, the doctors will assess and treat you accordingly. We have not discussed this topic further in this book.

PECULIARITIES OF MANAGEMENT OF ECTOPIC PREGNANCY IN A LOW-INCOME SETTING OF DEVELOPING COUNTRIES

In developing countries where the health budget is small, the expenses required in order to adequately manage patients cannot be met. Therefore, the services that are obtainable in developing countries are far less than that in the developed world.

The peculiarities of ectopic pregnancy and its management in the low-income setting of developing countries are as following:

- The prevalence of ectopic pregnancy is likely to be higher in developing countries than in developed ones
- Pelvic inflammatory disease PID is likely to be the main cause of it. This is because of incomplete treatment of PID by non-medical personnel.
- People are likely to present late with ruptured tubal pregnancy and associated shock.
- EPAU is unlikely to be available in developing countries, and therefore, follow-up is likely to be poor.
- Test for pregnancy hormones (HCG) and good ultrasound assessment
- may not be offered.
- Diagnosis like pregnancy of unknown location PUL may not exist, and therefore, management will not be appropriate.
- Conservative and medical treatments are almost not offered. What is offered is open surgery. Minimal access surgery which is the gold standard in developed countries is rarely performed.

Regarding the causes of ectopic pregnancy, one must admit that pelvic inflammatory disease is likely to be the main cause of ectopic pregnancy in developing countries. This is because of incomplete treatment of the disease by non-medical personnel. The prevalence of ectopic pregnancy is likely to be higher in developing countries.

The presentation of ectopic pregnancy is also likely to be different in developing countries. People are likely to present late with ruptured tubal pregnancy and associated circulatory instability (low BP and high pulse rates). Furthermore, a dedicated EPAU is unlikely to be available in developing countries, and therefore, follow-up is likely to be poor.

Diagnostic capabilities in developing countries are so poor that testing for pregnancy hormones (HCG and progesterone) and good ultrasound assessment may not be offered. Diagnosis like pregnancy of unknown location PUL may not exist in many of the countries, and therefore, management will not be appropriate. In the developing countries, conservative and medical treatments of ectopic pregnancy are almost not offered. What is offered is open surgical. Minimal access surgery which is the gold standard in developed countries is rarely performed.

So if you believe that you are likely to have ectopic pregnancy, discuss with your doctor about the options available in your local hospital, and if you are interested in other specific management procedure, you could ask for a referral to a unit where such service is offered.

SOURCES

- RCOG Green-top Guideline No. 21. The management of tubal pregnancy. May 2004, reviewed 2010.
- Ectopic pregnancy. Frequently asked questions. American College of obstetricians and gynecologists ACOG. 2011
- Information for you. Ectopic pregnancy, RCOG, August 2010.
- The Pregnancy Book, UK, 2009.
- www.patient.co.uk
- Ectopic pregnancy, Clinical Knowledge Summaries, February 2010.
- Nama V, Mayonda I. Tubal ectopic pregnancy: diagnosis and management. Arch Gynecol Obstet. 2008 Jul 30 [abstract].

NAUSEA AND VOMITING IN PREGNANCY

DEFINITION AND PRESENTATIONS

Nausea (feeling sick) and vomiting (being sick) in pregnancy (NVP) affect 50-90 out of 100 pregnant women.

PRESENTATION

- It presents with nausea, vomiting, and spitting with or without ptyalism (inability to swallow saliva).
- It typically starts in the first trimester. In 11-18 out of 100 women, it is confined to the morning hours.
- It resolves by 12 weeks gestation (60%) or by 16 weeks gestation (90%) but may persist throughout pregnancy in 1-3% of women.
- It can interfere with household activities, restricting interaction with children.
- It is associated with greater use of health care resources and time lost off work.

HYPEREMESIS GRAVIDARUM HG

This is a severe form of NVP and occurs in approximately 1 out of 100 pregnant women. Presentations of HG are as follows:

- severe and persistent NVP
- weight loss
- dehydration
- muscle wasting
- inability to keep down liquid and solid food when eating.
- disturbance of the normal functions of the kidneys, liver and other body systems

CAUSES OF NVP

The causes are not completely understood. It is probably caused by hormonal changes in the first 3 months of pregnancy, but other medical conditions may cause nausea and vomiting and should be excluded. You have more chance of developing NVP and HG if you have any of the following:

- increased body weight
- multiple gestation
- trophoblastic disease (disease of the placenta)
- HG in a prior pregnancy

WHEN TO GET HELP

If you are sick all the time and cannot keep anything down, tell your midwife or doctor.

ASSESSMENT

Diagnosis of HG is made after excluding other causes of nausea and vomiting.

- The aim of assessment is to identify
  - Mild cases, which do not require admission.
  - Severe NVP or HG, which requires admission. It presents with dehydration, ketosis (plenty of ketones in your urine), deranged liver and kidney function.

- – Atypical presentations of HG: Nausea and vomiting that continues beyond the twentieth week of pregnancy and cases that start after 10 weeks. Other causes of nausea and vomiting should be looked for.
- Your doctor will assess you, and the likely findings are as follows:
  - – high pulse rate
  - – dehydration
  - – low BP in some positions that you take (postural hypotension)
  - – urine test showing ingredient called ketone, which indicates that you are dehydrated
- Other conditions that cause vomiting will be ruled out, and they include
  - – water infection
  - – kidney failure
  - – molar pregnancy
  - – bowel problems such as ulcer, obstruction
  - – pancreatitis, inflammation of the pancreas
  - – adrenal problem (Addison's disease)
  - – high function of the thyroid gland
  - – diabetic complication
  - – brain tumour
  - – ear problem
  - – others
- Serious complications of HG will be looked for.

INVESTIGATIONS

- Blood tests to check for the following:
  - – signs of infection (full blood count and CRP, which is a marker of infection)
  - – functions of the kidney, liver, and the thyroid gland
  - – blood glucose levels to rule out diabetes
- Urine tests to check for dehydration and infection.
- Pelvic ultrasound to rule out multiple pregnancy and molar pregnancy.

HOW TO AVOID NAUSEA AND MORNING SICKNESS

- Give yourself time to get up slowly if you feel sick first thing in the morning. If possible, eat something like dry toast or a plain biscuit before you get up.
- Get plenty of rest and sleep whenever you can. Feeling tired can make the sickness worse.
- Eat small amounts of food rather than several large meals, but don't stop eating.
- Drink plenty of fluids.
- Ask those close to you for extra help and support.

- Distract yourself as much as you can. Nausea gets worse the more you think about it.
- Avoid food and smell that make you feel worse. It helps if someone else can cook. If not, go for bland, non-greasy foods, such as baked potatoes, pasta, and milk puddings, which are simple to prepare.
- Wear comfortable clothes. Tight waistbands can make you feel worse.

TREATMENT

CRITERIA FOR ADMISSION
- HG.
- If you cannot keep down liquid nor solid food.

In these circumstances, if you are less than 18 weeks pregnant, you will be admitted on the gynaecological ward; if more than 18 weeks, you will be admitted on the antenatal ward.

ACTUAL TREATMENT
- Drugs that may cause nausea and vomiting, for example iron supplements, will be stopped.
- Intravenous fluid will be given.
- Fluid balance chart will be maintained. The amount of fluids given to you and the amount that you pass out in the form of urine or vomiting will be recorded. You should be given a measuring jug with your name on it each time you go to the toilet to pass urine.
- Mouth care should be encouraged at this time as breath will smell bad (ketotic).
- Blood clots formation, which can be caused by dehydration, will be prevented by giving you heparin injections; you will also wear a pair of special stockings (page 356).
- Vitamin supplements.
  - Folic acid will be continued.
  - Thiamine (vitamin B1): Normal stores of thiamine are depleted after 2 weeks of persistent vomiting. The abnormal liver function that can occur when you are vomiting too much may reduce its production and storage. Therefore, you will be given thiamine supplements, if tolerated, by mouth; if not tolerated, then a solution called Pabrinex containing a mixture of vitamins B and C will be transfused once a week.
- Treatment that will stop the vomiting (anti-emetic treatment)
  - You will receive this on a regular basis.
  - A single anti-emetic drug will be prescribed regularly, with a second one given if you need it (pro re nata, PRN). After 24 hours,

if the second anti-emetic is being used regularly, 2 anti-emetics will be given regularly with another one on PRN basis. A third regular anti-emetic agent may be required.

- o If you fail to improve after admission despite three regular anti-emetics from three different groups of drugs and adequate fluid and electrolyte replacement, you will be given other medications such as ondansetron or corticosteroids.
- Alternative treatments for nausea and vomiting are as follows:
  - ginger
  - physiotherapy

Both treatment options have been shown to be effective in improving symptoms.

- Antacids (Ranitidine or omeprazole)—These are the drugs which neutralise the acid that is normally produced in the stomach. Prolonged vomiting can result in symptoms of severe heartburn, which should respond to these drugs.
- Nutrition and nutritional support
  - A light diet may be prescribed on day 2 of the treatment.
  - All the measures itemised above to avoid NVP should be observed.
  - If you are vomiting continuously, despite having drip and appropriate injections, a tube may be passed through your nose into the stomach (nasogastric tube) in other to decongest the later.
  - A record of your bowel movements will be kept as constipation worsens the symptoms.
- You will be referred to a dietician if
  - your prepregnancy diet is poor.
  - your prepregnancy BMI is less than 20.
  - your weight loss is more than 5% of prepregnancy weight.
  - you are vomiting at home for longer than 2 weeks.
  - your symptoms are unresolved after 5 days in hospital.
  - 'you decide against a nasogastric tube.
- Psychological support: You may require emotional and psychological support from both the medical and nursing teams through encouragement, explanation, and reassurance.

CRITERIA FOR DISCHARGE AND FOLLOW-UP

- There should be no ketones in your urine.
- You should be tolerating fluids and food for 24 hours.
- You should not need intravenous fluids for 24 hours.
- You are prescribed appropriate anti-emetics and multivitamins to be taken at home.
- Your follow-up is arranged for 1-2 weeks' time.

SOURCES
- Protocol of Barts and the Royal London Hospital on nausea and vomiting in pregnancy, 2013.
- Nausea and vomiting of pregnancy. American College of Obstetricians and Gynaecologists (ACOG); 2004 Apr. 13 p. (ACOG practice bulletin; no. 52). [94 references]
- The obstetrician and gynaecologist, RCOG TOG.
- Protocol of King's College Hospital on nausea and vomiting in pregnancy, 2009.

Development of Your Baby Stage by Stage

IMPORTANT DEFINITION

Gestational age is the age of your baby from the first day of your last period. Fertilisation is believed to occur 2 weeks after the first day of your last period. Embryonic age is the age of your baby from the date of fertilisation. Therefore, the first week of embryonic age is the third week of GA. However, the actual duration between last menstruation and fertilisation may differ from the standard 2 weeks by several days.

PERIODS OF DEVELOPMENT

The development of your baby is divided into two periods:
- The embryonic period, which begins at fertilisation (penetration of the egg by the sperm) and continues until the end of the tenth week of pregnancy, that is eighth week by embryonic age. During this critical period when the organs and systems are forming, the developing embryo is also susceptible to toxic exposures such as
  - alcohol, certain drugs, and other toxins that cause birth defects
  - infections, for example rubella
  - radiation from X-rays or radiation treatment
  - nutritional deficiencies such as folate and iodine
- The foetal period, which begins at the tenth week of pregnancy and continues till delivery.

THE EMBRYONIC PERIOD

DAY 1 OF FERTILISATION

At fertilisation, the male reproductive cell called the 'spermatozoa or sperm cells or sperm' and the female reproductive cell called the 'ovum' join together to form a single cell called the 'zygote'. Sperm cell is very tiny and has a head, neck, and tail (fig. 8). The tail moves from side to side so that the sperm can swim up the vagina into the uterus and fallopian tubes.

During sex, sperm is ejaculated from a man's penis into a woman's vagina. In one ejaculation, there may be more than 300 million sperm cells. Most of the sperm leak out of the vagina, but some begin to swim up through the neck of the womb. Only about 400 sperm will survive the arduous 10-hour journey from the vagina to the cervix, uterus, and then the fallopian tube, and only one sperm will succeed in burrowing through the outer layer of the egg, a process called fertilisation. This occurs during the next 12-24 hours after ovulation. It takes about 20 minutes for the lucky winner to burrow its way into the egg (Figure 19).

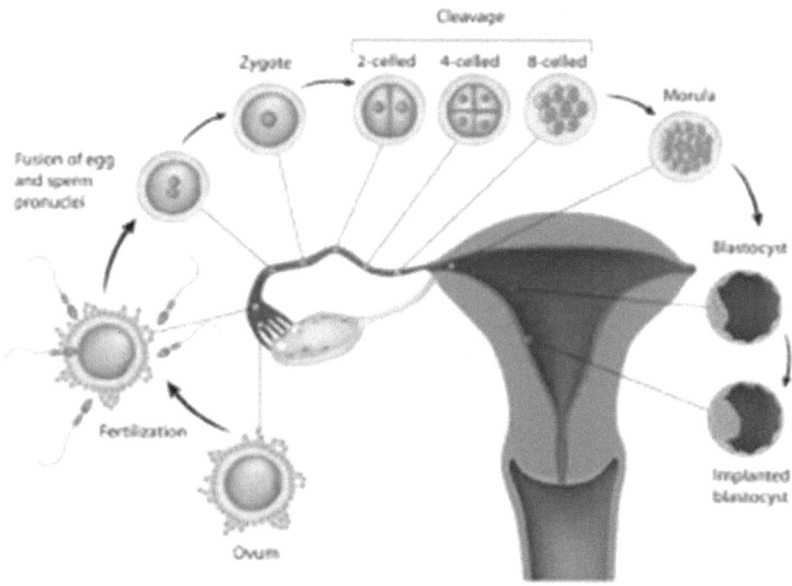

Day 1—I cell stage (zygote)	Day 3—8 cell stage
Day I.5—2 cell stage	Day 4—16 cell stage (Morula)
Day 2—4 cell stage	Day 5—Blastocyst

Figure 19. Fertilisation and development of the fertilised egg (zygote)

Upon penetration, the covering of the egg cell undergoes a change and becomes impenetrable, preventing further fertilisation from another sperm. Once the centre (nucleus) of the egg and the nucleus of the sperm fuse (within 11 hours of fertilisation), the final product is called 'a zygote', which is a single cell with a complete set of chromosomes (46), 23 from the egg and 23 from the sperm.

Day 1-5 of Fertilisation

The zygote now called an embryo spends the next few days travelling down the fallopian tube to the uterus. If a zygote doesn't move down to the uterus and implants itself in the fallopian tube, it is called an ectopic or tubal pregnancy. During its journey to the uterus, the embryo divides; the 16-cell stage is called 'morula' (figures 19). The morula undergoes further division to form a blastocyst, which contains a space within it (Fig. 20).

The morula undergoes further division to form a blastocyst, which contains a space within it. The blastocyst undergoes further development a day or two later after its formation. It contains only a thin rim of cells called the trophoblast cells and a clump of cells at one end known as the 'embryonic pole'. It is important to note that the developmental stages from the zygote to the blastocyst occur in the fallopian tube, and during this period, there is no growth in the overall size of the embryo as it is confined within a shell called zona pellucida. The cells become smaller with each division.

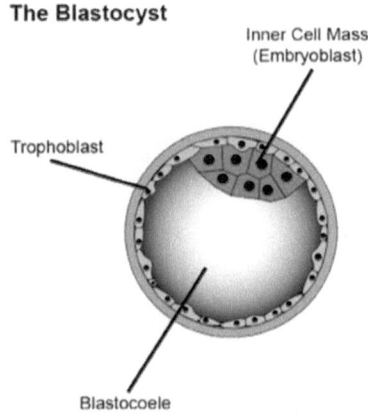

Figure 20. The blastocyst

Day 5-6 of Fertilisation

The blastocyst reaches the uterus, and the zona pellucida breaks away. This allows the trophoblasts to come into contact with the inner lining of the womb, the endometrium.

Week 4 (22-28 Days from the First Day of Your Last Menstruation)

The trophoblast of the blastocyst burrows into the lining of your uterus and forms the following:

- a structure called 'chorion' from which the placenta will develop
- a fluid-filled space that will become the bag of water surrounding your baby (amniotic sac)

This process in which the blastocyst attaches itself to the lining of your womb is called implantation. The blastocyst is fully implanted by day 12 after fertilisation. The embryonic pole of the blastocyst flattens into a disk that is two-cell thick. The process that begins with the fertilisation of an egg and ends with the implantation of the fertilised egg into a woman's uterus (womb) is called *conception.* If separation into identical twins occurs, two-third of the time it will happen between days 5 and 9 of fertilisation. If it happens after day 9, there is a significant risk of abnormality.

CHANGES IN YOU FROM THE DATE OF FERTILISATION TO THE END OF THE FOURTH WEEK OF PREGNANCY

During ovulation, the egg is expelled from the follicle, which is in the ovary; what is left in the ovary after that is the yellow body or corpus luteum. The yellow body does not disappear after fertilisation but continues to produce hormones, oestrogen and progesterone. The oestrogen enables the lining of the womb to build up and enrich it with blood vessels while the progesterone induces its relaxation in other to make room for the incoming blastocyst. Blood supply to your breasts is also enhanced by the hormones, making them feel heavy.

During the third week after your period, you will probably not know you're pregnant yet, but you may notice a little spotting by the end of this week. This is called 'implantation spotting'. It may be caused by the blastocyst burrowing into the blood-rich uterine lining. Only a minority of pregnant women experience it.

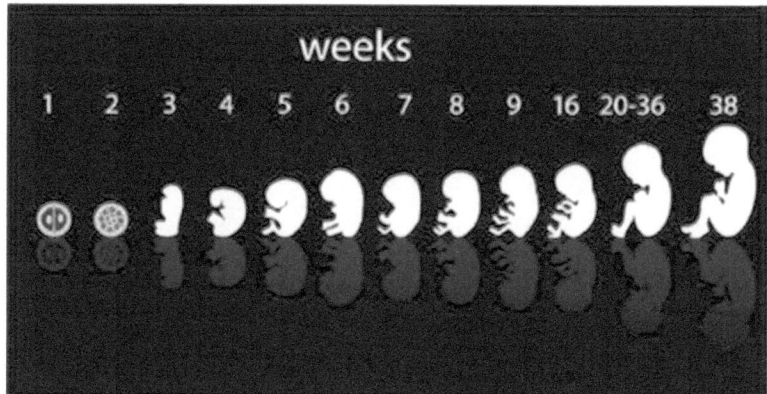

Figure 21. Foetal development week by week (from Fotolia)

The chorion (formed from the trophoblast) produces hormone called HCG, which prevents your ovaries from releasing eggs and triggers the increased production of the hormones oestrogen and progesterone by the corpus luteum. Later in pregnancy, the function of production of these hormones will be undertaken by the placenta. The increased levels of progesterone may make you feel depressed, tearful, have mood swings, or be easily irritated; these symptoms should get better after the first 3 months of your pregnancy.

The HCG induces a pregnancy test to be positive by the end of the second week after fertilisation; if your test is negative and you still haven't seen your period 2 or 3 days later, do it again.

WEEK 5 (4 WEEKS AND 0 DAYS TO 4 WEEKS AND 6 DAYS FROM THE FIRST DAY OF YOUR LAST PERIOD.)

GROWTH OF YOUR BABY

The organs will begin to develop. The two-cell thick disc of the embryonic pole of the blastocyst develops into three layers.

- The outer layer (ectoderm) will become the brain, spinal cord, skin, eyes and the ears. Typically at this stage of pregnancy, the neural tube which forms your baby's nervous system (brain and spinal cord) is already growing.
- The middle layer (mesoderm) will develop into the heart and blood circulatory system. Typically at this stage, the heart has started forming, and your baby already has some blood vessels. A string of these blood vessels connects your baby to you—this will become the umbilical cord.
- The inner layer (endoderm) forms the lungs, intestines, and the beginnings of the urinary system.

ULTRASOUND FINDINGS

A small pregnancy sac (2-5 mm) is seen within the lining of the womb. The sac is round, regular in shape, and located towards the top of the womb. The embryo can be seen in the sac.

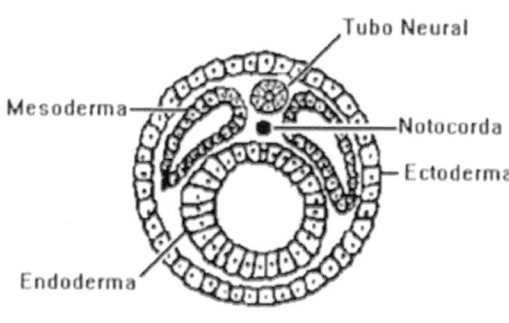
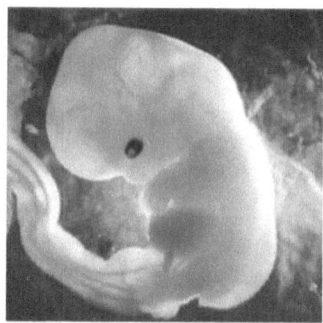

Figure 22. Early development of the embryo, 5-6 weeks

CHANGES IN YOU

You have probably just missed your period. Sometime this week, you may be able to confirm that you are pregnant by doing a pregnancy test. The mood swings that were present during the previous week may persist. You may start feeling the signs and symptoms of early pregnancy as enumerated on pages 29-30.

WHAT TO DO NOW

- Call your doctor or midwife in order to arrange your first prenatal appointment when a pregnancy test is positive. Most practitioners won't see you until you're about 8 weeks unless you have a medical condition, had problems with a previous pregnancy, or are having symptoms that need to be checked out.
- Find out about your health and safety at work, especially if you work with X-rays or chemicals or have a strenuous job.
- Start a gentle exercise routine (pages 162-174).
- Take folic acid daily. If your BMI is higher than 30, see your doctor, as she'll need to prescribe a higher dose of it.
- Find out about healthy eating in pregnancy and adapt to it.
- Ask whether it's safe to continue with any medication, prescription or over-the-counter, which you are taking.
- See your doctor if you suffer from early pregnancy symptoms or complications of early pregnancy, for example vomiting.
- Be sure to alert your caregiver to any other issues of concern.
- Go for a prepregnancy check, generally, if you have not done that already.

WEEK 6 (5 WEEKS AND 0 DAYS TO 5 WEEKS AND 6 DAYS AFTER THE FIRST DAY OF YOUR LAST PERIOD.)

GROWTH OF YOUR BABY

He or she measures about 4 mm in length in average and begins to curve into a C shape. The heart bulges and begins to beat regularly and is divided into chambers. The neural tube will close this week. Limb buds, a small opening from which the mouth will develop and the grooves which will form the face and neck will develop. The positions of future ears, yet to be formed, are marked by dimples on the side of the head. Trace of the lungs and the liver appear. Primitive internal organs like the gall bladder, pancreas, ureter, and the spleen also appear. Separate passages to pass faecal matter and urine are formed.

ULTRASOUND FINDINGS

A yolk sac becomes visible within the pregnancy sac. This should be seen in all pregnancies with a mean pregnancy sac diameter of more than 12 mm. The embryo measures 4 mm in length.

CHANGES IN YOU

There will be not much difference when compared with week 5. You may notice queasiness or go off certain foods. This is very common. You may have more pregnancy symptoms.

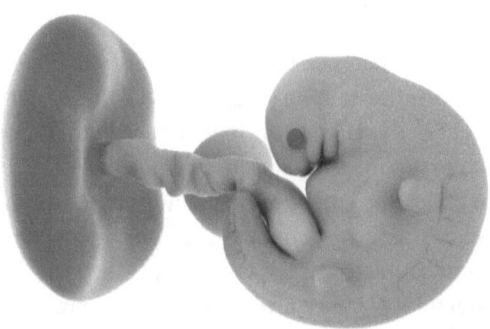

Figure 23. Week 6 of foetal development

WHAT TO DO NOW
- Do the same as at week 5.
- Get plenty of vitamin C every day, especially now, when your baby's cells are growing fast. Good sources include oranges, red peppers, blackcurrants, and kiwi fruit.

WEEK 7 (6 WEEKS TO 6 WEEKS AND 6 DAYS)

GROWTH OF YOUR BABY
The head is big because the brain is developing. Heart rate now is 100-160 bpm, and blood is beginning to course through his or her body. The position of the heart is indicated by a large bulge. Two dark spots which indicate the position of future eyes and two dimples for future nose appear. The brain divides into 5 parts. Future muscles and bones in the form of bumps on the body are forming, and the limb buds are becoming more prominent.

ULTRASOUND FINDINGS
The embryo becomes more kidney bean-shaped and the yolk sac is separated from it by a tube called the vitelline duct. The length of the baby (crown-rump length, CRL) is about 10 mm.

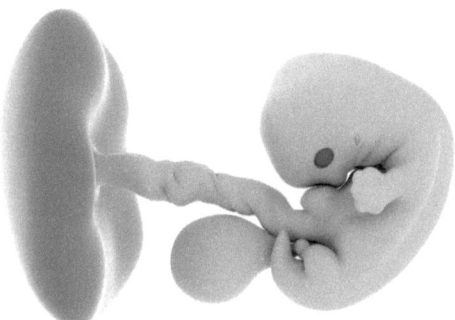

Figure 24. Week 7 of foetal development

CHANGES IN YOU
You may find yourself developing a bit of a split personality—feeling moody one day and joyful the next. This has continued from about 3-4 weeks of pregnancy. Unsettling as this is, what you're going through is normal.

WHAT TO DO NOW
- Involve your partner in your pregnancy.
- Try to get some rest as much as possible.
- Guide against constipation by eating more vegetables and drinking water.

WEEK 8 (7 WEEKS TO 7 WEEKS AND 6 DAYS)

GROWTH OF YOUR BABY
The embryo measures 13 mm. Lungs begin to form. The brain continues to develop. Arms and legs have lengthened with foot and hand areas distinguishable,

with digits but may still be webbed. Development of the vulva begins. Your baby is still considered an embryo and has a small tail. Eyelid folds partially covering her peepers, which already have some colour. Tiny veins beneath parchment thin skin have formed. Tooth buds, palate, and tongue are forming, while his ears continue to develop. The liver is producing red blood cells until her bone marrow forms and takes over this role. The umbilical cord now has distinct blood vessels to carry oxygen and nutrients to and from her tiny body.

Ultrasound Findings
The CRL measures 11-16 mm. The head part of the baby becomes distinguishable as a diamond-shaped space, enabling distinction of upper and lower part of the baby. The spine is seen as double bright parallel lines. The amniotic membrane, which is the bag that contains the amniotic fluid, becomes visible. The umbilical cord can also be seen.

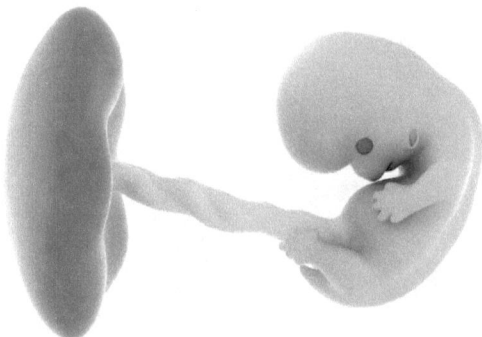

Figure 25. Week 8 of foetal development

Changes in You
Your uterus is expanding to accommodate your growing baby. Before pregnancy, it was the size of a clenched fist. Now it's as big as a grapefruit. As your uterus grows, you may feel mild cramps in your tummy and the odd twinge. Always check with your midwife to rule out ectopic pregnancy. The mood swings may persist. A combination of surging hormones and worries about pregnancy and parenthood can also result in vivid dreams or sleeplessness.

Morning sickness by now may be in full swing. If you're feeling fine, don't worry; you're lucky. You may pee more than usual, thanks to your increasing blood volume and the extra fluid being processed through your kidneys. Furthermore, as your uterus grows, pressure on your bladder will send you to the bathroom as well. Both the frequency and volume of urine tends to increase over the course of pregnancy. Other symptoms of early pregnancy may continue.

WHAT YOU NEED TO KNOW

- Prevent morning sickness by applying the measures that are itemised on Pages 45-46.
- Inform your midwife or doctor if peeing is becoming unbearable so that other problems can be ruled out.

WEEK 9 (8 WEEKS TO 8 WEEKS AND 6 DAYS)

GROWTH OF YOUR BABY

In his or her brain, nerve cells are branching out to connect with one another, forming primitive neural pathways. His or her eyelids cover more of his or her eyes. The tongue is present, and taste buds have just started forming. Nipples and hair follicles begin to form. Location of the elbows and toes are visible. The hand can now bend at the wrist, and feet have just started losing their webbed appearance. The internal organs and muscles are all developing and functioning. The heart has finished dividing into four chambers, and the valves have started forming. The external sex organs are there but won't be distinguishable as male or female for another few weeks. The embryonic 'tail' has completely gone.

Generally, she or he is starting to look more and more human. Her or his essential body parts are accounted for, though they'll go through plenty of fine-tuning in the coming months. At the end of the ninth week, your baby is called 'foetus'. The placenta has developed enough now to take over most of the critical job of producing hormones. Now that your baby's basic physiology is in place, she's poised for rapid weight gain.

THE UMBILICAL CORD, PLACENTA, AND AMNIOTIC SAC

These structures are responsible for transport and exchange of nutrient in the growing foetus. The umbilical cord is a baby's lifeline. It is the link between you and your baby. Blood circulates through the cord, carrying oxygen and food to the baby and carrying waste away from her.

The placenta is attached to the lining of the uterus and separates your baby's blood circulation from your own. In the placenta, oxygen and food from your bloodstream pass into your baby's bloodstream and are carried to your baby along the umbilical cord. Antibodies that give your baby resistance against infection, alcohol, nicotine, and other drugs can also pass to your baby this way.

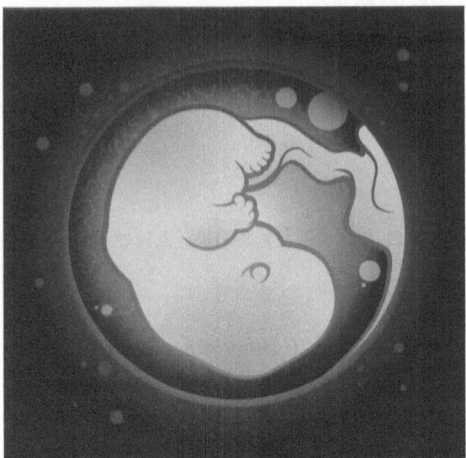

Figure 26. The umbilical cord, placenta, and amniotic sac

Inside the uterus, your baby floats in a bag of fluid called the amniotic fluid. It has a number of purposes, including protecting the foetus from trauma and infection, allowing lung development, and facilitating the development and movement of the limb and other skeletal parts. Before or during labour, the bag of fluid breaks, and the fluid drains out.

ULTRASOUND FINDINGS
The CRL is 17-23 mm. The forebrain, midbrain, hindbrain, and skull are all distinguishable. Limb buds are also visible. Midgut hernia, whereby the bowel appears outside the abdomen, can also be seen. The fluid bag, the umbilical, and movement of your baby can be seen.

CHANGES IN YOU
Your breasts are growing, and by now, it's likely your old bras are getting uncomfortable, so you should get a couple of bigger ones. You may notice your waistline expanding as well, forcing you to pack away your favourite jeans until next year. The amount of blood circulating around your body is steadily increasing. Your body is doing a wonderful job of helping your baby to grow, but the extra demands on your circulation can make you prone to varicose veins and piles. Discuss with your doctor about them.

Headache and backache are both common if you're expecting. Hormones flooding your body can also help to create the perfect environment for vaginal thrush. Being pregnant may affect your choice of destination for holidays. You need to think about insurance, how you're going to travel, and vaccinations before you decide where to take your holiday. If you have morning sickness, you may be worried that it will get worse at high altitudes.

What You Need to Do

- Continue with a balanced diet. The bad news is that you may not feel like eating it. Try not to worry. If you have morning sickness, it should soon pass.
- You are at risk of experiencing constipation, so you need to increase the amount of fibre-rich foods that you eat. Relaxin which is produced in your body during pregnancy loosens your joints, so you are at a risk of straining or falling over.
- Try to increase your calcium levels. Take milk, calcium-fortified soya milk, and a daily vitamin D supplement.
- Try to get plenty of rest.

The Foetal Period

Week 10 (9 weeks to 9 weeks and 6 days after the first day of menstruation)

Growth of Your Baby

Congratulation! Your baby is now called a foetus which means 'offspring'. His or her eyelids are now completely covering his or her eyes and won't open until week 26. Tiny earlobes are now visible. Your baby's essential body parts have already formed. His or her wrists are more developed; ankles have formed. Fingers and toes are clear to see. His arms are growing longer and bend at the elbows.

Ultrasound findings

The CRL is 23-32 mm. The limbs and other body parts are seen. Heart rate peaks at 170-180 bpm.

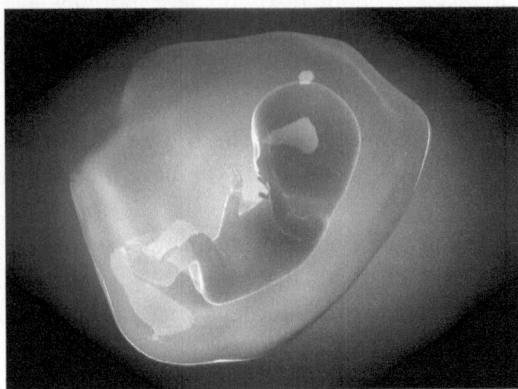

Figure 27. Weeks 9-12 of foetal development

CHANGES IN YOU

As your baby grows, your uterus (womb) is expanding to accommodate him or her. Your uterus is now big enough to fill your pelvis. The signs and symptoms of early pregnancy persist.

WHAT YOU NEED TO KNOW

- Around now, you should have your first antenatal appointment; this is when your midwife takes your booking blood samples.
- Make sure that your dating and first-trimester anomaly scan is booked for 11-13^{+6} weeks.
- Travelling by car may be a part of your daily life, but it is safe to use a seat belt during pregnancy.

WEEKS 11-12 (10 WEEKS TO 11 WEEKS AND 6 DAYS)

GROWTH OF YOUR BABY

The CRL is 4-5.4 cm and weight slightly less than 14 g. The development of the brain and spinal cord continues—your baby can squirm if you prod your belly, clench the fingers, curl the toes, and clench the eye muscles. The head comprises nearly half of the length of his or her entire body. Tooth buds, which will form the teeth, appear. Your baby's face is changing. The eyes, which started out on the sides of her head, have moved closer together, and his or her ears are almost in their final position.

Your baby's bowel is no more outside the abdomen; it has already moved into the abdomen. His or her vital organs—liver, kidneys, intestines, brain, and lungs—are fully formed and functional. The liver is producing bile, and his or her kidneys are secreting urine into his or her bladder. Red blood cells are also produced in the liver. The outline of his or her spine is clear to see.

Changes in You

You're getting close to the end of the first trimester. A dark vertical line of pigmentation, called the linea nigra, may appear on your belly. You may be having stress incontinence, that is leakage of urine when coughing, sneezing, or laughing; try not to worry. As soon as you become pregnant, hormones cause your pelvic floor tissues and muscles to stretch. This can lead to weakness in the sphincter muscles that control the release of wee from your bladder.

Doing regular pelvic floor exercises (pages 167-168) will strengthen these muscles. Your gums may bleed; therefore, you should floss carefully, as well as brushing. The top of your womb can now be felt at the bottom of your belly.

What You Need to Know

- Occasionally, stress can trigger domestic violence within a relationship. Find out from your doctor or midwife what to do if it happens to you.
- In the developed countries, you will be entitled to paid time off work for all antenatal appointments and classes. You may want to tell your employer you're pregnant.
- You must attend your first-trimester ultrasound scan for dating and different screening tests.
- You may start to notice stretch marks appearing, particularly on your breasts. Wearing a supportive bra may help. At least you'll be more comfortable.
- You can stop taking folic acid supplements from the end of this week because your baby's neural tube will be fully formed. Take good care of your skin.

WEEKS 13-16 (12 WEEKS TO 15 WEEKS AND 6 DAYS)

GROWTH OF YOUR BABY

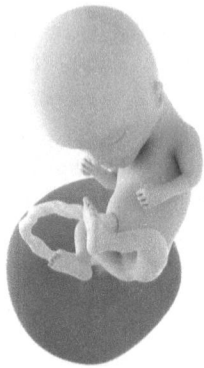

Figure 28. Weeks 13-16 of foetal development

The CRL ranges from 6.7 cm at week 13 to 10 cm at week 16, while the weight is 23 g at week 13 and 100 g at week16. The sucking muscles have appeared in the cheek. Girls have approximately 2 million eggs in their ovaries, but only a million will be present at birth. At week 14, the skin will start to be covered with ultra-fine hair, and on top of the head, the downy hair (lanugo hair) will be sprouting. Your baby can now grasp, squint, frown, grimace, and suck his or her thumb.

At week 15, your baby gets the hiccups, but he or she does not make any sound because their windpipe (trachea) is filled with fluid rather than air. The legs are longer than the arms, and the genitals have so much developed that they can be seen on an ultrasound scan. From the week 16, your baby will be playing, pulling, and grabbing the umbilical cord. The head is more erect than it has been, and the eyes are closer to the front of the future face. The blood vessels, heart and the urinary systems are all functioning at full capacity. Baby's poo called meconium is made in the bowel and the liver and pancreas produce their own secretions.

CHANGES IN YOU

The third trimester starts from the end of 13 weeks of pregnancy. You now have less early pregnancy symptoms, and you are more energetic. You may feel sexier than ever during the second trimester. Your short-term memory and concentration may be affected. Your immune system is slightly impaired when you're pregnant so you may have noticed that you've had more coughs and colds than you normally would. You may be prone to other infections, but the good news is that you are likely to be already immune to them before pregnancy.

From the week 16, sometimes, when you move suddenly, you may feel a slight pain in your sides. This is because the structures that hold the womb in place called 'ligaments' are stretching as your baby grows.

WHAT YOU NEED TO DO

- You should try chatting with other mums-to-be and find out how they are feeling at your stage of pregnancy.
- If you are having twins, find out what difference this will make to your antenatal care.
- If you're finding your job more of a challenge now, speak to your employer.
- It's good to keep active, but make sure you know when not to exercise.
- If you're single, this is also a good time to enlist support. You could ask your midwife about one-to-one antenatal sessions if you'd rather not go to couples' classes.
- From the second trimester, do not sleep on your back; you should rather lie on your left which is best for your baby. This position helps the flow of blood and nutrients to the placenta and also helps your kidneys to get rid of waste products and fluids from your body. This in turn helps to reduce swelling in your ankles, feet, and hands.
- You need to drink more fluid every day, at least 1.5 L.

WEEKS 17-19

GROWTH OF YOUR BABY

Your baby's weight ranges from 140 g at week 17 to 240 g at week 19. At week 17, baby's skeleton is mostly rubbery cartilage but will start to become bony as the pregnancy progresses. Sweat glands are starting to develop all over the body. The chest moves up and down to mimic breathing, blood vessels are visible through the skin, and the ears are now in their final position. The genitals are now clearly distinguishable. Baby swallows amniotic fluid, and his or her kidneys continue to make urine. Sensory centres in the brain for taste, smell, hear, see, and touch are developing.

CHANGES IN YOU

Your expanding uterus (womb) has distorted your balance, so wear flat slippers so that you do not fall. At week 18, you may have started feeling your baby's movements. The darkish circle of skin around your nipples, called the areola, may get larger as your breasts expand; this is perfectly normal and may last as long as 12 months after your baby is born.

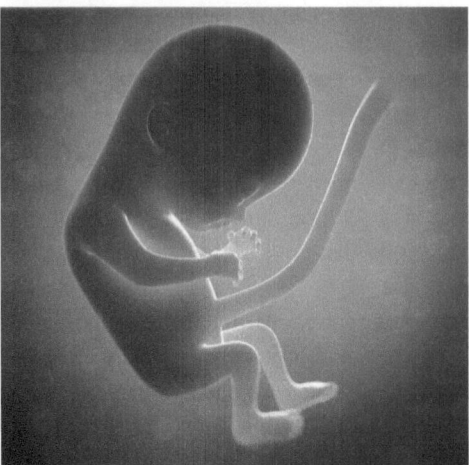

Figure 29. Weeks 17-20 of foetal development

The dark vertical line called the linea nigra at the middle of your tummy will be more prominent. You may develop darker pigmentation on your face; they will fade away after birth. Your growing bump probably means you need to be wearing larger sizes now. The top of your uterus (womb) may be reaching your belly button at week 19. From now on, your womb will be expanding at a rate of about a centimetre a week and ligament pain may get worse.

WHAT YOU NEED TO DO
Keep eating as healthy as you can, to make sure that you get the nutrients that your baby needs. You will need more calcium and vitamin D to help your baby grow strong teeth and bones. Do not forget about exercise in pregnancy.

WEEKS 20-23

HOW YOUR BABY IS GROWING
The weight of your baby ranges from 300 g at week 20 to 500 g at week 23. From week 20, whitish coat of fatty substance called vernix caseosa begins to cover your baby, protecting his or her skin during its long immersion in amniotic fluid and also easing childbirth. Your baby's swallowing more these week, good practice for his or her digestive system. After swallowing the amniotic fluid, his or her body absorbs the water in it and sends the rest into the large bowel where a sticky by-product called meconium accumulates. It'll appear in his or her first nappy after he or she is born.

Your baby's eyebrows and eyelids are fully developed, and he or she can now blink. The lips and the eyes have completely formed, but the coloured part of the eyes (the iris) still lacks pigment. The first signs of teeth appear in the form of tooth buds beneath her gum line. If you're having a boy, testes will descend from the pelvis into the scrotum in the coming weeks. From week 23, baby's hearing is established and can recognise your voice, the beating of your heart, and your stomach rumblings. So in the coming months, you could play classical music which foetuses like and read loud for your baby.

CHANGES IN YOUR LIFE

You're now halfway there! The top of your uterus (womb) now reaches your belly button and will grow about a centimetre a week. The pregnancy symptoms are almost all gone by now. You've probably gained between 5.5 and 7 kg so far. You may crave certain foods and feel clumsy because of the protruding abdomen. Your gums may bleed when you brush, and your belly button may now stick out.

Your fingers, toes, and other joints may be loosening, thanks to the effect of pregnancy hormones. There may be nosebleeding too. You may feel slightly breathlessness over the rest of your pregnancy as your expanding uterus pushes up against your lungs; if it gets worse, seek medical attention. From week 22, your breasts will start to produce colostrums, which is the first milk, full of protein and antibodies, which your baby will need in her first few days after birth. You may have more vaginal discharge and pass urine more often than before.

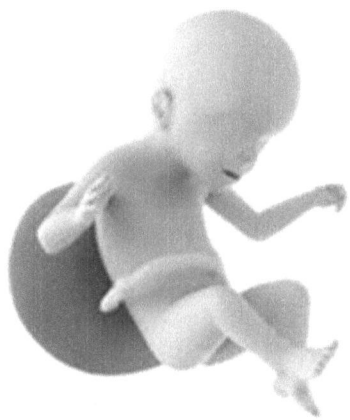

Figure 30. Weeks 21-24 of foetal development

What You Need To Do

- Read your pregnancy book.
- Go for your anomaly scan from 21 to 23 weeks.
- See your doctor if you notice any unusual symptoms like vagina discharge, passing urine too much, nosebleeding, bleeding gum, and so on.
- Discuss with your partner about his worries.
- Think about choosing name for your baby and whether your mother-in-law or your mother will help you to take care of your baby.
- Massage your bump (you or your partner can do that) as long as you use gentle strokes that glide over the contours of your body. It's one of the ways to be close to your baby.
- Inform your employer about your pregnancy and propose the date for your maternity leave. Your partner should also sort out his own paternity leave this time.

Weeks 24-25

How Your Baby is Growing

Your baby weighs 600-660 g. The skin is thin and fragile, but the body is well proportioned. At week 25, his or her wrinkled skin will begin to smooth out, and he or she'll start to look more like a newborn. Footprints and fingerprints are forming. Baby's lungs are developing branches of the respiratory tree as well as cells that produce surfactant. This substance will help baby's air sacs inflate once he or she is born, and therefore, from week 24, your baby has a chance of survival if delivered. At week 26, your baby responds to touch, and if you shine a light on your belly, your baby will turn his or her head, which confirms further development of a nerve in the brain called optic nerve.

Changes in Your Life

Stretch marks are prominent on the belly, hips, and breasts (page xxx). Your eyes may be light-sensitive and may feel gritty and dry. Try to rest your eyes as much as possible and keep them clean with cotton wool and warm water. If your dry eyes are bothering you, see your doctor to rule out infection and scarring. Other problems that can occur at this stage of pregnancy are gestational diabetes and carpal tunnel syndrome (page 188).

What You Need to Do

You should contact your doctor if you develop any of the obstetric problems that occur at this stage of pregnancy.

WEEKS 26-27

HOW YOUR BABY IS GROWING

Your baby weighs 760-875 g. He or she sleeps and wakes at regular intervals, may suck his or her finger or thumb, and responds to sound more as the pregnancy progresses. At first, your baby will only hear low-frequency sounds from inside your body, such as your heartbeat and your tummy rumbling but later, high-pitched noises from outside your body will be heard. He or she may be able to hear you and your partner chatting.

Your baby continues to practise breathing movements; this is a form of preparation for that critical moment of first breath at birth. At week 27, the characteristic grooves on the surface of his or her brain start appearing, and more brain tissue develops. Your baby can now dream. Hiccups are common this week and throughout the remaining pregnancy.

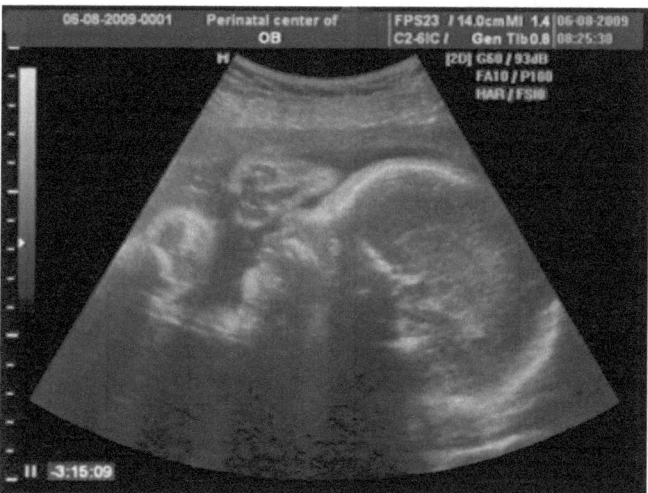

Figure 31. Ultrasound picture of the fetus at week 27

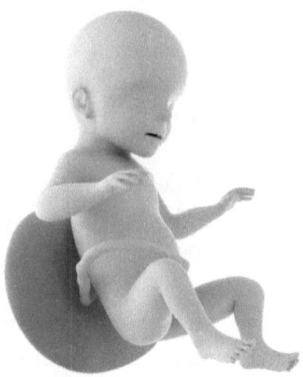

Figure 32. Weeks 25-28 of foetal development

CHANGES IN YOUR LIFE

Since your baby is now growing very fast and brain development is so intense at this stage, your nutrition is very important. Your third trimester starts when you've completed 27 weeks of pregnancy. Around this time, you may see a slight increase in your BP, which is normal but your midwife should be vigilant about PE by monitoring your BP and urine dipstick at each antenatal visit.

If you develop symptoms of PE namely headaches, blurred vision, and swollen hands and feet, you should call your midwife or doctor immediately. Starting from week 27, leg cramps, haemorrhoids, varicose veins, and an itchy belly may be plaguing you (page 178). You will be tested for anaemia at weeks 27-28, and if you are rhesus negative, a blood test will be done at the same time and repeated at week 34.

WEEK 28

HOW YOUR BABY IS GROWING

Baby's weight is just more than 1 kg, and length from top to toe is 38 cm. There are eyelashes, and baby can blink the eyes. The fat layers of the body are continuing to form, but bones are still soft and pliable.

HOW YOUR LIFE'S CHANGING

You can sing and read to your baby. The nerve pathways to your baby's ears are complete now. You may feel an unpleasant 'creepy-crawly' sensation in your lower legs and an irresistible urge to move them while trying to relax or sleep.

Try stretching or massaging them and cut down on caffeine, which can make the symptoms worse. Iron supplements can sometimes relieve this problem.

WHAT YOU NEED TO DO

Find out about antenatal classes and read real-life birth stories to help you prepare for the big day. Your partner should read tips from other people who've been a birth partner to find out more. Make a list of the things you need to put in your hospital bag just in case you need to go in early and also find out what should go in a dad's bag too. If you have young children, it's good to talk to them about the new baby. Make sure your shoes are comfortable, and if you get tired, try to rest with your feet up.

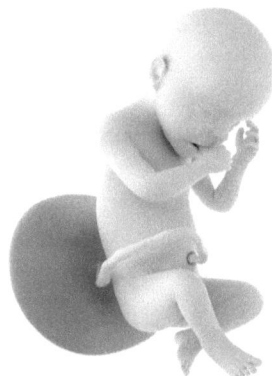

Figure 33. Weeks 29-32 of foetal development

WEEK 32

HOW YOUR BABY IS GROWING

Your baby now weighs about 1.7 kg and is around 42 cm long from head to toe. Your baby gains a third to half of his or her birth weight during the next 7 weeks as he or she fattens up for survival outside the womb. Although baby's lungs won't be fully developed until just before birth, babies born from this week have good chance of survival. For boys, the testicles should have descended from the abdomen into the scrotum by now. Sometimes, however, one or both testicles won't move into position until after birth. In two-thirds of all baby boys who have undescended testicles at birth, the condition corrects itself by their first birthday.

HOW YOUR LIFE'S CHANGING

You may be feeling breathless, tired, suffer from heartburn, and back pain (pages xxx). Speak to your midwife or doctor about them. If you're feeling closer than ever, you should not be worried; having sex in the final months will not harm your baby, but you should not have sex if your waters have gone.

Your expanding uterus shifts your centre of gravity and stretches out and weakens your abdominal muscles, changing your posture and putting a strain on your back. Hormonal changes in pregnancy loosen your joints and the ligaments that attach your pelvic bones to your spine. This can make you feel less stable and cause pain when you walk, stand, sit for long periods, roll over in bed, get out of a low chair, bend, or lift things.

WEEK 36

HOW YOUR BABY IS GROWING

Your baby weighs nearly 2.7 kg and is about 47 cm long from head to toe. At the end of this week, your baby will be considered full-term which is 37-42 weeks. Babies born before 37 weeks are pre-term and those born after 42 are post-term. Most likely, he or she's in a head-down position. But if he or she isn't, your practitioner may suggest scheduling an 'external cephalic version', which is a fancy way of saying she'll try to coax your baby into a head-down position by manipulating his or her from the outside of your belly.

HOW YOUR LIFE'S CHANGING

Now you should have less heartburn and breathe easier since your baby has probably started to 'drop' down into your pelvis. This process is called 'lightening'. You may also feel increased pressure in your lower abdomen and in the vagina, which may make walking increasingly uncomfortable, and you'll probably find that you have to pee even more frequently. Some women say it feels as if their baby is going to fall out. Practising your pelvic floor exercises can help. If you've given birth before, 'lightening' probably won't happen before labour starts, especially if you are of African descent because of the nature of African women's pelvis.

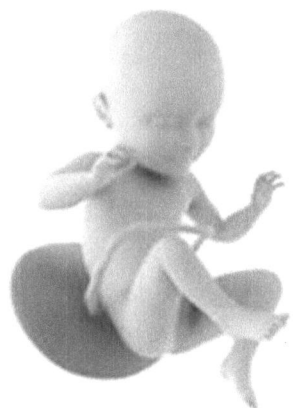

Figure 34. Weeks 33-36 of foetal development

You might also notice that your Braxton Hicks contractions are more frequent now and your breasts are leaking a little. This is quite normal. They are producing the rich first milk called colostrum that will give your baby a great start in life.

WHAT YOU NEED TO DO

You should know the signs of labour and when to go to the hospital (page xxx). Even if you're enjoying an uncomplicated pregnancy, it's best to avoid flying or any travel far from home during your final month because you can go into labour at any time.

WEEK 40

HOW YOUR BABY IS GROWING

He or she is getting a little heavier and may grow a bit more in length. It's hard to say for sure how big your baby will be, but a weight between 2.5 and 3.8 kg is normal and so is a length of about 51 cm. Your baby's head has probably 'engaged'. Engagement means the major part of the presenting part (PP), probably the head is in the pelvis. Sometimes, the head doesn't engage until labour has started. In Africans, it may not engage until the second stage of labour.

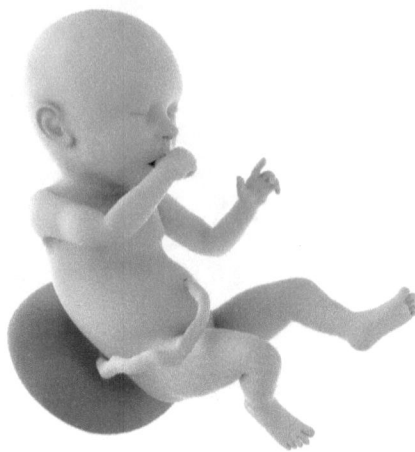

Figure 35. Weeks 37-40 of foetal development

Skull bones are not yet fused, which allows them to overlap a bit if the head cannot fit into the birth canal properly during labour.

Your baby sheds the greasy white substance (vernix caseosa), which has been protecting her skin. If she shows no sign of making an appearance after another week, she may have a dry skin when she arrives. Your baby has mastered all the skills that she'll need after birth. She can instinctively search for her thumb and suck it, just as she will search for your breast for a feed soon after birth.

How Your Life's Changing

After months of anticipation, your due date has finally arrived and you're still pregnant. It's frustrating, but lots of women find themselves in this situation. If your waters break or you start to feel contractions, do call your doctor or midwife straightaway. At about week 41, your doctor may assess you and send you for scan to check for well-being of your baby.

Sources

- How your baby grows during pregnancy. Frequently asked questions. American College of obstetricians and gynecologists ACOG. 2012
- Baby Centre Internet Service.
- Jurkovic D, et al. Landmarks for diagnosis ultrasound features of normal early pregnancy development. Curr Opin Obstet Gynaecol. 1995;7:493).
- The Pregnancy Book. NHS, UK, 2009.
- UK NHS Choice, Your health, your choices. Pregnancy Guide, 2012.

Emotional and Social Aspects of Pregnancy

FEELINGS DURING PREGNANCY

Pregnancy changes how you feel—about yourself, baby, family, and your surrounding in general. People expect you to be excited, but sometimes, you may find yourself sad for no apparent reason. Coping with these changes can be challenging. Hormonal changes taking place in your body are responsible for these feelings. Talk to your midwife about it.

RELATIONSHIP DURING PREGNANCY

Pregnancy can cause changes in your relationship with your loved ones, especially your partner or husband, especially in a first pregnancy. Your children, parents, and friends may be affected. You may or may not cope with these changes easily. You may quarrel or argue with your partner for things that are insignificant. Thought of uncertainty and how to cope as a mother or father can also ignite argument. These problems can be resolved by discussing with your partner about the matters concerning the pregnancy, for instance your next antenatal appointment, labour, the part that your partner is going to play, and so on. If there is issue of domestic violence, you should ask your midwife how to get help.

Your parents, siblings, and friends may be offering you help. Sometimes, you may feel that they are controlling you. In that situation, it should be appropriate to tell them that there are some decisions that only you and your partner can take and others that only you can take.

SEX IN PREGNANCY

SAFETY

If your pregnancy is of low-risk category, that is pregnancy without anticipated complication, you can have sex throughout the pregnancy. Your baby is protected by the amniotic fluid and the sac, the muscles of your womb including the cervix with its thick mucus plug which prevents infection from going into the womb from the vagina. Furthermore, your partner's penis during sex can penetrate only into the vagina; it does not go into the cervical canal. So you will not hurt your baby during sex; he or she will not know what is going on.

You may feel some abdominal cramps or tightening called Braxton Hicks during or immediately after intercourse; this is caused by orgasm, nipple stimulation, and the prostaglandins in semen. It is temporary and harmless. Lying quietly in bed till the contractions pass is advisable in that situation. You will have to call for help in the following circumstances:

- persistent contractions that do not go away during or just after intercourse or orgasm
- significant abdominal pain after sex
- bleeding during or after sex

The only situations in pregnancy when you have to say 'no' to sex are as follows:
- When your waters break.
- When you are bleeding.
- When you have abnormal discharge.
- When you have a low-lying placenta.
- When you have premature labour.
- When you have threatened premature labour (even if it has stopped).
- When you go into labour.
- If you have very short cervix or cervical incompetent in your previous pregnancy.
- If you have a dilated cervix.
- When you and your partner have active genital herpes or feel one coming on.
- If your partner has a history of genital herpes (and you don't) whether or not he has symptoms, you should not have sexual contact with him during the third trimester. The same applies to receiving oral sex if he has oral herpes (cold sores) or previous history of the disease.
- If your partner has other sexually transmitted diseases, for example HIV, then having unprotected sex is dangerous. Research has shown that HIV can be transmitted through tiny wound in the mouth. So use some sort of protection during oral sex, for example a dental dam, which is a sheet of latex that you place between your genitals and your partner's mouth.

Regarding oral sex during pregnancy, you partner can give you 'licking' but blowing into your vagina is not allowed because it can force a bubble of air into your blood circulation. Although this situation is rare, it can constitute a serious problem for you and your baby. If you are a single mother and not in a relationship, it is safe to abstain from sex during pregnancy. If you do engage in a sexual act, it is advisable to always use a barrier contraceptive measure, male or female condoms for penetrative sex and dental dams for oral sex.

SEX DRIVE

You may find out that sex feels different during pregnancy. Your libido in most cases may be higher than other time, and therefore, sex can be very enjoyable; in some cases, it may be low and you may be turned off completely. These feelings are dictated by what is happening in your body and the complications that can occur in pregnancy.

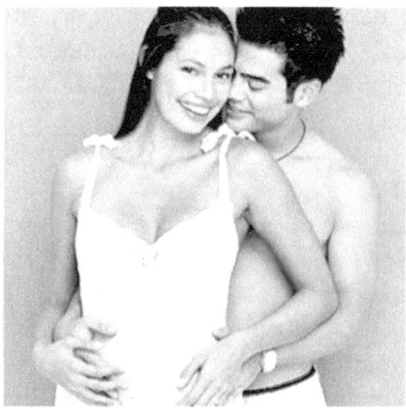

Figure 36. Increased libido during pregnancy

During pregnancy, there is increased blood flow to your genital organs including the uterus, cervix, and vagina; this will give rise to increased sensation and therefore increased libido and also increased vaginal discharge or moistness which will add to the heightened sensation. For some women, the genital engorgement during pregnancy may be a source of uncomfortable feeling of fullness and therefore have decreased libido. Furthermore, the tenderness in your breast in the first trimester will pass and what will remain will be increased tingly and sensitivity to touch. In most cases, this will make sexual act pleasurable, while for others, it will not be pleasant, and they may prefer that their breasts are not touched.

Your emotional and physical feeling can determine what happens to your sex drive. Tiredness, negative emotional changes, nausea, and vomiting can turn you off sex, especially in the first trimester. Things should get better in the second trimester after these problems have eased up. Furthermore, your libido can dip again in the third trimester, particularly in the last month. You may be too big, too tired, having backache, preoccupied with the thought of labour and birth, and problems associated with motherhood, and all these may turn you off sex.

Regarding your partner, in most cases, he will find you more attractive during pregnancy. Again, his sexual desire may fluctuate based on the prevailing circumstances. His libido may be decreased because of the following reasons: thought of what you will be through during labour and childbirth, responsibilities as a father, fear that intercourse could hurt the baby, and so on. One way of addressing his anxiety is for him to attend the antenatal clinic with you, and his questions can be answered there.

So your libido and that of your partner can fluctuate in pregnancy; that is perfectly normal. Let your partner know how you feel and reassure him that you still love him. At this crucial time, communication is important as you go through these changes together. If you are turned on but not enjoying intercourse, you can consider other erotic activities, such as self-stimulation, hugging, kissing, caressing each other, and oral sex.

POSITION DURING SEX

The conventional sexual position with the man on top is not recommended in the second and third trimesters. Even in the first trimester, it can become uncomfortable to have sex with your partner on top. Generally, 'man-on-top' position is not good because of the following reasons: your bump, tender breasts, and it can also be uncomfortable if your partner penetrates you too deeply. If you do use this position after the first trimester, wedge a pillow under you so you're tilted and not flat on your back, and make sure your partner supports himself so his weight is not on your abdomen.

You will have to explore other positions with your partner. Possible conducive sexual positions during pregnancy are as follows:

- Lie on your side with your partner facing your back and entering from behind. In this position, penetration should be shallow, and this is good for the pregnancy.
- Place your legs on both sides of your partner's pelvis as he lies on his back or sits on a chair. In this position, you will have no weight on your womb and you can control the depth of penetration.
- Lie on your back with your side supported with a pillow wedge, shift your bottom to the side or foot of the bed and bend your knees and feet with the sole of your feet resting on the mattress. Your partner will then kneel or stand and enter you from the front.
- Place yourself in all fours position, that is on your knees and elbows, and your partner enters you from behind while he kneels down.

WORK

You may have mixed feelings when you go on maternity leave. The leave is a good opportunity to make some new friends. You may meet other mothers at antenatal classes, or you may get to know more people living close by. You may think about spending some time at home with your baby, or you may be planning to return to work soon.

If you will be going back to work, you need to start thinking about childcare in advance. Possibilities are

- having a relative
- contacting information service for a list of registered childminders and nurseries

- organising care in your own home, either on your own or sharing with other parents

If you are to claim financial help with the costs as in developed countries, the carer must be approved through the Government's Childcare Approval Scheme.

BONDING WITH YOUR BABY WHEN YOU ARE PREGNANT

You should regularly bond with your baby when you are advance in your pregnancy by reading, singing, and talking to your bump.

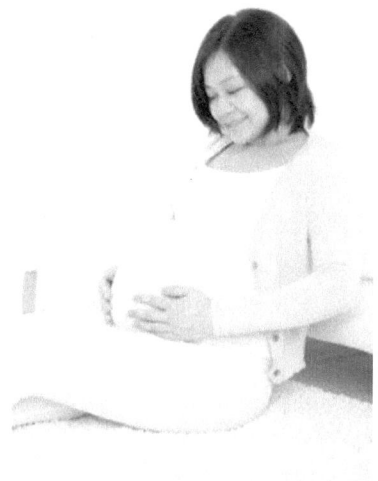

Figure 37. Bonding with your bump

SOURCES

- Routine Postnatal Care of Women and Their Babies. The UK National Collaborating Centre for Primary Care. July 2006.
- Antenatal Care: Routine Care for the Healthy Pregnant Woman. National Collaborating Centre for Women's and Children's Health. Commissioned by the UK National Institute for Health and Clinical Excellence. March 2008. This is a partial update of the 2003 guideline.
- www.patient.co.uk
- Baby Centre website.

Antenatal Care

Antenatal care is defined as a specialized healthcare service that should be received by pregnant women during the antenatal period of pregnancy. Antenatal period starts from conception and ends with delivery of your baby. Healthcare professionals will check you and your baby to confirm that you are well, give you useful information about you and your baby, and answer your questions at different stages of your pregnancy. So make sure that you book early for your antenatal care.

YOUR CARE PROVIDERS

Your care providers are the medical personnel who will take care of you on regular basis during your pregnancy. Even if you see different staff at different time, the continuity of care will be maintained since everything about you will be written in your medical record.

The medical personnel who you will meet during your pregnancy are listed below.
- Midwife
- Supervisor of midwives
- Obstetrician
- Feto-maternal medicine specialist
- Anaesthetist
- Paediatrician
- Sonographer
- Obstetric physiotherapist
- Health visitors
- Theatre nurses
- Dietician
- Health care assistant
- Medical research students
- Students (medical students, student midwife)

MIDWIFE
A midwife is a medical personnel who is trained to care for women during pregnancy, labour, and up to 28 days after delivery.

SUPERVISOR OF MIDWIVES
A supervisor of midwives provides care as a midwife and also supervises other midwives having had additional educational training. They will support you if you are having any problems with your care or if you feel that your wishes and requests are not being considered.

OBSTETRICIAN
An obstetrician is a doctor who has already specialised or specialising in the care of pregnant women including antenatal care, care in labour and 6 weeks after delivery. You will see trainee obstetricians at different levels of their training, who are supervised by their respective consultants.

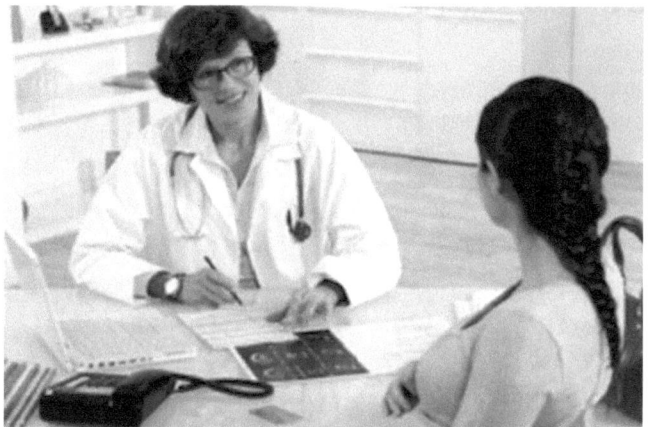

Figure 38. Your consultation with your obstetrician

FETO-MATERNAL MEDICINE SPECIALIST

A feto-maternal medicine specialist is an obstetrician who focuses on the medical and surgical management of high-risk pregnancies. Management includes monitoring and treating you, ultrasound assessment of your baby at different stages of pregnancy, invasive diagnostic procedures (page 103), and foetal surgery or treatment. Depending on your circumstances, you may come in contact with a feto-maternal medicine specialist during your pregnancy.

ANAESTHETIST

An anaesthetist is a doctor who specialises in providing pain relief. It is the anaesthetist who sets up your epidural in labour, during instrumental delivery or caesarean section. During the antenatal period, your doctor may refer you to an anaesthetist if you have any medical condition that can affect appropriate pain relief in labour, for example heart problem, lower back problem at the level where epidural is normally inserted, and so on.

PAEDIATRICIAN

A paediatrician is a specialist who takes care of babies and children. He or she checks your baby after birth to make sure all is well and will be present when your baby is born if you have had a difficult labour. If your baby is born at home or your pregnancy is of low risk, you may not see a paediatrician at all. Your midwife or GP will check that all is well with you and your baby.

SONOGRAPHER

A sonographer will perform all your scans during pregnancy. This service is also offered by a specialist in feto-maternal medicine.

OBSTETRIC PHYSIOTHERAPIST

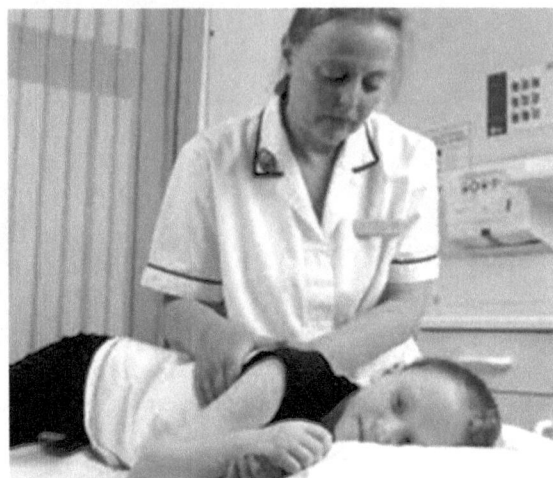

Figure 39. Obstetric physiotherapist at work

An obstetric physiotherapist helps you cope with physical changes during pregnancy, childbirth, and afterwards. They teach antenatal exercises, relaxation and breathing, and other ways you can keep yourself fit and healthy during pregnancy, labour, and post-natal. Your midwife also helps with these exercises.

HEALTH VISITORS

You may meet your health visitor before the birth of your baby, and you will be visited by a member of the team in the first few weeks after your baby is born. You may continue to see your health visitor or a member of the health visiting team at home, at your child's health clinic, at children's centre, at health centre, or at your doctor's clinic.

THEATRE NURSES

These are nurses who work in theatre.

DIETICIANS

They give advice about healthy eating or special diets, for example if you develop gestational diabetes.

HEALTH CARE ASSISTANT

They help with cleaning the wards and changing the beddings. They are not directly involved in your care.

MEDICAL RESEARCH STUDENTS

Research students may ask you to participate in a research project during your care. Such projects improve maternity care. The student will explain the research to you and you are free to say yes or no; your answer will not affect your care.

STUDENTS

These are medical students and student midwives. They will be at various stages of their training and will observe how care is provided. Sometimes, they may take history from you. You can say no, but if you let a student be present during your care, it will help their education.

ANTENATAL APPOINTMENTS

Your antenatal appointments should take place in a conducive environment where you should feel comfortable to discuss sensitive problems that may affect your pregnancy (such as domestic violence, sexual abuse, mental illness, or recreational drug use). This may be at a primary health care unit, your doctor's clinic, district general or teaching hospital, and sometimes at your home.

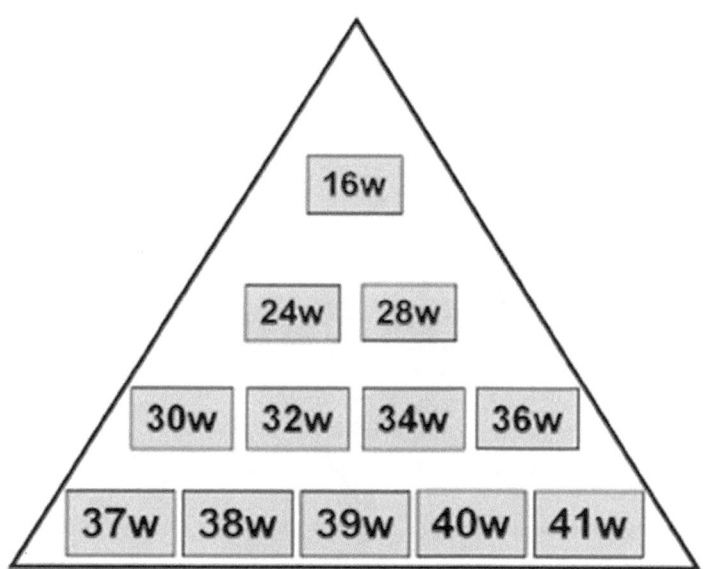

Figure 40. The pyramid of antenatal care from 1929 till now

HISTORICAL BACKGROUND TO ANTENATAL
APPOINTMENTS AND THE PYRAMID OF CARE

In the nineteenth century, pregnancy care was confined to the time of delivery and reserved for the wealthy. In the beginning of the twentieth century, the high maternal and infant deaths stimulated the establishment of institutions for provision of antenatal care. In 1929, the Ministry of Health in the UK issued a memorandum on antenatal clinics, recommending that women should first be seen at the sixteenth week of pregnancy and then 24 and 28 weeks, fortnightly until 36 weeks and then weekly until delivery (figure 40). This guideline established the pattern of antenatal care that is still followed throughout the world today.

In the last 20 years, the following have become possible at an integrated antenatal clinic at 11-13[+6] weeks:

- More than 95 out of every 100 cases of all major chromosomal abnormalities can be identified.
- The chance of you developing certain complications of pregnancy can be determined, for example miscarriage and stillbirth, PE, diabetes during pregnancy, PTD (delivery before 34 weeks of pregnancy), small-for-age babies, and large-for-age babies.

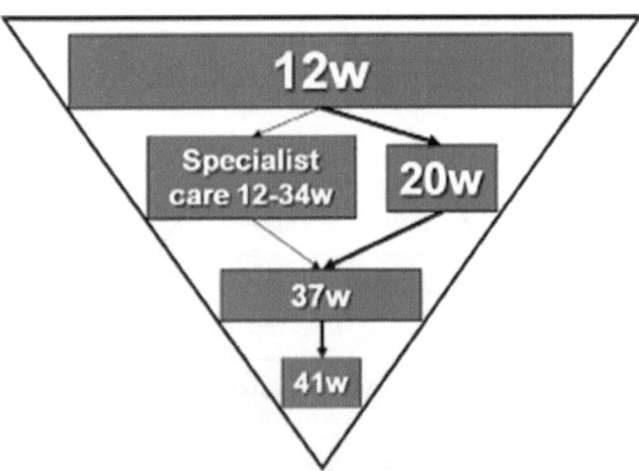

Figure 41. Pyramid of antenatal care turned upside down (Kypros Nicolaides, 2011)

Early estimation of your specific risks for these pregnancy complications would improve pregnancy outcome by shifting antenatal care from a series of routine visits to a more individualised patient and disease-specific approach both in terms of the schedule and content of such visits. The small proportion of women identified as being at high risk for a variety of pregnancy complications can have close surveillance in dedicated clinics dealing with each of these pregnancy complications. This information is illustrated in the pyramid above—'Turning the pyramid of care upside down' (Prof. Kypros Nicolaides, 2011).

The great majority of women identified as being at low risk for pregnancy complications can have less antenatal appointments and managed solely by midwives unless problems develop when they will be referred to a doctor. Therefore, the 11-13 weeks antenatal assessment is likely to be the basis for a new scientific approach to antenatal care by turning the 80 years pyramid of care upside down. This new approach has been adopted by many hospitals in Asia, America, Europe, including King's College Hospital, London, where the concept was first highlighted.

ANTENATAL SCHEDULES AND MANAGEMENT

Irrespective of the overwhelming evidence supporting turning the pyramid of care upside down, it has not been fully implemented in clinical practice. We have illustrated in this book a modified guideline which was approved by the National Institute of Clinical Excellence (NICE), United Kingdom. The antenatal schedule in the guideline does not differ much from what is obtainable in developed and developing countries.

A. First contact with your midwife or doctor (4-8 weeks)

As soon as you miss your period, you should take a pregnancy test; if this is positive, you should make an appointment to see your midwife or GP. At the appointment, the following will be done:
- The pregnancy will be confirmed with a urine pregnancy test.
- If you have not had a prepregnancy care, this will be an opportunity for your doctor to go through it with you, including taking folic acid and Vitamin D.
- You will be introduced to antenatal appointments and screening tests.

B. Booking appointment (11-13^{+6} weeks)

At this clinic, a full history will be taken from you, including personal, family, past obstetric and gynaecological, medical, and so on. You will be asked a lot of questions to build up a picture of you and your pregnancy. The rationale will be to identify those factors that are likely to affect the management of your pregnancy in order to assign you to either a low—or high-risk group (next chapter). The first is managed by the midwife and GP, while the later is managed by your obstetrician.

Your midwife or doctor should give you information about
- development of your baby stage by stage—page 48
- nutrition and diet—page 139

- exercise in pregnancy—page 162
- antenatal screening tests—page 99
- antenatal education—page 131
- planning your labour
- your options for where to have your baby
- breastfeeding, including workshops and
- maternity benefits

Your midwife or doctor should
- measure your height and weight and calculate your BMI.
- measure your BP and test your urine.
- identify any potential risks associated with any work you do.
- find out whether you are at increased risk of gestational diabetes or PE.
- offer you screening tests and make sure that you understand what they involve before embarking on any of them.
- take your booking blood tests.
- offer you an ultrasound scan at 11-13^{+6} weeks for reasons stated below under 'C'.
- define your risk and plan the care you will get throughout your pregnancy if you belong to the low-risk category.
- refer you to an obstetrician if you belong to the high-risk category.
- give you your hand-held notes and plan of care.
- make a dental appointment, free in the UK during pregnancy and for a year after birth.

C.   Ultrasound scan at 11-13^{+6} weeks

Indications or reasons are as follows:
- to date the pregnancy and confirm the expected date of delivery (EDD)
- to check for foetal abnormalities
- to screen for chromosomal abnormalities
- to screen for preterm labour, that is labour before 37 weeks of pregnancy
- to screen for PE, which is high blood pressure in pregnancy (HIP)
- to screen for slow growth of the baby as pregnancy progresses
- to check the position of the developing placenta

D.   Review with results (16 weeks)

Your midwife or doctor should
- measure your BP and test your urine for protein.
- help with any concerns or questions you have.

- discuss and record the results of booking blood tests, Down's syndrome test, and screening for abnormalities in the baby.
- plan your care based on the new information received.
- give you information about anomaly scan at 20-32 weeks.
- consider giving you iron and folic acid supplements if you are anaemic.

E. Anomaly scan and review (20-23 weeks)

Indications or reasons are as follows:
- to check for the reasons listed under 'C' above
- to check placental position
- to confirm the number of blood vessels in the umbilical cord of your baby
- to find out the sex of your baby if you want to know it

F. 25 weeks

This clinic is mainly for women expecting their first children. Your midwife or doctor should
- measure your BP and test your urine for protein.
- check the size of your uterus.
- review the screening tests done at 20-23 weeks if not already reviewed.
- From this stage of pregnancy, you should start planning about your maternity leave.
- If you live in the UK,
  - you should get your maternity certificate (form MAT B1) from your doctor or midwife.
  - you can claim for Statutory Maternity Pay (SMP) and the Health in Pregnancy Grant at the same time from 26 weeks of pregnancy; in order to collect your SMP, you must inform your employer at least 28 days before you stop work.
  - you should also ask your partner to inform his employer if he plans to take paternity leave.

G. 28 weeks

Your midwife or doctor should
- measure your BP and test your urine for protein.
- use a tape to measure the size of your uterus.
- do full blood count to screen you for anaemia; if you have a rhesus negative blood group, blood test will be taken for its level and you will be given anti-D.

- offer more screening tests, namely
    - blood tests for HIV, syphilis, and malarial parasite if you live in an endemic region
    - cervical swabs for chlamydia and gonorrhoea

Ultrasound is indicated if any of the following is applicable to you:
- Low level of placental hormone pregnancy- associated plasma protein-A (PAPP-A) at 11-13+6 (high risk of having a small babies)
- Screened positive for PE and small babies at the 20-23 weeks scan
- Early PE or fetal death before labour or preterm labour before 34 weeks in your previous pregnancies.
- Medical condition (diabetes, etc.) or you are on any medication that can affect you or your baby, e.g. heparin.
- You live in sub-Saharan Africa or other parts of the world that are endemic for malaria.

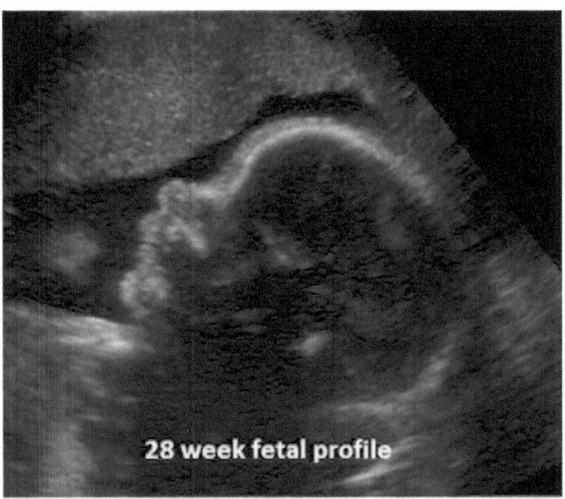

Fig. 41A. Growth scan at 28 weeks

H. 31-32 weeks

Your midwife or doctor should
- review, discuss, and record the results of any screening tests or ultrasound report from the last appointment if not already done.
- measure your BP and test your urine for protein.
- measure the height of your womb.

You will be offered a repeat ultrasound scan for the same reasons that were outlined for 28 weeks.

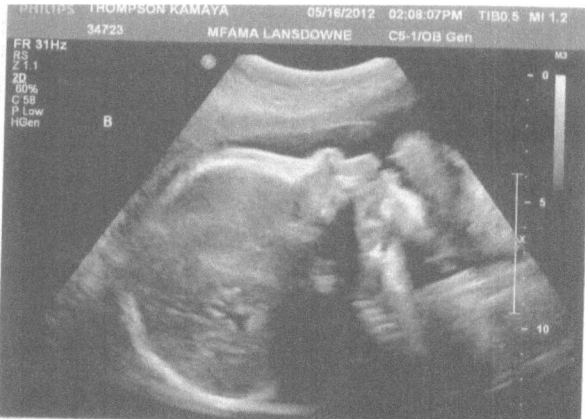

Fig. 41B. Growth scan at 31-32 weeks

I.   34 weeks

Your midwife or doctor should
*   give you information about preparing for labour and birth, including how to recognise active labour, ways of coping with pain in labour, and your birth plan.
*   review and discuss the results of the scan at 31-32 weeks if not already done.
*   measure the size of your uterus.
*   measure your BP and test your urine for protein.
*   offer your second anti-D treatment if you are rhesus negative.

You should
*   make arrangements for the birth.
*   make childcare arrangements for children, if you have children already, when you go into labour.
*   make sure you have all your important telephone numbers handy in case labour starts.
*   plan to take a tour of maternity facilities for birth.
*   think about who you would like to have with you during labour.
*   get your bag ready if you are planning to give birth in hospital or in a primary health centre.
*   be attending antenatal classes now.
*   be more aware of your uterus tightening from time to time. These are mild contractions known as Braxton Hicks contractions.

J. 36 weeks

Your midwife or doctor should give you information about
- feeding and caring for your newborn baby
- vitamin K and screening tests for your newborn baby
- 'baby blues' and post-natal depression Your midwife or doctor should
- measure your BP and test your urine for protein.
- measure the height of your womb.
- check whether baby's head is engaged or not.
- offer you a scan if any of the following is applicable to you:
  - abnormal findings on the scan at 31-32 weeks
  - suspected abnormal on clinical examination findings, e.g. small baby.
  - medical condition e.g. diabetes
  - living in the Sub-Saharan Africa or other parts of the world endemic for malaria
  - screened positive for PE at 20-23 weeks scan
  - history of previous PE or small baby or previous fetal death before delivery

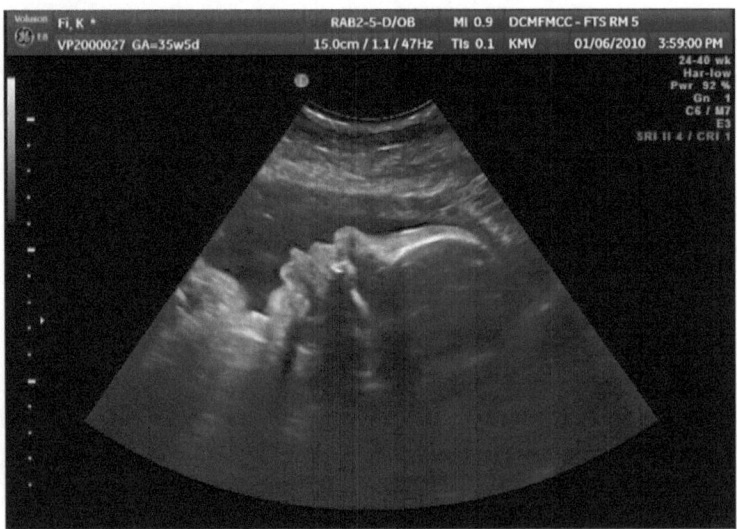

Fig. 42. Growth scan at 36 weeks

Your midwife or doctor should
- discuss the options available if your pregnancy lasts longer than 41 weeks. Most women will go into labour between 38 and 42 weeks.
- measure the size of your uterus.
- measure your BP and test your urine for protein.

L. 40 weeks

This is an extra appointment if you are expecting your first baby. Your midwife or doctor should

- measure your BP and test your urine for protein.
- measure the size of your uterus.
- offer you a postdate scan to check growth and amniotic fluid level. Not offered in every hospital

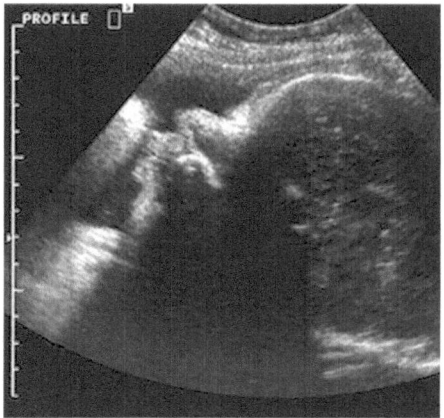

Fig. 43. Growth scan at 40 weeks

M. 41 weeks

Your midwife or doctor should

- measure your BP and test your urine for protein.
- measure the size of your uterus.
- do internal examination and a membrane sweep, which may help in getting you into labour soon.
- discuss IOL with you.
- offer you extra appointment if this is your first baby.

It is important to note that the above antenatal schedule is based on the practice in developed countries generally and recommendations of the NICE guideline, United Kingdom. So the practice and antenatal schedule in your hospital may be slightly different from this guideline, but the content and principle should be about the same.

The practice in developing countries follows the same principle as enumerated above, but the content may be different; for instance, it is unlikely that anomaly scan in the first and second trimesters will be offered. So speak to your doctor and ask for a referral if any of the services that you need is not available in your local health care facility.

SOURCES

- Nicolaides KH. A model for a new pyramid of prenatal care based on the 11 to 13^{+6} weeks' assessment. Prenatal Diag. 2011;31:3-6.
- The current American Congress of Obstetricians and Gynecologists (ACOG) Guidelines for Perinatal Care, Seventh Edition. October 2012. available at http://www.acog.org/resources_and_publications/ 1
- Antenatal Care: Routine Care for the Healthy Pregnant Woman. NCCWCH Commissioned by the UK NICE, March 2008. Partial update of the 2003 guideline.
- Ministry of Health Report. 1929. Memorandum on Antenatal Clinics: Their Conduct and Scope. London: His Majesty's Stationery Office; 1930.
- The NHS Pregnancy Book, UK, 2009.

FIRST TRIMESTER ANTENATAL RISK ASSESSMENT

INTRODUCTION

Risk assessment is carried out at 11-13+6 weeks by your midwife or doctor (GP and/or obstetrician). Its purpose is to classify you into low or high-risk category, which will determine the content of your care.

The risk assessment will include the following:
- Medical history
- Examination
- Screening for obesity (overweight)
- Booking tests, including screening for infection
- Screening for genetic conditions in you and your partner
- Screening for foetal abnormalities, PE, preterm labour, and small baby

MEDICAL HISTORY

- History of the present pregnancy: Whether there has been any problem or not, obstetric history and whether your pregnancy is spontaneous or assisted conception.
- Past obstetrics and gynaecological history.
- Ethnic background: It will determine your risk of certain genetic condition e.g. sickle-cell disease (SCD) in Africans.
- Family history of inherited conditions, for example sickle cell or cystic fibrosis, other abnormalities, PE, diabetes, heart disease, and so on.
- Past medical, including mental health history.

- History of domestic violence, sexual abuse, or genital tract mutilation.
- Past surgical history generally.
- Social history, for example smoking, alcohol, and so on.
- Environmental and workplace hazards.
- Drug history.

EXAMINATION

The doctor will examine you from head to toe.

SCREENING FOR OBESITY (OVERWEIGHT)

Your weight and height will be taken and your body mass index BMI will be calculated. Most women put on between 10 and 12.5 kg (22-28 lb) in pregnancy, most of it after the twentieth week.

BOOKING TESTS

All the blood tests are performed with a single needle inserted into your vein at booking. Blood is taken for the following tests:

- Full blood count to rule out anaemia. Anaemia makes you tired and less able to cope with any loss of blood when you give birth. If tests show you are anaemic, you will probably be given iron and folic acid supplements.
- Blood group and rhesus group. People who are rhesus positive have a substance known as D antigen on the surface of their red blood cells. Rhesus negative people do not have that. A woman who is rhesus negative may carry a rhesus positive baby if the baby's father is rhesus positive. During pregnancy or birth, small amounts of baby's blood can enter into mother's bloodstream. This can stimulate maternal blood to produce antibodies; that is, she becomes sensitised. Therefore, if she gets pregnant in the future with another rhesus positive baby, much more antibodies will be produced if baby's blood enters into her own blood The antibodies can cross the placenta, attach themselves to baby's red blood cells and destroy them, causing anaemia in the baby. Anti-D injections prevent rhesus negative women from producing antibodies against their own babies and reduce the risk of a rhesus negative woman becoming sensitised. This is why rhesus negative mothers who are not sensitised are offered anti-D injections at 28 and 34 weeks as well as after the birth of their baby.
- Screening for infections. Blood will be taken for rubella, hepatitis B and C, syphilis, HIV infection and malaria if you live in endemic region. Routine antenatal blood test for toxoplasmosis will not be offered. However, in France, pregnant women are routinely screened for the infection.

In addition to the blood test, your urine and swab from the vagina will be tested for infection

- Screening for genetic conditions such as: SCD and thalassaemia, (Africans, the Caribbeans, Italians, Maltese, Portuguese, and Spanish, Indians, and the Chinese), cystic fibrosis and Tay-Sachs disease, depending on your ethnic origin.

SCD and thalassaemia: If you and/or your husband has the disease or is a carrier and you are pregnant, the status of your baby can be determined by a technique called chorionic blood sampling at 11-14 weeks of pregnancy (pages 104-106).

You will then have the choices of continuing with the pregnancy if the baby is not affected or terminating or continuing with it if the baby is affected.

Cystic fibrosis: It affects vital organs in the body, especially the lungs and digestive system, by clogging the organs with thick sticky mucus. The sweat glands are also affected. The disease is inherited, and both parents must be carriers of the gene variation for their baby to be born with cystic fibrosis. Testing is offered if there is a family history of cystic fibrosis.

Tay-Sachs disease: Testing for Tay-Sachs disease will be offered if you or your partner is of Ashkenazi Jewish origin and you consider yourself or your partner to be at risk.

CERVICAL CANCER SCREENING TEST

If you are due to have a cervical smear (i.e. you have not had one in the last 3 years), you will probably be told to wait until 3 months after your baby is born unless you have a history of abnormal smears.

COMBINED RESULTS OF THE RISK ASSESSMENT AND PLAN OF CARE

If you are in the high-risk group, you should have a joint care by an obstetrician and your GP or midwife, and delivery should occur in a hospital (private or government owned) that is well equipped to deal with possible complications. Those in the low-risk category will be cared for by midwives and delivery should occur either in a hospital, midwifery unit or primary health centre.

Your risk will be reassessed each time you are admitted to hospital and also when seen at the antenatal or the post-natal ward. If you develop any risk factor, you should be referred to an obstetrician (or another appropriate specialist) who will take care of you during your pregnancy.

CRITERIA FOR MIDWIFERY-LED CARE

All women are suitable for midwifery-led care except those in the following categories, who should be in a high-risk category:

- Pre-existing medical conditions, for example brain, lung, heart, bowel urinary tract problems, obesity. Talk to your doctor about them.
- Relevant infections, for example HIV, active genital herpes, active malarial infection.
- Drug abuse such as alcohol and drugs called opiates, for example morphine, cocaine, tobacco (more than 15 cigarettes a day).
- Obstetric history, for example previous stillbirth or neonatal death, previous baby with a birth defect, previous preterm labour, that is before 37 weeks, PE, small baby. Talk to your midwife and doctor.
- Previous anaesthetic problems.
- Previous surgery or trauma to genital tract, for example removal of fibroid, surgery on the cervix.
- Screened positive at the first-trimester risk assessment for the following conditions:
    - fetal abnormality
    - early onset of PE
    - small-for-age baby
    - preterm labour
    - gestational diabetes (diabetes that develop during pregnancy) in previous pregnancy

SOURCES

- Nicolaides KH. A model for a new pyramid of prenatal care based on the 11 to 13^{+6} weeks' assessment. Prenatal Diag. 2011;31:3-6.
- Screening tests for birth defects. Frequently asked questions. ACOG. 2013
- California Prenatal Screening Program to include noninvasive testing. Monica Flessel, PhD, and Sara Goldman, MPH, Genetic Disease Screening Program, California Department of Public Health ACOG, 2014
- Antenatal Care: Routine Care for the Healthy Pregnant Woman. NCCWCH Commissioned by the UK NICE, March 2008. Partial update of the 2003 guideline.
- The Pregnancy Book, UK, 2009.

THE 11-13^{+6} WEEKS SCAN

PURPOSE OF THE SCAN

- Demonstrate that your baby (the foetus) is alive by seeing the heart beating.
- Date the pregnancy.
- Diagnose multiple pregnancy.
- Screen for chromosomal abnormalities.
- Screen for the following conditions: major abnormalities in the baby, preeclampsia, small baby, and preterm labour.

HOW ULTRASOUND SCAN WORKS

Ultrasound scan uses sound waves to build up a picture of your baby in your uterus. The scan is completely painless, has no known serious side effects on mothers or babies, and can be carried out at any stage of pregnancy. If you have any concerns about having a scan, talk it over with your midwife, GP, or obstetrician.

ULTRASOUND PROCEDURE

The sonographer will introduce himself or herself and any other person in the room. He or she will ask you some basic questions, for example your name, age, about your pregnancy, and obtain verbal consent for the scan.

You may be asked to drink plenty of water before you have the scan if the scan will be performed through your abdomen (transabdominal scan). A full bladder pushes your uterus up, and this gives a better picture; it also acts as a window through which the ultrasound wave passes to your womb. Sometimes, drinking water before the procedure leads to poor images, and therefore, you may be asked to empty your bladder. You will then lie on your back and some jelly is put on your abdomen.

The ultrasound probe is passed backwards and forwards over your abdomen, and image is achieved on the screen. It can be very exciting to see a picture of your own baby moving about inside you. Ask for the picture to be explained to you if you cannot make it out. Ask if it's possible to have a copy of the picture. There may be a small charge for this.

Sometimes, it may not be possible to get all the necessary information through the abdominal scan. In that situation, you would be offered *transvaginal scan,* which involves you emptying your bladder completely. You would then remove your underwear, lie on the back, and an ultrasound probe will be passed into the vagina. This will give a better view of your baby. It is safe and does not pose any harm to you or your baby. There will be a chaperon, preferably a woman, present during the examination.

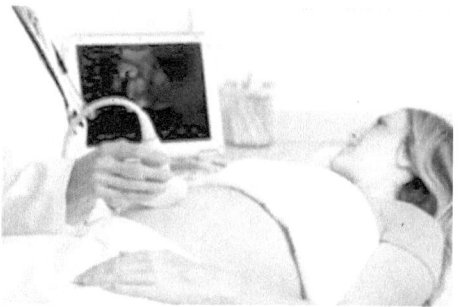

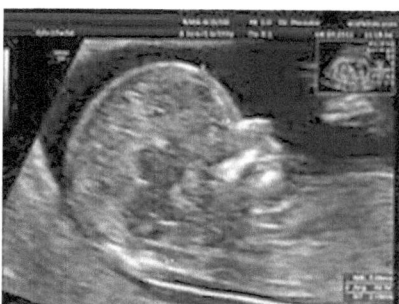

Figure 44a. Transabdominal ultrasound   **Figure 44b. Nuchal scan at 11-13^{+6} weeks**

Specific Features and Measurements During the Scan

The operator who may be a sonographer or a doctor will examine the following structures in your baby:

- skull and brain
- face
- spine and overlying skin
- heart
- ribcage, (thorax) to demonstrate the lungs, heart, and upper gut or oesophagus
- abdomen, to demonstrate the stomach, bladder, and insertion of the umbilical cord into the abdomen
- limbs

Abnormalities of these organs can be detected at this stage of pregnancy. Measurements that will be taken are as follows:

- Brainstem diameter—to predict the risk of baby having spina bifida.
- Blood flow in the vessels that supply blood to your womb—to predict the risk of early onset PE before 32 weeks and small baby.
- Heart rate and blood flow in other foetal vessels.
- Cervical length, that is the length of the neck of the womb—to predict the risk of preterm labour before 34 weeks.

If screening for Down's syndrome is offered in your hospital, the sonographer should assess the markers (signs) associated with or used in screening for it, namely

- nuchal translucency (NT), that is the thickness of the fluids at the back of the baby's neck
- nasal bone (NB, present or absent)
- foetal heart rate (FHR), that is the number of baby's heartbeat per minute
- blood flow in the heart and liver

The inclusion of the last three measurements into Down's syndrome screening may give almost 100% chance of detecting the condition (page xxx). The last two assessments will also help in predicting the risk of baby having heart problems.

MANAGEMENT OF THE FINDINGS AT THE SCAN

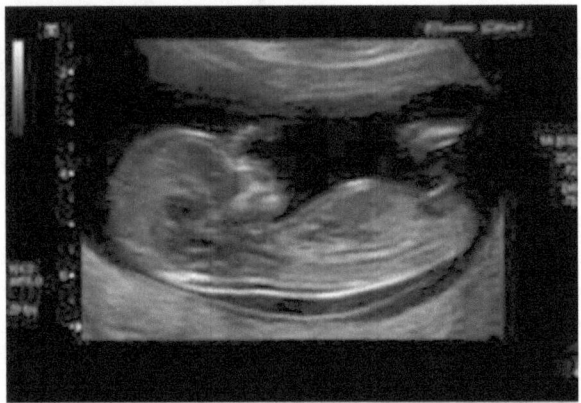

Figure 45. Scan picture for the measurement of crown-to-rump length

PREGNANCY DATING AND EXPECTED SIZE OF YOUR BABY

Dating your pregnancy accurately helps us to know the following:
- when your baby was conceived
- your EDD
- when you are overdue.
- when to start you off (induce labour),
- etc.

Pregnancy is dated by the CRL or HC if the CRL is more than 84 mm or you are 14 weeks and more. Scan dating of pregnancy is better than using the first day of your last period.

In IVF pregnancies, dating is from the date of egg collection. In cases where frozen eggs are used, dating will be by embryo transfer date. If a frozen blastocyst (page 50) was transferred, dating will still be by the blastocyst transfer date, but this will be reduced by 5 days. It takes a fertilised egg about 5 days to develop into the 'blastocyst' stage.

BABY'S OR FOETAL HEART RATE

Very high or low heart rates in early pregnancy may be associated with chromosomal abnormalities (page 101).

OTHER ASPECTS OF MANAGEMENT OF THE
FINDINGS AT THE FIRST-TRIMESTER SCAN

Ultrasound finding	Management plan
CRL less than 45 mm.	You will be rebooked for scanning in 1 week when the result of the scan can be used to calculate the risk of chromosomal anomaly. At week 11, the CRL should be 45 mm.
CRL more than 84 mm.	Thickness of the fluid at the back of baby's neck (NT) will not be used to screen for Down's syndrome. You will be offered a test called quadruple test (see page xxx) to screen for chromosomal anomaly.
Pregnancy sac visible but no baby in it and no smaller (yolk) sac. Mean pregnancy sac diameter equals or is greater than 25 mm.	You will be referred to the EPAU, where you will be reassessed. It is likely to be a miscarriage. If there is any doubt or you request for another scan, this will be done a week later in the EPAU.
Pregnancy sac visible but no baby in it and no smaller (yolk) sac. Mean pregnancy sac diameter less than 25 mm.	This is likely to be a very early pregnancy. You will be referred to the EPAU. You will have rescan a week later there.
CRL equals or more than 7 mm and no heartbeat. Findings confirmed by a second sonographer.	You will be referred to the EPAU since it is a miscarriage. If there is doubt or you request for another scan, this will be done a week later in the EPAU.
CRL less than 7 mm and no heartbeats.	This is likely to be a very early pregnancy. You will be referred to the EPU. You will have rescan a week later there.
Pregnancy sac not seen and pregnancy hormone free beta-HCG more than 5.	You will be referred to the EPAU. Another blood test will be repeated 48 hours later.
Pregnancy hormone free beta-HCG less than 5.	You will be referred to the EPAU. This means you are not pregnant. No more action needed.

Suspected molar pregnancy. This means precancerous condition, which can be cured completely.	You will be referred to a consultant with special interest in early pregnancy management and also gynaecological oncologist, who deals with gynaecological cancer.
NT > 3.5. Suspicion of heart defect. Previous history of child with severe heart defect.	Scan of the baby's heart (echocardiogram) by a heart specialist should be performed and also at 20-24 weeks in order to rule out heart problem. Also full screening for Down's syndrome is recommended.
Reverse blood flow in the right part of the heart (tricuspid regurgitation). Reversed blood flow in the liver in a blood vessel called 'ductus venosus'.	Scan of the baby's heart (echocardiogram) by a heart specialist should be offered at 20-24 weeks of pregnancy.
You want chorionic villus sampling (CVS) (page xxx) having screened positive for chromosomal abnormality.	The CVS will be done, and the pieces of placenta collected will be sent to the laboratory. The result will either confirm or refute chromosomal abnormality, and further counselling will follow.
Foetal anomaly detected.	You will be referred to a specialist in a branch of obstetrics called foetal medicine or to an obstetrician with special interest in foetal medicine, and there, you will be given the available options.
Multiple pregnancy found.	Please see page 235.
The length of the cervix is less than 15 mm (page 229).	You are better managed by a foetal medicine consultant or an obstetrician or doctor with special interest in dealing with short cervix.

Table 2. Some aspects of management at the first-trimester scan

SOURCES
- The NHS Pregnancy Book, UK, 2009.
- Antenatal Ultrasound Scans. Information for pregnant women. www.kch. nhs.uk. July 2010.
- The website of Fetal Medicine Foundation, London.
- Guideline for Practice. Harris Birthright Research Centre for Fetal Medicine, King's College Hospital, London, 2011, 2012.

SCREENING AND DIAGNOSTIC TESTS FOR CHROMOSOMAL ABNORMALITIES

INTRODUCTION

The need for screening for chromosomal abnormalities came in the 1970s in developed countries. The idea was to identify chromosomal abnormal babies early in pregnancy and terminate such pregnancies instead of carrying it to term. The chromosomal abnormalities under question are

- Down's syndrome or trisomy 21 (T21)
- Edwards' syndrome or trisomy 18 (T18)
- Patau's syndrome or trisomy 13 (T13)

Others are Turner's syndrome, triploidy, and sex chromosomal abnormalities. Over the years, the primary motive has been to identify and subject those few women who screen positive for chromosomal abnormalities to invasive diagnostic tests such as CVS or amniocentesis (page xx).

SCREENING METHODS USED IN THE FIRST TRIMESTER

MATERNAL AGE AS A SCREENING TOOL

The risk for many of the chromosomal defects increases with maternal age, and because babies with these defects are more likely to die in the womb than normal ones, the risk decreases with the increasing age of your pregnancy.

Maternal age (years)	Chance of Down's syndrome	
	At 12 weeks	At birth
20	1 in 1,070	1 in 1,530
25	1 in 950	1 in 1,350
30	1 in 630	1 in 900
32	1 in 460	1 in 660
34	1 in 310	1 in 450
35	1 in 250	1 in 360
36	1 in 200	1 in 200
38	1 in 120	1 in 170
40	1 in 70	1 in 100
42	1 in 40	1 in 55
44	1 in 20	1 in 30

Table 3. Maternal-age-associated risk for Down's syndrome

The effects of maternal age on the risk assessment are as follows:
- The risk for trisomies 21, 18, 13 increases with maternal age.
- The risk for Turner's syndrome and triploidy does not change with maternal age.
- The rate of foetal death in trisomy 21 between 12 and 40 weeks is about 30%.
- The rate of foetal death between 12 and 40 weeks is about 80% in trisomies 18, 13 and Turner's syndrome.

NT AS A SCREENING TOOL
NT is the sonographic appearance of accumulation of fluid behind baby's neck in the first trimester of pregnancy.
- Foetal NT normally increases with gestation (CRL) in the first trimester. The larger the NT, the higher the risk. In contrast, the smaller the NT, the smaller the risk.
- During the second trimester, NT usually resolves, but in a few cases, it evolves into a swelling on baby's neck called cystic hygromas with or without generalised swelling of the baby.

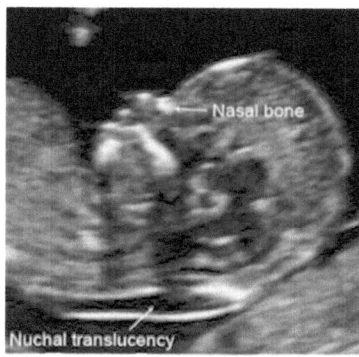 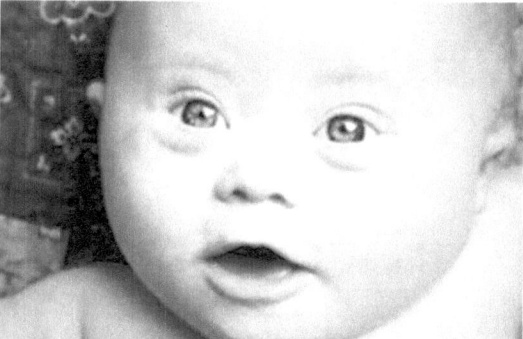

Figure 46. Increased nuchal fold   **Figure 47. Down's syndrome features**

- In the first trimester, in those cases where the NT is high but invasive diagnostic test has ruled out chromosomal abnormalities, there is still high risk of other problems namely
  - foetal death
  - heart problem
  - other major abnormalities in the baby

SUBSTANCES IN YOUR BLOOD AS SCREENING TOOLS IN THE FIRST TRIMESTER

The biochemical substances measured in your blood are HCG and PAPP-A and are produced by the placenta.

- The higher the level of HCG and the lower the level of PAPP-A, the higher the risk for trisomy 21.
- In trisomies 18 and 13, the levels of maternal serum free HCG and PAPP-A are decreased.

ABNORMAL FHR AS A SCREENING TOOL

In normal foetus, the heart rate is as follows:
- 110 bpm at 5 weeks
- 170 bpm at 19 weeks
- 150 bpm at 14 weeks

In babies with T21 and T13, the heart rate is on the upper limit of the norm, especially in T13, while in T18, the heart rate is very low.

NASAL BONE, BLOOD FLOW IN THE LIVER AND THE HEART

The NB is absent and the blood flow in baby's liver and heart is abnormal in babies with Down's syndrome.

Method of screening	Detection Rate DR in %
Maternal age (MA)	30
Combined MA, free HCG and PAPP-A at 11-13+6 wks	50-70
Bart's test at 15-18 wks (page 103)	50-70
Combined MA and NT at 11-13+6 wks	70-80
Combined MA, NT, free or total HCG and PAPP-A at 11-13+6 wks	85-90
Combined MA, NT, an NB at 11-13+6 wks	90
Combined MA, NT, NB, free or total HCG and PAPP-A at 11-13+6 wks	95
Combined MA, Ultrasound findings (NT, NB, blood flow in baby's liver and the heart and heart rate of the baby), free HCG and PAPP-A at 11-13 weeks	98. Cut-off risk at which invasive test can be offered is 1:150. This is the practice at King's College Hospital, London, where most of the research was performed

Table 4. Comparison of the detection rates DRs for Down's syndrome, for a false positive rate (FPR) of 5%.

SCREENING TEST RESULT AND MANAGEMENT

The results of a screening test for chromosomal abnormalities are as follows:

- 'Low risk or screen negative': This means the risk of the baby having Down's syndrome is lower than the recommended cut-off point, for instance less than 1:250. It does not mean there is no risk.
- 'High risk or screen positive': This means the risk of the baby having Down's syndrome is greater than the recommended cut-off point, for instance greater than 1:250. It means that you are at a high risk of having a baby with Down's syndrome, but it does not indicate that your baby definitely has Down's syndrome. In that situation, you will be offered two options:
  - do a diagnostic confirmatory test
  - do nothing and continue with the pregnancy
- If PAPP-A is low and the foetus has no Down's syndrome, there is a small increase in the chance that the growth of the baby may be slow later in the pregnancy. In that situation, it is recommended that you have a growth scan for your baby at 28, 32, and 36 weeks.

Bart's or quadruple test

This test is normally offered to patients who present after 13^{+6} weeks and can therefore not have the nuchal scan. A sample of your blood is taken, and the concentration of four substances produced by the placenta and secreted into your blood will be measured. The substances are as following:

- Alpha-fetoprotein (AFP)
- HCG
- Oestriol (uE3) and
- Inhibin-A

On the basis of these four substances you will be categorized into a positive or negative test group for chromosomal abnormalities. If the test result is negative, you will be reassured. If positive, you will be offered amniocentesis (page 107).

Among women in the screen-positive group, 1 out of 21 will have a pregnancy with Down's syndrome.

If the level of AFP is two and a half times the average level for gestation age or higher, you will be categorized as being at high risk of having a baby with Neural tube defect. You will therefore be offered detailed ultrasound scan at different stages of pregnancy. Detection rate is 85 out of 100 cases of open spina bifida and nearly all cases of anencephaly (baby without a head).

Invasive (Diagnostic) Tests for Chromosomal Abnormalities and Other Genetic Disorders

The tests under consideration are

- CVS
- Amniocentesis

CVS is performed between 11 and 14 weeks and involves taking a small amount of tissue from the placenta. It means that if abnormality is detected and you decide to have a termination, this can be done easily in the first trimester. Amniocentesis involves taking fluid from around the baby and is usually done after 15 weeks. This means if abnormality is detected and you decide to end the pregnancy, it has to be done by IOL.

Both methods provide a sample that contains tissue that has the same genetic make-up as the baby. But the problem with these invasive tests is that they can cause a miscarriage, even if the baby is entirely normal. The risk of miscarriage is about 1 in 100.

Indications for CVS and amniocentesis are as following:

- High risk or positive test for chromosomal abnormality.
- To check for rare inherited disorders
- High risk for having a child with SCD, thalassaemia, or cystic fibrosis.
- Previous pregnancy affected with a genetic disorder.
- One or more of your relatives are affected with a genetic disorder.
- To determine the sex earlier, which may be important in conditions such as haemophilia (a blood disorder) and muscular dystrophy (a group of inherited disorders that involve muscle weakness, loss of muscle tissue, affects only boys, although girls may carry the disorder in their chromosomes and pass it on to their sons.)
- To test for fetal infection.

TECHNIQUES OF THE PROCEDURES

TRANSABDOMINAL (THROUGH THE ABDOMEN) CVS

First, you will be counselled on the indication, technique, risks, and expectation afterwards, and if you choose to have the procedure, you would be expected to sign a consent form. Second, gel is applied over your abdomen and you will be scanned to check the positions of both the baby and the placenta (afterbirth) and determine the safest point where to insert the needle.

Third, your skin will be cleaned and local anaesthetic will be injected to numb the area where the needle will be inserted, after which the area will be cleaned again. Under ultrasound guidance, as shown in Figure 48, a fine needle to which a tube with a syringe is attached or syringe attached directly as above is pushed through your abdomen and the wall of the womb into the placenta. A small amount of placental tissue is sucked up into the syringe by moving the needle in and out of your abdomen. The needle is then taken out and your baby is checked on ultrasound.

The whole procedure is done under ultrasound guidance to make sure that the needle does not injure internal organs or the baby, and it takes about 5 minutes to complete it. After the procedure, the placental tissue will be sent to the laboratory for testing.

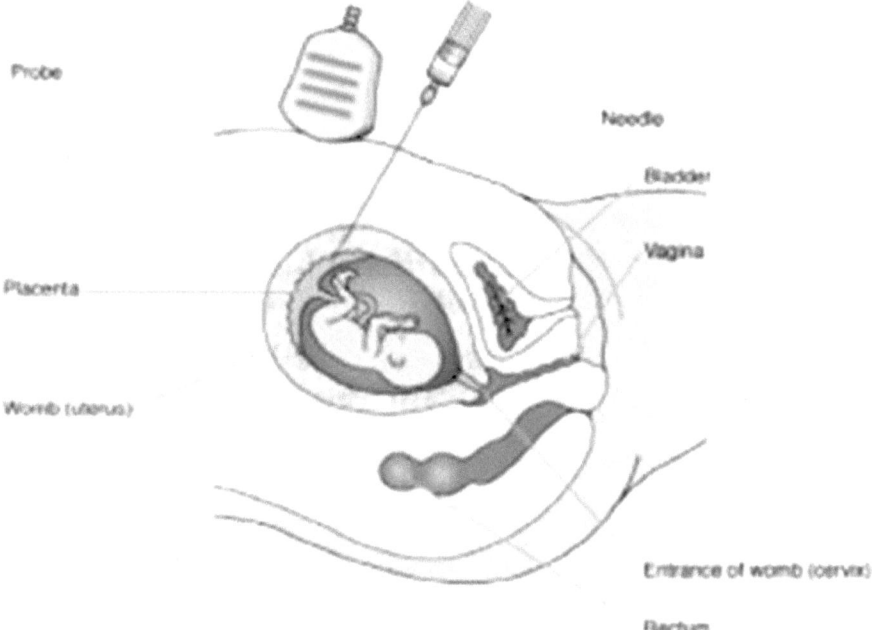

Probe

Needle

Bladder

Vagina

Placenta

Womb (uterus)

Entrance of womb (cervix)

Rectum

Figure 48. CVS through the abdomen

TRANSVAGINAL (THROUGH THE VAGINA) CVS

A speculum (a plastic or metal instrument used to separate the walls of the vagina and also used for vagina swab test) is inserted into your vagina to enable the doctor to see your cervix. The vagina and cervix are cleaned. Under ultrasound guidance, a fine needle is passed through the cervix to the placenta. A tiny amount of placental tissue is removed. Baby is then observed on ultrasound to confirm that he or she is alright. After the procedure, the placental tissue will be sent to the laboratory for analysis.

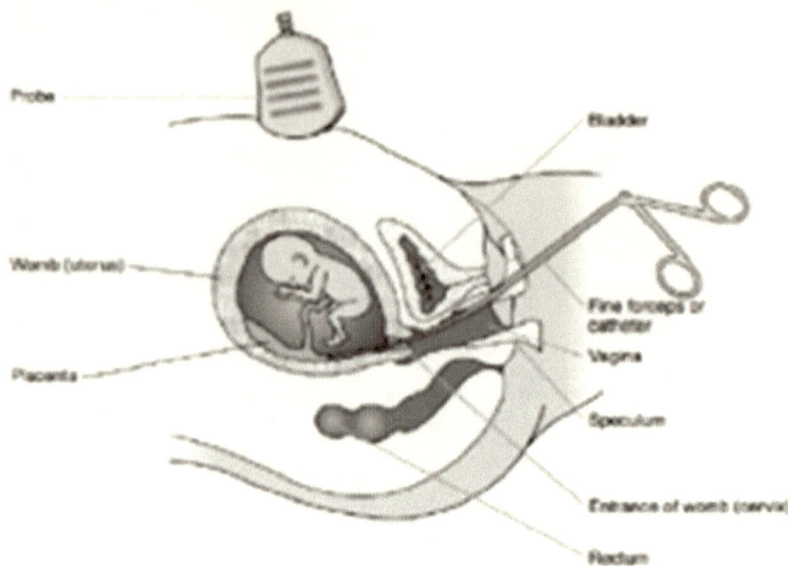

Figure 49. CVS through the vagina

AMNIOCENTESIS

First, the operator will counsel you about the procedure such as indication, technique, risks, and expectation afterwards, and if you choose to have the procedure, you would be expected to sign the consent form. Second, gel is applied over your abdomen and you will be scanned to check the positions of both the baby and the placenta (afterbirth). Third, your skin is cleaned where the needle will be inserted. You do not usually need a local anaesthetic before amniocentesis is performed, but sometimes, it is given.

Fourth, under ultrasound guidance, to ensure that your baby is not injured, a fine needle is inserted into your skin, through your abdomen and womb into the fluids surrounding your baby. Usually, the placental site is avoided when inserting the needle. Sometimes, the needle will go through the placenta as this might be the only way to get the fluid. This is unlikely to cause you or your baby any harm.

Fifth, a small sample of the fluid surrounding the baby is aspirated using a syringe. This fluid is foetal urine, and the amount lost should be reformed within a few days. This fluid should be in amber/or yellow colour but may be stained with blood from the procedure. This is not harmful but may affect the accuracy of the result. The needle is then withdrawn from your abdomen, and your baby will be

106

checked on ultrasound. The amniotic fluid, which contains baby's cells, will then be sent to the laboratory for testing.

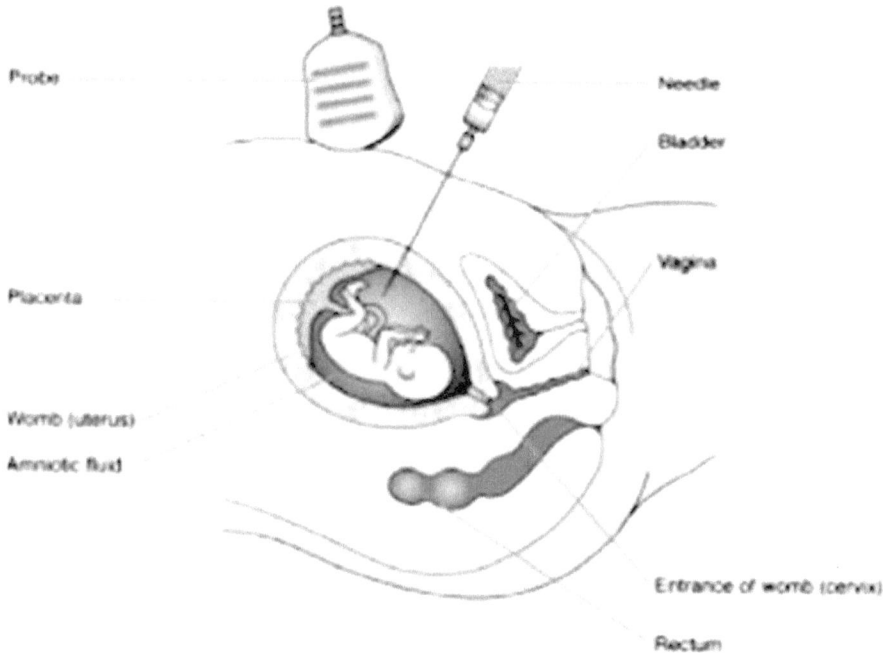

Probe

Needle

Bladder

Vagina

Placenta

Womb (uterus)

Amniotic fluid

Entrance of womb (cervix)

Rectum

Figure 50. Amniocentesis

THE RISKS OF CVS AND AMNIOCENTESIS

- Mild abdominal, a bit like a period pain. The trans-cervical CVS is like having a cervical smear test.
- Risk of miscarriage is 1-2% for CVS and 1% for amniocentesis.
- Risk of infection of less than 1 in 1,000 women.
- If CVS is done before 10 weeks, there is a small risk of abnormalities of the fingers and/or toes. It is therefore performed after 11 weeks of pregnancy.
- For amniocentesis, there is less than 1% chance of having blood-stained amniotic fluids and also a 1% risk of repeating the procedure due to inadequate fluids been collected.
- You may notice some 'spotting' of blood and cramping for a few hours afterwards. This is normal, and it is safe to take paracetamol.

Precautionary Measures During CVS and Amniocentesis

- If your blood group is rhesus negative, you will be given an injection of anti-D after the procedure to prevent you from developing antibodies against your baby's red blood cells.
- If you are HIV positive and you decide to have amniocentesis, this might increase the risk of passing HIV on to your baby. You may be offered treatment with highly active antiretroviral therapy (HAART) if you are not already taking it. This reduces the risk of the HIV virus infecting your baby.
- It is important to know that if you carry hepatitis B or hepatitis C viruses, there is, in theory, a possibility that amniocentesis might increase the risk that you pass this on to your baby.

Laboratory tests

The specimens (placenta tissue or amniotic fluid) are analyzed by using the following tests: a rapid test which gives the preliminary result within 4 days and karyotype which gives the full result within 2 weeks.

Test Results And Management

The most likely result of the laboratory test is that no abnormality is detected. Abnormal result means baby has the disorder that has been tested for. If that is the case, you will probably be shocked when you are first told the diagnosis and may find it hard to take in the information. Think things through and talk to your partner and your loved ones.

If you decide to continue with the pregnancy, you will have appropriate support from health care professionals to help you and your family prepare for the birth and aftercare of your baby. If you decide to end the pregnancy, you will be counseled about what this involves.

Very occasionally, the test is done to detect Down's syndrome but another disorder is detected.

First-Trimester Screening for Down's Syndrome in developing countries

Screening tests are performed in some developing countries. The situation in the Sub-Saharan Africa is different. The tests are not performed, except in South Africa and sporadically in Kenya.

Although medical practitioners in Sub-Saharan Africa may be overwhelmed with infectious diseases, the prevalence of chromosomal and other structural abnormalities is likely to be more in Africans than in any other race. This is because of uncontrolled environmental hazards in different parts of the continent and lack of genetic counseling, which should prevent the occurrence of some of those disorders. Research carried out in some Sub-Saharan African countries, for example Nigeria, confirmed this assumption.

The question to answer now is how can the developing countries introduce a screening programme in their country, given that financial resources are limited. Even if screening is not made universal for all pregnant women, it should be offered to women at significant risk of having baby with Down's syndrome. This includes women of more than 35 years of age, women who have had baby with Down's syndrome in the past, and those with Down's syndrome baby in their family.

It must be noted that some women actually travel from developing countries, for example Nigeria, to developed ones, the primary motive being to have a screening test for chromosomal abnormalities; this is particularly so in young educated patients.

Given the growing demand for screening tests for chromosomal abnormalities in some of the developing countries, for example Nigeria, we think it is quite feasible to introduce a screening programme which uses only ultrasound screening tools. The ultrasound criteria that can be used are as follows:
- Maternal age
- Foetal NT
- Foetal NB
- FHR
- Blood flow in the liver

Screening period will be 11-13+6 weeks. This combined screening test should be affordable, and it can detect more than 90% of babies with Down's syndrome with a false-positive result of 5% (Kypros Nicolaides, 2004).

So if you live in a developing country and choose to have a screening test for chromosomal abnormality, speak to your doctor, who should arrange a referral for you.

NEW DEVELOPMENT IN SCREENING FOR CHROMOSOMAL ABNORMALITIES

Cell-free DNA tests for chromosomal abnormalities have been introduced in the USA and the UK. The big question about the tests is whether they should be offered to patients at high risk of having a baby with chromosomal abnormalities or to every pregnant woman.

SOURCES
- FMF UK website: www.fetalmedicine.com/fmf/
- Screening tests for birth defects. Frequently asked questions. ACOG. 2014
- California Prenatal Screening Program to include noninvasive testing. Monica Flessel, PhD, and Sara Goldman, MPH, Genetic Disease Screening Program, California Department of Public Health ACOG, 2014
- Guideline for Practice. Harris Birthright Research Centre for Fetal Medicine, King's College Hospital, London, 2011, 2012.
- Information for patients. The Barts and the London School of Medicine and Dentistry. Quadruple test.
- Patient information leaflet. CVS and amniocentesis. Harris Birthright Research Centre for Fetal Medicine, King's College Hospital, London.
- RCOG guideline. Amniocentesis and chorionic villus sampling, June 2010.
- RCOG patient information leaflet. Information for you. Chorionic villus sampling and amniocentesis. RCOG, 2011.
- Screening test for you and your baby. www.screening.nhs.uk, 2010.
- The NHS Pregnancy Book, UK, 2009.

THE 20-23 WEEKS SCAN

THE PURPOSE OF THE SCAN

The scan will check and confirm the following:
- The growth of your baby and how far you have gone in the pregnancy (GA).
- Baby's anatomy
- Signs of chromosomal and other defects
- Fetal tumours (abnormal growths)
- Placental position
- The amount of liquor surrounding your baby
- The risk of preterm labour by measuring cervical length.
- The risk of developing preeclampsia or fetal growth restriction(FGR)

SCANNING PROCEDURE

The scan is divided into two parts:
- Transabdominal scan, that is through your abdomen
- Transvaginal scan, that is through the vagina

TRANSABDOMINAL SCAN

In most cases, the scan starts with the sonographer checking the following:
- Number of babies
- How baby is lying and the part that is presenting towards the birth canal
- Heartbeat of your baby
- Placental localisation

- Amniotic fluid volume (AFV)
- Number of blood vessels in the umbilical cord

MEASUREMENTS

From 20 weeks of pregnancy, foetal size is assessed by the following parameters, which are measured with ultrasound:
- Distance around the top of the head or HC.
- Abdominal circumference (AC) at the level of the stomach.
- Thigh bone length (FL).
- Estimated foetal weight, that is determined by a formula which incorporates the first three parameters. This is the most accurate assessment of foetal size.

Other measurements are as follows:
- Length of the NB
- Length of the arm bone (humerus length)

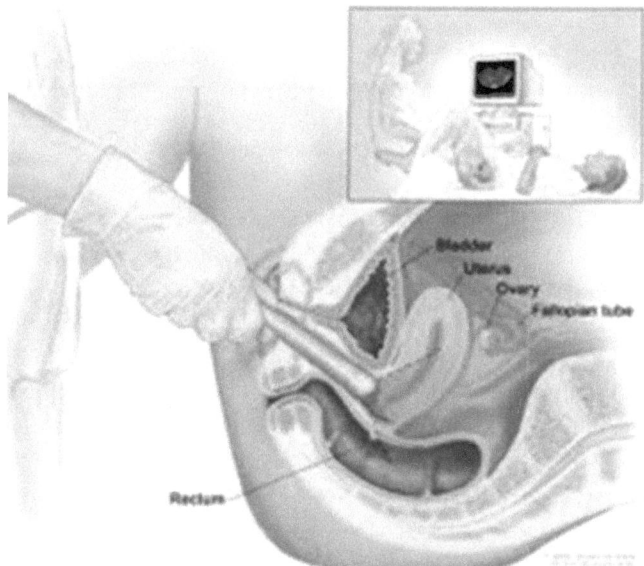

Figure 51. Transvaginal ultrasound

The sonographer will also check different organs and systems of your baby in order to rule out abnormalities.

TRANSVAGINAL SCAN

This is used to check the following:

111

- blood flow from you to your baby in order to assess your risk of developing PE and having a small baby
- length of the cervix in order to predict your risk of having preterm labour (delivering your baby before 37 weeks)

MANAGEMENT OF THE FINDINGS

LOW-LYING PLACENTA

This means that the placenta covers the internal cervical (the inner mouth of the cervix) or the lower edge of the placenta is within 6 cm of it.

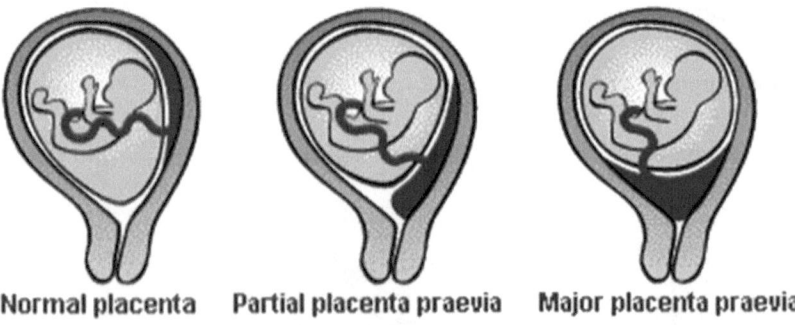

Normal placenta   Partial placenta praevia   Major placenta praevia

Figure 52. Low-lying placenta

In this situation, the placental position should be determined again at 32 weeks by doing transvaginal scan. As the pregnancy progresses, the placenta normally grows away from the inner mouth of the cervix.

TWO BLOOD VESSELS IN THE UMBILICAL CORD

Normally, the umbilical cord has 2 arteries and 1 vein, that is three blood vessels. If the cord has only one artery, it means it has only two blood vessels (one artery and one vein). Isolated finding without any associated abnormality is found in 1 in 200 normal pregnancies but in about 10% of cases, it is associated with SGA babies in the last 13 weeks of pregnancy. You would be offered scan at 28, 31-32, and 36 weeks to check growth and liquor volume.

THE CERVIX AND PREVENTION OF PRETERM BIRTH (PAGE 226)

HIGH RESISTANCE TO BLOOD TO YOUR WOMB

This predicts
- your risk of developing PE.
- your risk of having a small baby (stunted growth).

You will be offered scan appointments at 28, 32 and 36 weeks to check fetal growth, liquor volume and blood flow in baby's blood vessels. You will also have regular checks for signs of PE, namely high BP and protein in your urine at each antenatal appointment.

ABNORMALITIES PICKED UP AT THE 20-23 WEEKS SCAN

Abnormalities of the following systems and organs can be detected at the 20-23 weeks scan

- Head and brain
- Neck and skin Spine Face
- Lungs
- Abdominal wall
- Stomach and bowel
- Urinary tracts
- Skeleton including Upper and lower limbs

The abnormalities which may be major or minor may be associated with chromosomal defects and therefore, they should modify the risk derived from the first-trimester screening tests for these defects. So if any abnormality is picked up, you should be referred to a specialist in fetal medicine who will manage the pregnancy.

FOETAL TUMOURS (ABNORMAL GROWTH)

These are abnormal swelling that can affect any organ or system of a baby from the head to the toe, for example, brain baby's neck heart, liver, etc. If any tumour is seen on ultrasound, you will be referred to a fetal medicine specialist who will manage the situation.

THE 20-23 WEEKS SCAN IN DEVELOPING COUNTRIES

Only few developing countries offer this scan to pregnant women. Specifically, in the sub-Saharan African countries, probably only South Africa offers it. In Nigeria, it is not offered at all; this is because of lack of trained specialists in fetal medicine. So if you live in Nigeria or any other developing countries of the world, speak to your doctor about this vital service. You could be referred to a clinic or hospital that may be able to offer the service.

SPECIALIZSED SCAN OF BABY'S HEART (FOETAL ECHOCARDIOGRAM)

This is practised under a specialised area of obstetrics called foetal medicine. It is a part of the 20-23 weeks anomaly scan that is normally carried out by a sonographer, but on this occasion, a more detailed assessment of baby's heart is carried out by a specialist called foetal echocardiologist or a foetal medicine specialist trained to do it. The indications for this type of scan are outlined below.

AT 11-14 WEEKS OF PREGNANCY

- Thickness of the fluid at the back of baby's neck (NT) equals to or is more than 3.5 mm (NT ≥ 3.5).
- Suspicion of heart (cardiac) malformation on scan.
- Previous history of child with severe heart defect.

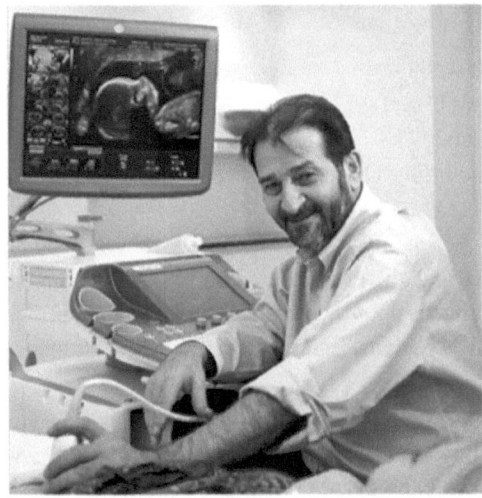

**Fig. 53. Prof. Kypros Nicolaides performing fetal medicine ultrasound
with the left hand at the FMF, London**

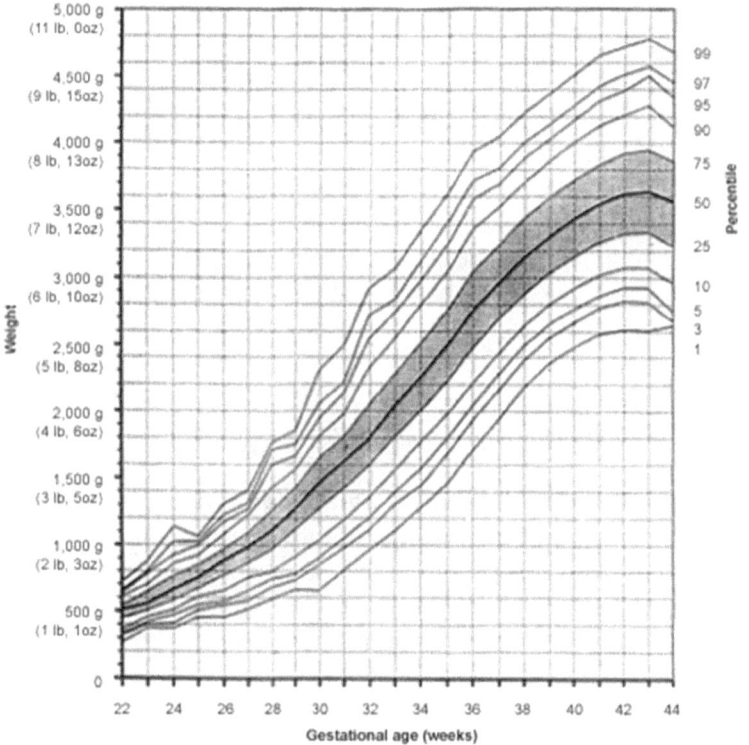

Fig. 54 showing fetal growth in centiles (Please see glossary of terms)

At 20-24 Weeks

- Suspicion of heart malformation on a scan performed by a sonographer.
- Non-cardiac abnormality found at the 20-23 weeks scan performed by a sonographer or a fetal medicine specialist
- The following findings at the 11-13[+6] weeks:
  - Significantly increased NT or leakage in the valve between the right chambers of the heart.
  - Your screening test at 11-13[+6] weeks shows that you are at high risk for chromosomal abnormality but you did not go for a diagnostic test (CVS or amniocentesis.) or you did not have Cell-free DNA test.
  - You did not have the screening for chromosomal abnormalities at 11-13[+6], but your age-related risk for Down's syndrome was more than 1 in 150.
  - Abnormal blood flow in baby's liver (ductus venosus).

- Foetal hydrops which is a condition characterised by accumulation of fluid in at least two compartments of the baby, for example the lung, abdomen, around the heart, and so on.
- Monochorionic (MC) twins (twins with 1 afterbirth and 2 sacs).
- Family history (mother, father, child) has heart defect.
- You have the following conditions:
    - Insulin-dependent diabetes mellitus (IDDM).
    - Epilepsy and you are on medication.
    - Your blood contains a substance called anti-Ro antibody which can pass into your baby's blood and adversely affect his or her heart.

AFTER 24 WEEKS OF PREGNANCY
- Any heart problem found in pregnancy

FETAL ECHOCARDIOGRAM IN DEVELOPING COUNTRIES
In developing countries, specialised scan of baby's heart is almost not offered. So if you live in those countries and any of the indications above is applicable to you, you should speak to your obstetrician about the service. Referral to a specialist, if available within the country or abroad, is possible options.

THE 31-32 WEEKS SCAN

Ultrasound scan at 31-32 weeks of pregnancy is routinely performed in many developed countries of the world, especially in Europe. The UK has not adopted the practice universally, except Harris Birthright Research Centre for Fetal Medicine in King's College Hospital and few others. We believe the 31-32 weeks scan is worth doing because of its purpose and content. We have adapted and modified the protocol used at King's College Hospital, London, as a model on which other protocols and guidelines will be based.

THE PURPOSE OF THE SCAN
- To assess the growth and wellbeing of your baby.
- To recheck for major structural anomalies in the baby.
- To confirm placental position.
- To confirm the number of umbilical arteries.
- To check for abnormal growth (fibroid of the womb or cyst of the ovary) that may be in the way of the birth canal or near to it and therefore may affect mode of delivery.

GROWTH AND WELL-BEING OF YOUR BABY

- Baby's growth will be assessed by measuring the following parts of the body:
    - HC, which is the distance around the top of the head
    - AC, which is the distance around the tummy at the level of the stomach
    - Length of the thigh bone (FL)
    - Expected foetal weight (EFW)
- The AC and EFW are used to diagnose small-for-gestational-age (SGA) babies (page xxx).
- Measurement of the deepest pool of the fluid surrounding your baby.
- Measurement of blood flow will also be conducted
    - from you to your baby.
    - in the umbilical artery.
    - in baby's brain in a blood vessel called the middle cerebral artery (MCA).
    - in a tiny blood vessel in baby's liver called ductus venosus.

MAJOR STRUCTURAL ABNORMALITIES

The foetal anomaly screening as performed at the 20-23 weeks scan will be conducted in all cases. This will enable the sonographer to identify those defects that are missed earlier. However, it may not be possible to conduct the full screening.

MANAGEMENT

Findings on the scan	Management plan
Normal 31-32 weeks scan—growth (EFW), amniotic fluid (deepest pool of amniotic fluid), and blood flow in baby's blood vessel are normal.	Reassurance and no more scan unless requested by your midwife or doctor.
Baby not growing as expected (SGA).	This finding can occur singly or in combinations with other problem. It is best managed by a specialist in fetal medicine. If your doctor has been trained to manage such a case, then he will do so.
Small amount of amniotic fluids around baby (oligohydramnios)—deepest pool of fluid less than 3 cm.	Your obstetrician, preferably a fetal Medicine specialist will manage the finding which may be associated with other problem.

Abnormal blood flow in the baby.	Your doctor, preferably an obstetrician, or better still a specialist in foetal medicine will plan the management.
Single umbilical artery which can be associated with SGA babies.	Your doctor, preferably an obstetrician, or better still a specialist in foetal medicine will plan the management.
Too much amniotic fluids around the baby (polyhydramnios)—deepest pool of fluid more than 8 cm.	You will probably require blood tests to rule out diabetes in pregnancy and viral diseases because these two conditions can be associated with too much fluids around baby (Page 219).
Large-for-date baby (LFD), which can be a sign of diabetes in pregnancy (gestational diabetes).	You will probably require blood tests to rule out diabetes in pregnancy and a further scan will be arranged to monitor fetal growth.
Foetal abnormalities.	Fetal medicine specialist will manage them
The placenta overlaps the inner mouth of the cervix (internal os) by more than 2 cm.	The placenta will remain within 2cm of the outlet of the womb at the end of the pregnancy and therefore vaginal delivery will not be possible. Your obstetrician will prepare you for caesarean section at 39 weeks.
The placenta covers the inner mouth of the cervix by less than 2 cm, or the lower border of the placenta is within 2 cm of it.	A further scan will be carried out at 37 weeks. If at 37 weeks the position of the placenta has not changed, your obstetrician will decide on the appropriate method of delivery which will be by Caesarean section.

Table 5. Management of abnormal findings

ADDITIONAL SCANS DURING PREGNANCY

These are the same in content to the 31-32 weeks scan and are carried out in selected cases. The indications and stages in pregnancy when the scan will be performed are itemised below.

- Foetal abnormalities detected at the 11-13, 20-23, or 31-32 weeks scans will be followed up as determined by your doctor or obstetrician or better still a foetal medicine specialist by further scans.

- Scan for growth, AFV, and blood flow in the baby will be performed at 28, 31-32, and 36 weeks of pregnancy for the following condition or situations:
  - Low levels of pregnancy hormone PAPP-A at 11-13 weeks. PAPP-A is part of the screening test for Down's syndrome, and its low levels may predict risk of having SGA baby in later pregnancy.
  - Single umbilical artery at the 11-13 or 20-23 weeks scan because of its association with poor fetal growth.
  - Poor blood flow to the womb at 20-23 weeks which predicts risk of developing PE and having small baby.

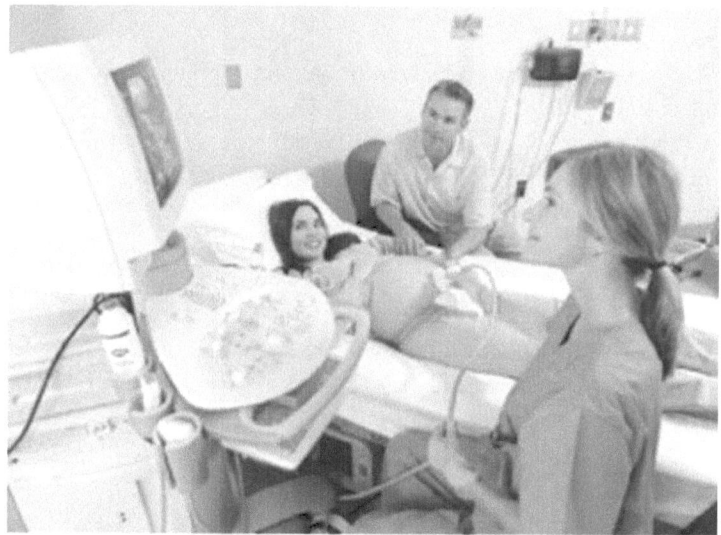

Figure 55. Performing a growth scan in the third trimester

  - Previous early onset of PE, that is PE before 32 weeks of pregnancy or SGA baby associated with abnormal blood flow.
  - Previous delivery before 34 weeks due to SGA and abnormal blood flow in the baby (fetal growth restriction, FGR).
  - Previous intrauterine death, that is baby's death in the womb after age of viability.
  - Pre-pregnancy diabetes and gestational diabetes.
  - Other significant medical conditions in pregnancy - heart or kidney disease, and so on.
  - Any medication you are taking can affect you or your baby during pregnancy. Some of these medications are drugs used for the treatment of low thyroid function, high thyroid function, diabetes, epilepsy, etc.

Other indications for scan appointment in pregnancy are enumerated below, and the schedules for the scans are determined by the doctor concerned.

- Suspected breech presentation at 36-37 weeks.
- Suspected SGA, large for gestational age (LGA), small or too much fluid around your baby.
- Identified fibroids or ovarian cyst at the 11-13 or 20-23 or 31-32 weeks scan—to check their growth and position with relative to birth canal.
- Reduced foetal movements (RFMs).
- Bleeding in pregnancy.
- Suspected leakage of amniotic fluid.

Sources

- Antenatal Ultrasound Scans. Information for pregnant women. www.kch. nhs.uk. July 2010.
- Ultrasonography in pregnancy. Washington (DC): American College of Obstetricians and Gynaecologists (ACOG); 2009 Feb. 11 p. (ACOG practice bulletin; no. 101). [44 references]
- Guideline for Practice. Harris Birthright Research Centre for Fetal Medicine, King's College Hospital, London, 2012.
- The 11-13+6 and the 18-23 weeks fetal anomaly scan, Fetal medicine, FMF UK website: www.fetalmedicine.com/fmf/
- The NHS Pregnancy Book, UK, 2009.
- UK NHS Choices, Your health, your choices. Last reviewed: 2011.
- UK NHS Fetal Anomaly Screening Programme 18+0 to 20+6 Weeks. Fetal Anomaly Scan, National Standards. January 2010.

Procedures at antenatal clinic and emergency assessment in pregnancy

Introduction

Having regular antenatal care is important for your health and that of your baby. Antenatal care in different countries of the world is different in its content and the place of provision, but the general principles of care remain the same. Generally, most antenatal services are now provided in easily accessible settings such as

- Primary health centres
- GP clinics or private hospitals
- Government district general hospitals
- Teaching hospitals

There may be the need for you to wait longer than planned at your antenatal clinic because doctors are overwhelmed by a large number of attendants and partly because of the thorough assessment that individual needs. So try to plan ahead to make your visits easier.

You may like to do any of the following:
- take a snack with you or buy something for refreshment at the clinic.
- prepare for the care of your other children few days before the appointment date.
- prepare your questions for your health care provider and make sure you get answers to them at the clinic.
- go to the clinic with your partner if he is free. This can help them feel more involved in the pregnancy.

HAND-HELD NOTE

Your pregnancy history will be documented in a hand-held note which should be given to you at your first antenatal clinic. You will have to take your hand-held note along with you to all your clinics and wherever you go to when you are pregnant. It will be referred to whenever you need medical attention. The note is designed to support comprehensive history taking and promote effective communication between you and the multidisciplinary care team and between members of the team. Each hospital has its own hand-held note, but the contents are about the same. It contains specific sections and subsections which are discussed below.

GP, patient, and partner's personal details: In this section, the following contact details are documented:
- Your GP—name, name of his or her surgery or clinic, address, and telephone number.
- Yourself, your partner, your next of kin—name, date of birth, address, telephone numbers, email address, religion and ethnic background.

Medical professional's section: In this section, each professional who sees you has to document his or her name, date when you are seen, and signature.

Appointment schedules: This section contains the appointment schedules for uncomplicated pregnancy. It also contains specific appointments booked for high-risk pregnancies to see obstetricians and other allied specialists, for example cardiologist, diabetologist, and so on.

Past pregnancy history: It contains data on your past pregnancies and outcome.

Gynaecological history: This contains details of your last menstrual period, regularity of your periods, whether your pregnancy was spontaneous or assisted conception, last smear test, previous gynaecological operations and problems, and so on.

Medical history: This will include history of medical conditions, allergy, social and family history, drug use, and sexually transmitted diseases.

Sensitive data: This section will contain data about you that will be kept in the hospital, and only you and your health care professional will have access to it. The data are as follows:
- Whether your partner is your baby's father; if not, information may be collected about the father of your baby.
- History of genital infection and dates, for example syphilis, gonorrhoea.
- Result of HIV screening.
- Social care involvement—whether you or any of your children has been in care.

Risk assessment and referrals: Details of your risk assessment.

Investigations and results: Details of investigations at booking and at 28-32 weeks.

A section on abbreviations used by midwives and doctors: These abbreviations will help you to understand better what is written in your hand-held note by your care providers.

Care plan of management of pregnancy, birth, and post-natal period: This section is divided into three subsections namely plan for antenatal period, labour/delivery, and post-natal period. Each subsection is based on your risk assessment.

Place and type of birth.

Birth plan: This is the space where you will indicate your wishes during labour.

Section on follow-up antenatal visits: This section contains details of what happens at each antenatal visit. The clinic is made easier by using a specifically dedicated proforma. For example, here is the modified one used at King's College Hospital, London. Meaning of the abbreviations is outlined.

Date	GA	SFH (cm)	Presentation	Engagement	Oedema	FH/ FM	BP	Urine	Wt (kg)	New risk and Mx	Signature

| 22/11/11 | 33 | 33 | Cephalic | 5/5 | + | FHH
FMF | 120/70 | 2+
Protein | 65 | Pre-eclampsia |

Table 6. Antenatal pro forma

Designation: Midwife consultant ST6/7 ST3-5 ST1-2 GP

GA—gestational age

SFH—Symphysis-fundal height

FM—foetal movements

FMF—foetal movements felt

BP—blood pressure

+—— some quantity, present or yes

GP—general practitioner

Date—date of the clinic

Wt—your weight

kg—kilogram

FH—foetal heart

FHH—foetal heart heard

ST6/7, ST3-5, ST1-2—These are hierarchy of training positions in the UK

UAlb—albumin, a name for one of the proteins detected in urine

Nil or NAD—Nothing abnormal has been discovered

Antenatal admission: In this section, management during each antenatal admission to hospital is documented.

Labour/delivery section: This section contains the following subsections:
- Labour risk assessment: This will be completed when you are admitted for induction or augmentation of labour or at the onset of labour. A specific proforma will be used for the risk assessment. The proforma will contain details of your initial risk assessment at booking, subsequent assessment during pregnancy, and new risk assessment at admission for labour. Again you will be categorised into low or high risk and that will determine the type of care that you receive in labour.
- IOL assessments.
- Parthogram which illustrates the events that are taking place in labour, including its progress.
- Foetal monitoring (page 136).
- Birth details.
- Checklist for maternal transfer to the post-natal ward.
- Checklist for newborn transfer to the post-natal ward.

Post-natal ward and discharge section: This section contains details of your care after transfer to the post-natal ward, checklist for fitness for discharge home, and your discharge summary.

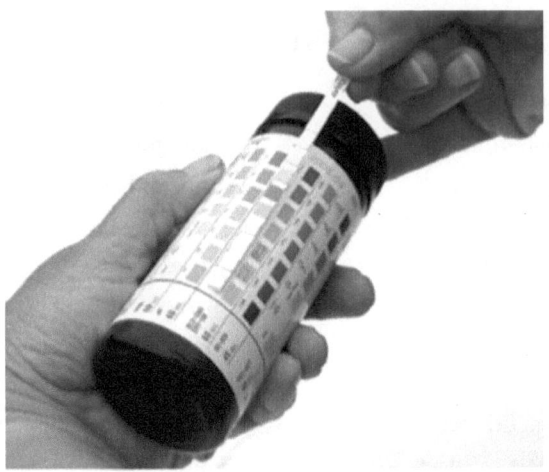

Figure 56. Urine dipstick

ANTENATAL EXAMINATIONS AND TEST

URINE TEST
At each antenatal clinic, your urine will be tested for a number of ingredients in it, each of which has its significance.
- Protein in the urine—sign of water infection or PE
- Glucose in the urine—sign of diabetes
- Nitrite in the urine—sign of water infection
- Blood in the urine—sign of water infection and kidney stones.

Ketones in the urine—normally, only small amount of ketone is excreted daily in the urine (3-15 mg), and this may not show on urine dipstick test. Increased values may be found and are displaced in pluses (1+, 2+, 3+, and 4+); they occur in the following situations:
- poorly controlled diabetes
- starvation, for example
  - ➤ not eating for 12-18 hours
  - ➤ alcoholism
- poisoning (e.g. with a drug called isopropanol)
- others

BLOOD PRESSURE

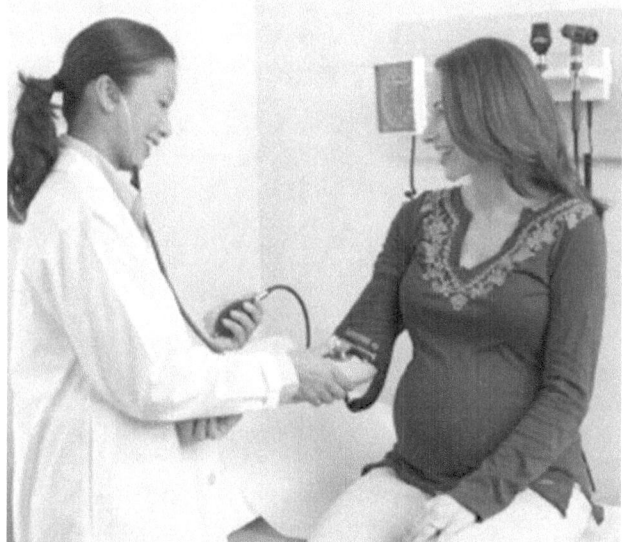

Figure 57. BP measurement in pregnancy

It is normally the same throughout pregnancy except in the middle of your pregnancy when your BP becomes lower than at other times. This is not a problem but may make you feel light-headed if you get up quickly. Talk to your midwife if you have any concern. High BP in the last half of pregnancy may be a sign of PE.

MEASUREMENT OF BP
- An automated or mechanical device will be used, and this should be calibrated at regular intervals.
- You should be in a sitting position with your arms supported at the level of the heart.
- A small (<22 cm), normal (22-32 cm), or large (33-42 cm) adult cuff should be used depending on the mid-arm size (circumference).
- The usual practice is that after rest for 5 minutes, BP is measured in one arm. It is likely that it will be more accurate if BP is measured in both arms simultaneously about 4 times at 1-minute intervals in order to rule out white coat BP increase. The average of the last two readings will be taken as your BP.

YOUR BMI
Your BMI will be calculated from the values of your weight and height at the first antenatal appointment in the first trimester.

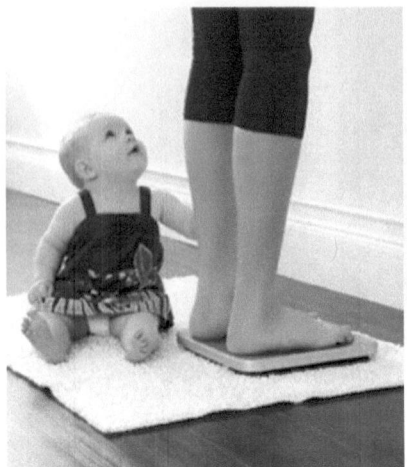

Figure 58. Taking your weight

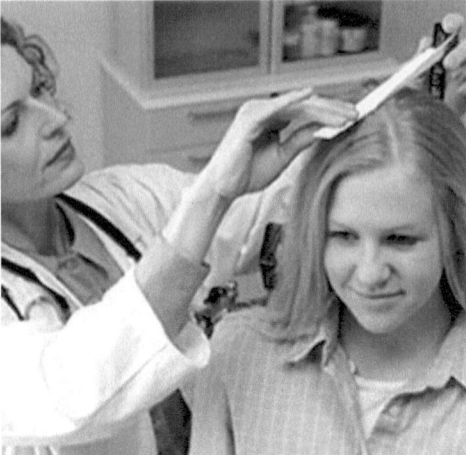

Figure 59. Taking your height

BABY'S GROWTH

This is done in the following ways:

• Measuring the symphysis-fundal height (SFH):
  To measure the SFH, a tape is passed from the bone low in front (pubic bone) to the top of your womb (fundus). Each centimetre of the tape is equivalent to 1 week of your pregnancy. If you are 30 weeks pregnant, the measurement should be about 30 cm.

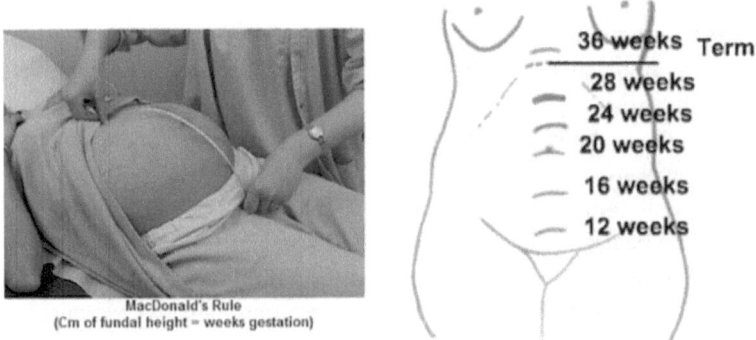

Figure 60. Symphysis-fundal height

PALPATION

By gently pressing on your abdomen, the midwife or doctor can feel your uterus. Within the first 12 weeks, the top of the womb is not felt through your abdomen, and at 20 weeks, the top of the womb is supposed to be at the level of the navel. With palpation, as few as 30% of SGA foetuses can be detected. The lie and presentation of your baby can also be assessed by palpation and confirmed by scan.

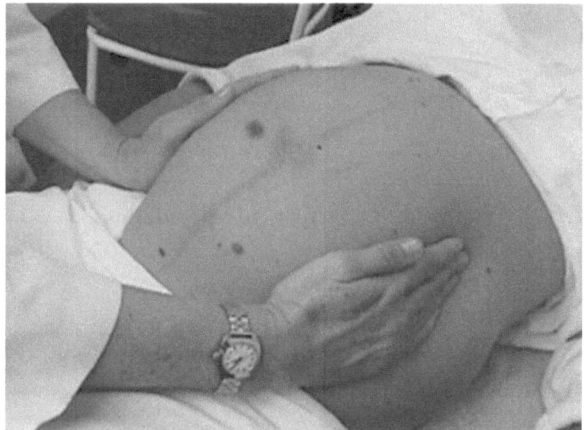

Figure 61. Palpation in pregnancy

FOETAL LIE AND PRESENTATION

FOETAL PRESENTATION

This refers to the part of baby that points towards the birth canal, that is the presenting part PP. The presentations are as follows:
- Head or cephalic presentation, head downwards.
- Breech presentation, bottom downwards.
- Transverse position, which means your baby is lying across your abdomen and the shoulder is presenting.

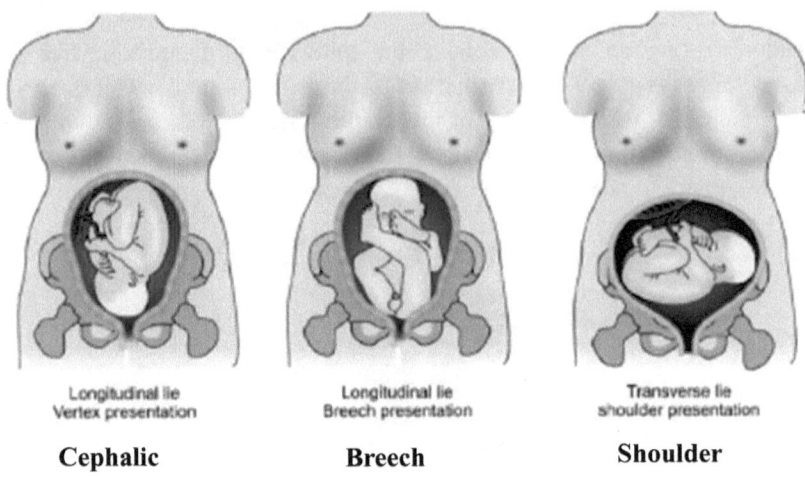

Longitudinal lie Vertex presentation	Longitudinal lie Breech presentation	Transverse lie shoulder presentation
Cephalic	**Breech**	**Shoulder**

Figure 62. Three types of presentations

FOETAL LIE

This is the relation of the long axis of the foetus to that of your own, the mother, and is either longitudinal or transverse.

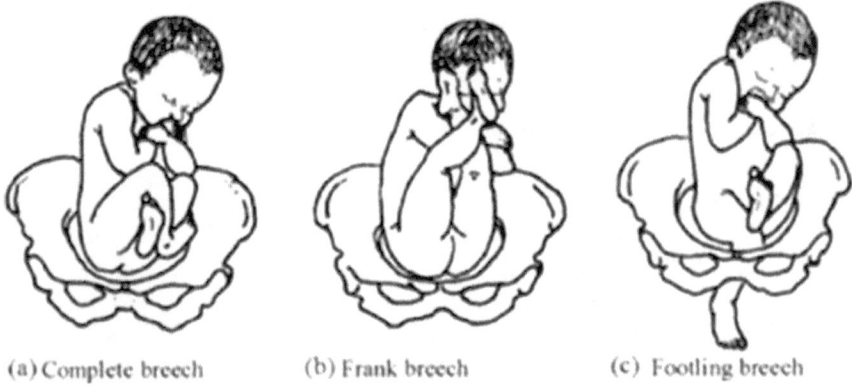

(a) Complete breech	(b) Frank breech	(c) Footling breech

Figure 63. Variation of breech

RELATION OF THE PP TO THE PELVIC BRIM

At the end of pregnancy, the PP of the baby will start to move into your pelvis. In order to assess the relationship of baby's head to the pelvic brim (the bone in front), the head is divided into 5 parts. The description of how far the head has gone down into the pelvis is achieved by judging how many 'fifths' of the head that can be felt above the pelvic brim. The descriptions are as follows:

- 5/5 of the head felt above the brim—all of your baby's head can be felt above the brim.
- 4/5 of the head palpable—head not engaged into the pelvis.
- 3/5 of the head palpable—the head is not engaged yet but going down into the pelvis.
- 2/5 of the head palpable—the head has engaged into the pelvis.
- 1/5 of the head palpable—the head has engaged more into the pelvis.
- 0/5 of the head palpable—this means no part of baby's head is felt above the pelvic brim. It is favourable for instrumental delivery.

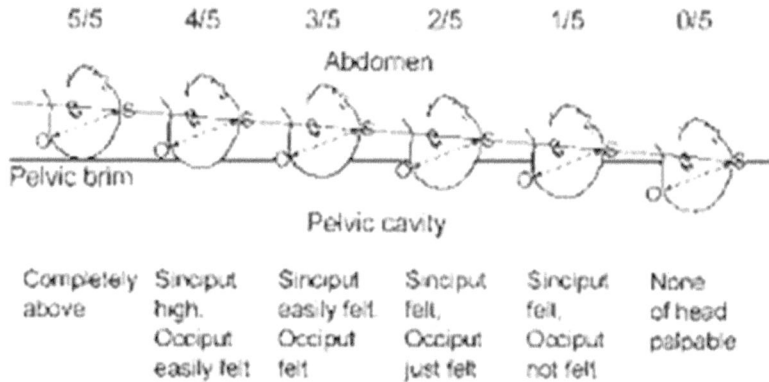

Figure 64. Diagram showing how much of the head that is felt through your tummy (sinciput—front of the head; occiput—back of the head)

FOETAL HEART ASSESSMENT

This confirms that your baby is alive. It is performed by listening to foetal heartbeat with a hand-held device. A Pinard stethoscope, with one end held against your bump at the position of baby's heart and the other end to the operator's ear, is used in listening to baby's heartbeat. Alternatively, a Doppler monitor called Sonicaid is also used for this purpose. It is switched on, placed on your bump at the level of baby's heart, and the heart rate is assessed. If the heartbeat is not heard, you will be referred for a scan.

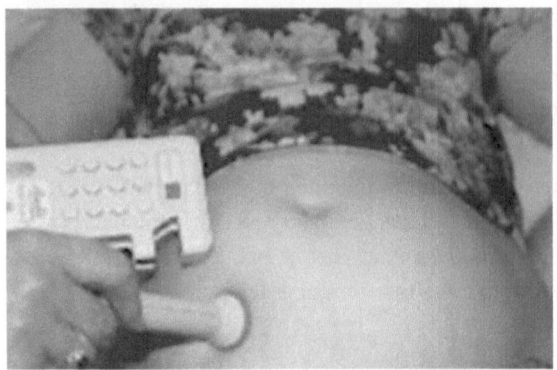
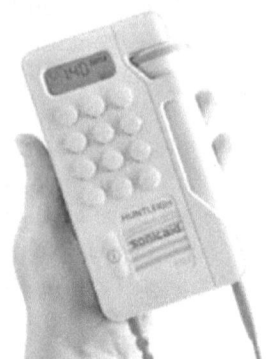

Figure 65a. Foetal heart assessment with a Sonicaid

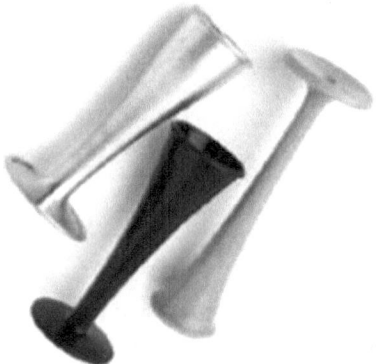

Figure 65b. Pinard stethoscopes

CARDIOTOCOGRAPHY

This is electronic FHR monitoring. It is not normally offered in the antenatal clinic if your pregnancy is straightforward. It is offered when there is concern about baby (page xx).

ULTRASOUND ASSESSMENT IN THE THIRD TRIMESTER

FOETAL MOVEMENTS

Foetal movement is checked by asking you whether you feel your baby move or not. Routine formal foetal-movement counting will not be offered. However, if you are happy with the movements of your baby, that is reassuring about his or her well-being. You will usually start feeling some movements between 16 and 22 weeks. Later in pregnancy, your baby will develop its own pattern of movements, which you will soon get to know. These movements will range from kicks and jerks to rolls and ripples, and you should feel them every day. A change, especially a less frequent movements or not feeling the movements, may be a warning sign that your baby needs further tests, cardiotocogram (CTG) and/or ultrasound. You should, therefore, inform your midwife if you are not happy with the movements of your baby.

OEDEMA

This means swelling, and it occurs in the feet and hands. It is common in pregnancy, and usually, it is nothing to worry about. However, if it is getting worse, it may be a sign of PE, so inform your midwife or doctor about it.

EMERGENCY ASSESSMENT IN PREGNANCY

The assessment will depend on how far you have gone in your pregnancy. If you are 16 weeks and less, you should call your GP, go to the A&E unit or to the EPAU. If you are more than 16 weeks pregnant, then you should go to the maternity assessment unit or the labour ward.

MATERNITY ASSESSMENT UNIT/LABOUR WARD

You should call your midwife and contact the maternity assessment unit or labour ward if you are over 16 weeks and are experiencing the following:
- You have vaginal bleeding that is not a show (small amounts of mucus blood).
- You have severe constant abdominal pain.
- You have severe headaches and/or spots in front of your eyes.
- Your waters have broken.
- Your baby is not moving as much as usual.
- You are concerned about some aspect of your pregnancy.
- You are in labour.

SOURCES
- The NHS Pregnancy Book, UK, 2009.
- The current American Congress of Obstetricians and Gynecologists (ACOG) Guidelines for Perinatal Care, Seventh Edition. October 2012. available at http://www.acog.org/resources_and_publications/ 1
- NHS Choices, Your health, your choices. Last reviewed: 2011.
- Protocol for maternity assessment unit, King's College Hospital, London, 2012.
- Hand-held-note, King's College Hospital, London, 2012

ANTENATAL EDUCATION

AIM OF ANTENATAL EDUCATION

The primary aim of antenatal education (sometimes called antenatal classes or workshop) is as follows:

- To keep you fit and well during pregnancy and give you confidence.
- To educate you about pregnancy, labour, birth, and the choices available to you.
- To promote confidence in you and your partner to meet the challenge of childbirth and early parenting.
- To acquaint you with the people who will look after you during labour, talk over any worries, and discuss your plans, not just with professionals but with other women and their partners as well.
- To make friends with other expectant parents.
- To reduce the incidence of complications during pregnancy, labour, and after childbirth, generally.

Classes or workshops	When it is run and duration	What it covers	Additional information
Early pregnancy class	• Starts from first signs of pregnancy to 20 weeks • Conducted once a week, lasting about 1 hour per session	• Healthy eating • Caring for yourself and your developing baby	• A midwife, dietician, and physiotherapist conduct the class • Your partner, parent, or friend are welcomed to attend with you
Teenagers' antenatal class	• Held at different stages of pregnancy.	• Aspects of antenatal education are discussed • It provides you time to talk openly about your specific needs • It allows greater choice to attend with fellow teenagers or join with a regular antenatal group	• The midwife, physiotherapist, and medical social worker run the class jointly • You, your partner, or companion can attend
Physiotherapy antenatal class	• Commences at 28 and ends at 36 weeks; conducted twice a month, about 2 hours each session	• Safe exercise in pregnancy • Promotion of continence • Care of your back	• The workshop is conducted by a physiotherapist

	• Conducted once a week in the post-natal period depending on demand	• General aches of pregnancy • Returning to fitness after birth	
Labour, birth, pain relief, and relaxation	• Commences between 28 and 32 weeks • Each class held once or twice a week • Consists of about three classes	• Signs of labour • Types of labour: low- and high-risk labour, home birth • Pain relief in labour • A video of a normal birth is presented • Stages and process of labour and coping strategies • Comfortable positions, basic massage, relaxation, and the role of your birth partner in labour • IOL • Assisted births with vacuum or forceps and Caesarean section	• Conducted by midwife, obstetrician, and anaesthetist • Your partner or parent or friend is welcomed to attend with you
Feeding your baby	• Commences between 28 and 32 weeks • Held once a week	• Breastfeeding • Expressing and storing milk • Positioning and attachment of your baby at the breast Where to get help and support for feeding your baby	• Conducted by a breastfeeding specialist midwife • Your partner, parent, or Child minder are welcomed to attend with you
Parenting	• Held once a week from 34 to 36 weeks	• The parenting role	• The classes will be conducted

		• Demonstration on caring for your baby, bathing and daily care • Car safety • Reducing the risk of cot death • Feeding will be revisited, how to store breast milk, sterilise bottles, and prepare all formula feeds • Emotional changes following childbirth, recovery, and support	by a midwife and a medical psychologist • Partners, parents, or friends are welcomed to attend
Multiple pregnancy	• Ideally between 24 and 34 weeks • Conducted once every 6 weeks	• The needs of women expecting more than one baby • A visit to the neonatal unit will be arranged during the workshop	• Conducted by a midwife • Partners can attend
Tour of maternity unit	• 34-36 weeks	• To view patient areas of maternity unit • Tour and photographs of the labour rooms, birthing pool, garden room, operation theatre, and post-natal areas	• Conducted by a midwife • To attend with your partner
Refresher classes	• Between 30 and 36 weeks • Conducted twice a month	• For mothers who have had a vaginal birth in the past • This class is for mothers only	• Conducted by a midwife
Refresher classes	• Between 30 and 36 weeks • Conducted once a month.	• For mothers who have had a previous Caesarean birth	• Conducted by a midwife • Partners are welcome

Individual antenatal class		• Classes are held on a one-to-one basis in certain circumstances • Booking is essential	
Yoga for pregnancy	• 2 classes a week • 1½ hours for each session • A programme consists of 6 sessions		• You can rebook for more than one programme, but there may be financial cost attached to it

Table 7. Antenatal classes' schedules

ANTENATAL CLASSES OR WORKSHOP

The number of different antenatal classes available varies from place to place and from hospital to hospital. If you are expecting a multiple pregnancy, try to start your classes at around 24 weeks, because your babies are more likely to be born earlier. Think about what you hope to gain from antenatal classes so that you can find the sort of class that suits you best. You need to start making enquiries early in pregnancy so that you can be sure of getting a place in the class you choose.

Some classes are for pregnant women only, while others will welcome partners or friends, either to all the sessions or to some of them. There are also classes for single mothers and those for teenagers. You can go to more than one class. Ask your midwife, health visitor, or GP about what is available. Speak to your community midwife if you cannot go to classes. She may have DVDs to lend you, or you may be able to hire or buy one.

YOGA

Yoga is an ancient and holistic system of harmonising body, heart, and mind, and it involves performing certain exercises. The content of the classes includes various breathing techniques, various postures and movements followed by deep relaxation and visualisation. It is an ideal form of exercise during pregnancy. It can also be practised during labour and the post-natal period. Most healthy women can join yoga class. Minor disorders of pregnancy generally do not pose a problem. In a hospital that offers yoga, you can access the service by self-referral or a letter from your doctor/midwife.

BENEFITS OF YOGA IN PREGNANCY
- Encourages focus on the pregnancy
- Deepens awareness of the baby
- Increases flexibility and strength

- Raises energy levels
- Helps minor pregnancy complaints
- Helps you to achieve deep relaxation
- Improves sleep

BENEFITS FOR LABOUR
- Helps with pain in labour
- Increases comfort and helps with birth positions
- Helps in physical and emotional grounding

SOURCES
- Antenatal classes at the National Maternity Hospital, Holles Street, Dublin, Ireland. Ph. (01) 637 3100.
- Antenatal education workshop of guys and St. Thomas Hospital, London.
- The NHS Pregnancy Book, UK, 2009.

FOETAL MONITORING IN THE ANTENATAL PERIOD

DEFINITION
This is a test of well-being of your baby which involves monitoring his or her heartbeat. The aim of the monitoring is to identify a baby who is likely to be short of oxygen or is already short of it (hypoxia) so that necessary action can be taken. The action will be the following:
- Look for the cause and treat it.
- Ask you to change position; for instance, if you are lying on the back, you may be asked to lie on the left side.
- Set up intravenous fluids (drip) for you.
- Perform Caesarean section immediately if the problem persists, or your waters will be broken if you are due.

INDICATIONS FOR FOETAL MONITORING
They are as follows:
- in the antenatal clinic for routine assessment of FHR
- in the community and GP surgery to monitor foetal heart
- in the maternity day unit to monitor foetal heart in low-risk patients and patients sent with different obstetric problems, for example RFMs
- on the labour ward for antenatal patients presenting with different obstetric problems

METHODS OF BABY'S WELL-BEING MONITORING
- Intermittent monitoring—listening to foetal heartbeat with a hand-held device (page xxx)

- Continuous electronic foetal monitoring (CEFM)

CONTINUOUS ELECTRONIC FOETAL MONITORING

This is a method of monitoring your baby by using two electronic sensors, called transducers, placed on your bump: one at the top of your uterus to measure contractions and the other close to your baby's heart to monitor his or her heart rate. Both sensors are connected to a machine called CTG and secured to straps, which are fastened firmly around your abdomen. The tracings are printed out on a paper from the machine as seen below.

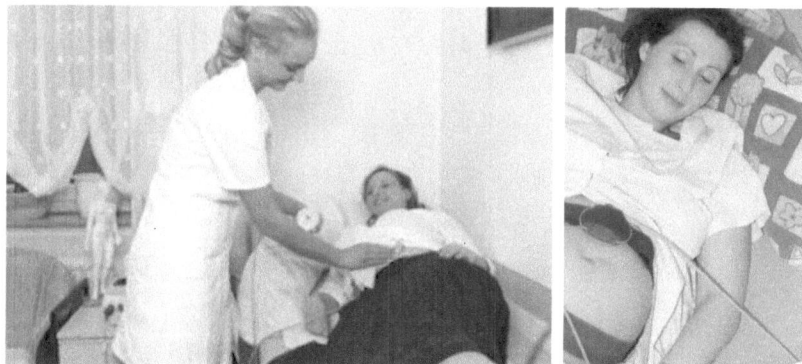

Figure 66a. Fixing the CTG monitor

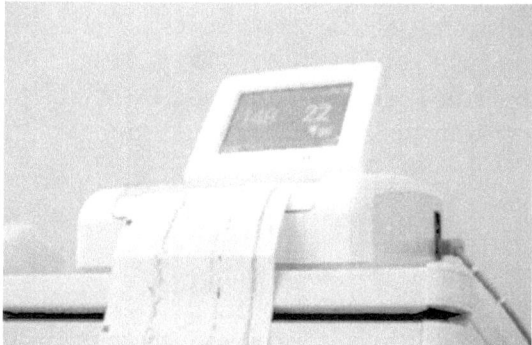

Figure 66b. CTG machine with the trace

Indications for CEFM in the antenatal period are as follows:
- if there is a suspicion of FHR abnormalities on intermittent monitoring
- if you have any obstetric problem presented in the maternity day unit or labour ward, for example abdominal pain, decreased foetal movements, or spontaneous rupture of membrane

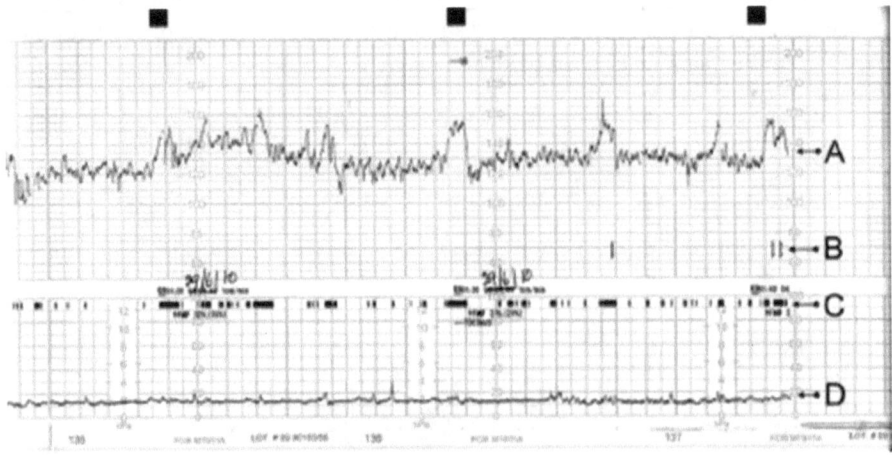

Figure 66c. CTG trace in the antenatal period

- if you are in the high-risk category and you have been reviewed in the maternity day unit
- if you are admitted to the antenatal ward

MANAGEMENT OF THE FINDINGS DURING CEFM

The CTG trace is categorised into the following groups:
- Normal
- Suspicious
- Abnormal (pathological)
- Grossly abnormal (bradycardia)

A normal trace means your baby is happy, and monitoring will be discontinued. A suspicious or pathological trace indicates that your baby may not be getting enough oxygen (which is necessary for normal working of different organs of the body) in his or her blood. In that situation, the actions outlined on page xxx above under 'definition' will be carried out.

SOURCES

- Clements RV. Safe Practice in Obstetrics and Gynaecology. Edinburgh: Churchill Livingstone; 1994:492.
- Laura Coughlin, Amber Huntzinger. ACOG Recommendations for Fetal Heart Rate Monitoring Am Fam. Physician 2005 Aug. 1;72(3):527.
- Gibb D, Arulkumaran S. Fetal Monitoring in Practice. 3rd ed., 2007.
- James DK, et al. High Risk Pregnancy. London: WB Saunders; 1994:1318.
- The Use of Electronic Fetal Monitoring: The Use and Interpretation of Cardiotocography in Intrapartum Fetal Surveillance (Guideline No. 8). London: RCOG Press; 2001. MDA SN2002(23) Cardiotocograph monitoring of the foetus-update.

Healthy Living in Pregnancy

HEALTHY EATING IN PREGNANCY

INTRODUCTION

A balanced diet is the basis of good health which will influence you, your partner's fertility, and your ability to become and stay pregnant. It provides enough energy and nutrients for your baby to develop and grow and for you to cope with the changes that take place during pregnancy. 'Eating for two' during pregnancy is not necessary. It is the quality of the food that you eat that is important and not the quantity. This chapter contains practical guides to help you make some healthy food choices while you are pregnant. The balanced diet plate shown below contains different types of food which should be eaten in different proportion as indicated by the size of the partitions.

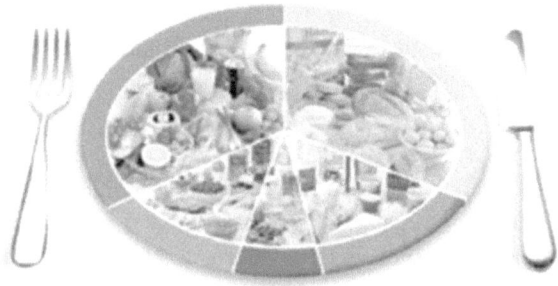

Figure 67. Balanced diet plate in pregnancy (NHS, UK)

CARBOHYDRATES

They are satisfying, do not contain too much calories, and are an important source of vitamins and fibre. Sources of carbohydrates are starch-based foods such as bread, breakfast cereals, potatoes, rice, and pasta. Other sources are oats, noodles, maize, millet, yams, and cornmeal. These foods should be the main part of every meal. Eat wholemeal bread or cereals when you can. Breakfast cereals are often fortified with extra vitamins and minerals, including iron.

FATTY AND SUGARY FOOD

Spreading fats, oils, salad dressings, cream, chocolate, crisps, biscuits, pastries, ice cream, cake, puddings, and fizzy drinks all belong to this group of food. You should eat a small amount of this food. Sugar contains calories without providing any other nutrients that the body needs. Sugary foods and drinks can cause tooth decay, especially if you have them between meals.

Eating more fatty foods and sugary food are likely to make you put on weight. Some fats called saturated fat can increase the amount of cholesterol in the blood, which increases the chance of developing heart disease. Try to cut down on food that is rich in saturated fat.

PROTEIN

Lean meat (except liver), fish, poultry, eggs, pulses (such as beams, peas, and lentils), seeds, and nuts all count towards your daily protein needs. They are good sources of nutrients and iron. Eat protein food in moderation about 2 portions a day.

MEAT

When choosing meat, choose low-fat or lean meats and poultry (chicken). Trim fat from meat and remove skin from poultry before cooking. Use cooking methods that needs little fat or do not add fat, such as grilling, broiling, or roasting. Avoid too much salt. Ensure that all meat, eggs, poultry, pork, burgers, and sausages are cooked thoroughly. Check that there is no pink meat and that juices have no pink or red in them. Remember to store cooked and raw meats separately.

MEAT ALTERNATIVES

Beans (including tinned baked beans), chickpeas, lentils, nuts, and seeds are particularly important in a vegetarian or vegan diet and so, too, are soya products and other meat alternatives, such as tofu, Quorn, and textured vegetable protein.

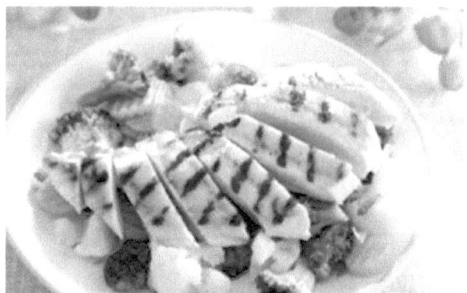 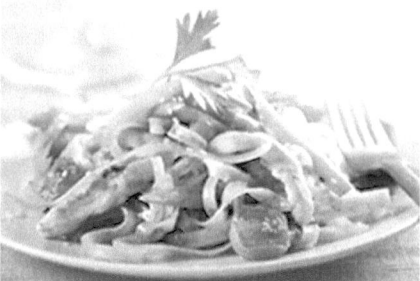

Figure 68. Healthy eating options

FISH

Aim to eat at least 2 portions of fish per week, with at least one portion being oily fish such as fresh tuna, salmon, mackerel, sardines, and trout. However, there are some important exceptions. Do not eat raw fish or uncooked shellfish, which may contain bacteria, viruses, or parasites.

Some types of fish may contain a small amount of dangerous chemicals from pollution, including substances called dioxins and polychlorinated biphenyls. If you eat a lot of these fish, these chemicals may build up in your body over time, which may be harmful. Therefore, it is advisable that you should have no more than 2 portions a week of any of the following fish:

- Sea bream, sea bass, turbot, halibut, rock salmon (also known as dogfish, flake, huss, rigg, or rock eel).
- Brown crabmeat.
- Oily fish, including mackerel, sardines, salmon, trout, and tuna.

Avoid swordfish, marlin, and shark because they may contain high mercury levels which can damage a baby's developing nervous system. Tuna may also contain mercury.

EGGS

Please see below.

FRUIT AND VEGETABLES

Fruit and vegetables are good sources of vitamins, minerals, and fibre which help digestion and prevent constipation. They probably reduce the risk of miscarriage. Try to eat 5 portions a day of fresh, frozen, canned, dried, or juiced fruit and vegetables, including a glass of pure fruit juice. Leafy green vegetables and yellow and red vegetables (such as peppers, tomatoes, and carrots) are good choices.

Frozen and tinned vegetables are usually as nutritious as fresh ones. It is best to choose fresh, frozen, or dried fruit rather than tinned fruit, which usually contains added sugar. Do make sure that your fruit and vegetables are washed thoroughly before eating. Eat them lightly cooked in a little water or raw to get the most out of them.

DAIRY FOOD

This includes milk, cheese yoghurt and fromage frais. They contain calcium and other nutrients needed for baby's development. Try to eat 3-4 portions a day of dairy products or plant-based alternatives before and during pregnancy using low-fat varieties whenever you can, for example, semi-skimmed or skimmed milk, low-fat yoghurt and half-fat hard cheese. It is important to avoid unpasteurised dairy products, such as raw (untreated) milk and soft or mould-ripened cheeses like Brie, Camembert, and blue cheeses. Cream cheese and cottage cheese are safe to eat.

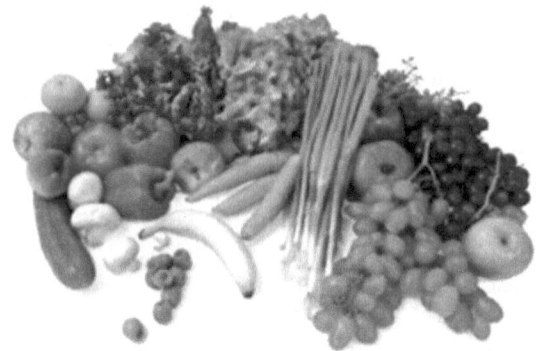

Figure 69. Some healthy eating options—fruits and vegetables

FOOD AND DRINK TO AVOID

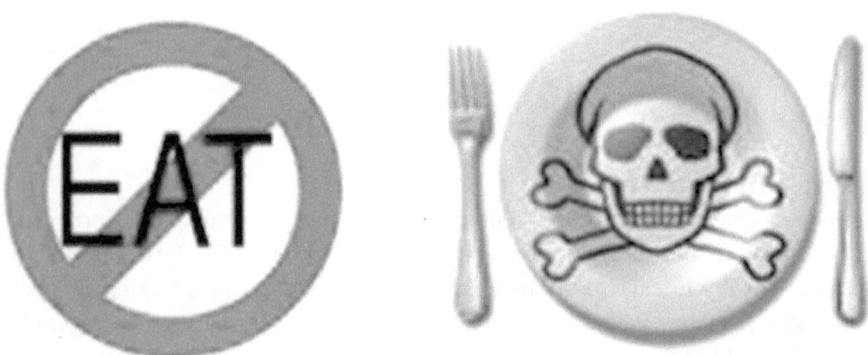

Figure 70. Food to avoid

You should not eat the following if you are pregnant or trying to become pregnant:

- Anything with a lot of vitamin A: It can cause severe birth defects if taken during pregnancy. So avoid vitamin A and food products that contain it, for example liver and its pate, cod liver oil.
- Food containing less iodine: Examples are fast food. Except most items containing milk and fish, fast food are not good sources of iodine, an integral component in the human body, especially for pregnant women.
- Food which may have high levels of germs, for example listeria; Listeria is a germ which causes miscarriage, stillbirth, and infections of babies after birth. The following food items are most at risk of carrying listeria and so avoid them:

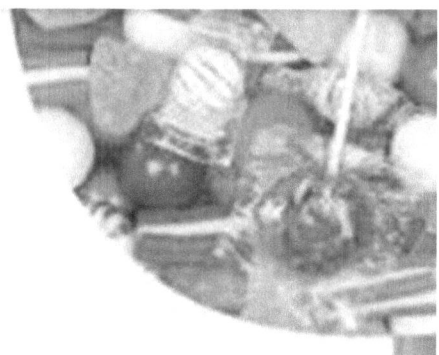
Figure 71a. Sweet

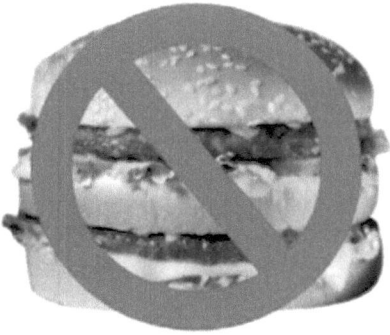
Figure 71b. Burger

- Undercooked meat and eggs. Make sure all meat foods are cooked until piping hot. Eggs should be cooked until the white and yolk are solid.

- Food that may contain raw eggs such as some types of mayonnaise and mousse.

- Mould-ripened and soft cheeses such as Brie, Camembert, and blue-veined cheeses.

- Patés including vegetable patés.

- Raw fish including shellfish.

- Unpasteurised milk. It is important to note that goat's milk is often unpasteurised, and its products such as cheeses are often made from unpasteurised milk.

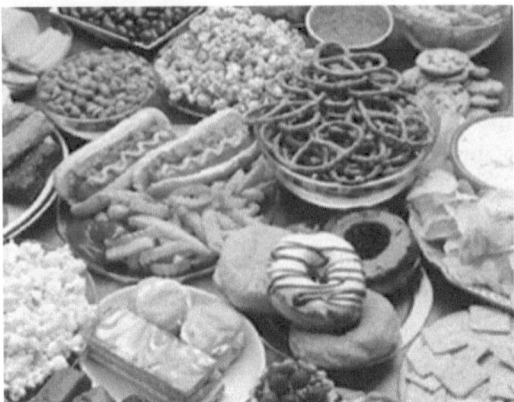

Figure 72. Other food to avoid

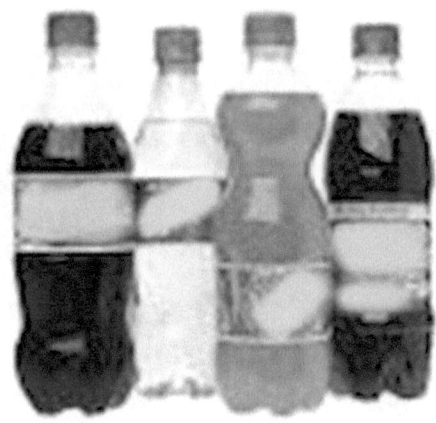

Figure 73. Other food to avoid—the junk drinks

- Certain fishes as described earlier.
- Peanuts: There is no evidence that you should exclude peanuts from your diet when trying for a baby, during pregnancy, and when you are breastfeeding.
- Foods containing sugar as stated above.
- Foods continuing fat as stated above.
- Liquorice should be avoided because it may be associated with having children with lower intelligence levels and more behavioural problems; further research is needed to clarify this issue.
- Caffeine: You should limit the amount of caffeine you have each day because high levels of it can cause LBW and/or miscarriage. Caffeine

occurs naturally in some foods and hot drinks such as coffee, tea, and chocolate, some soft and energy drinks, certain cold and flu remedies. It is important to have no more than 300 mg of caffeine a day.

Each of the following items contains roughly 300 mg of caffeine:
- 3 mugs of instant coffee
- 4 cups of instant coffee
- 3 cups brewed coffee
- 6 cups of tea
- 8 cans of coke
- 4 cans of energy drink
- 8 bars of chocolate

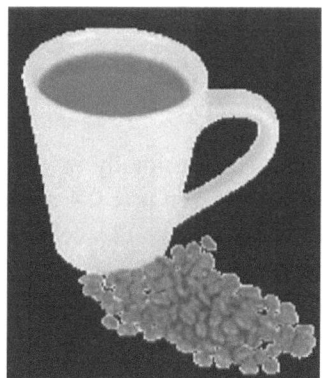

Figure 74. Caffeine (from NHS Pregnancy Book, 2009)

Try decaffeinated tea, coffee, fruit juice, or mineral water.

PREVENTION OF GERMS
There are certain precautions that you have to take in order to safeguard your baby's well-being and yourself. In addition to the precautions already discussed above, the following are also important:
- Measures to prevent toxoplasma infection (Page 291).
- You should practice general hygiene.
    - Wash your hands before and after handling any food.
    - Make sure that raw food is stored separately from ready-to-eat one.
    - Keep leftovers covered in the fridge and use within 2 days.

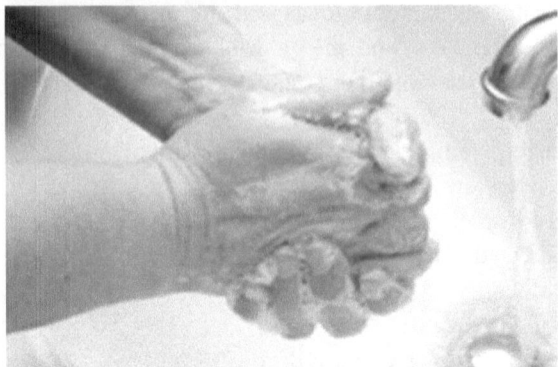

Figure 75. Wash your hand before and after handling any food

VITAMIN AND MINERAL SUPPLEMENTS

FOLIC ACID

Folic acid is a vitamin which occurs naturally in certain food products that are listed below. It is recommended that you take 0.4 mg of folic acid daily from the time you start trying for baby until you are 12 weeks into your pregnancy because of its benefit which are as following:

- Folic acid reduces the risk of having a baby born with spina bifida (a spinal cord problem).
- It also significantly decreases the chance of occurence of PTD (page 226) if taken for 1 year prior to pregnancy.
- It reduces the risk of having a baby born with a cleft lip and palate and a heart defect.

Because of its substantial benefits, some countries routinely fortify staple foods such as wheat, cornflour, or rice with folic acid.

A higher dose of the drug (5 mg daily) is required in the following situations:

- You have had a previously affected baby with spina bifida.
- You or your partner has a spinal cord defect.
- You are obese.
- You are taking medication for epilepsy.
- You have certain illness such as coeliac disease, diabetes, sickle-cell anaemia, or thalassaemia.

You are also advised to eat food that contains folic acid, which are as follows:

- dark leafy greens and vegetables such as spinach, collard and turnip greens, romaine lettuce, broccoli, and asparagus

- enriched breads and cereals
- citrus fruits and juices such as strawberries, oranges, and orange juice
- brown rice
- dried peas and beans such as pinto, chickpeas, and black-eyed peas
- folic acid-fortified breakfast cereals

IRON

Your iron levels can be low during pregnancy, and this can lead to anaemia and tiredness. To prevent that happening, the following advice is given:

- Eat plenty of iron-rich foods, which are red or lean meat (eat it well cooked), pulses, fortified cereals, bread, green and dried vegetables, liver (don't eat it), dried fruits and nuts (not peanuts).
- Take iron supplements, which come in tablet or liquid forms.
- Avoid drinking tea or coffee when eating iron-rich foods because the drink could make it harder for the body to absorb iron.

VITAMIN C

Food rich in vitamin C are citrus fruits, tomatoes, broccoli, peppers, blackcurrants, potatoes, and some pure fruit juices. You need vitamin C as it may help you to absorb iron from food. So if your iron levels are low, it may help to drink orange juice with an iron-rich meal.

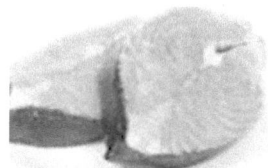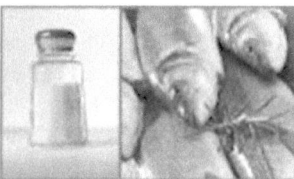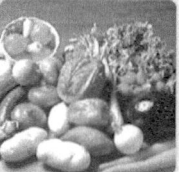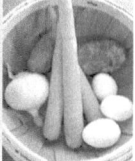

Figure 76. Good sources of iodine

IODINE

Iodine mainly comes from milk, yogurt, eggs, and fish. Because iodine intake can be variable, some countries routinely fortify cereals and bread with iodine, but not the UK. Iodine is essential for the brain development of a baby in the womb. Its deficiency may lead to reduced brain development in the fetus and consequently, baby may be less intelligent than he or she would otherwise have been. Cauliflower, broccoli, cabbage, mustard, tapioca, and corn can interfere with the absorption of iodine and therefore their intake should be reduced or avoided in pregnancy.

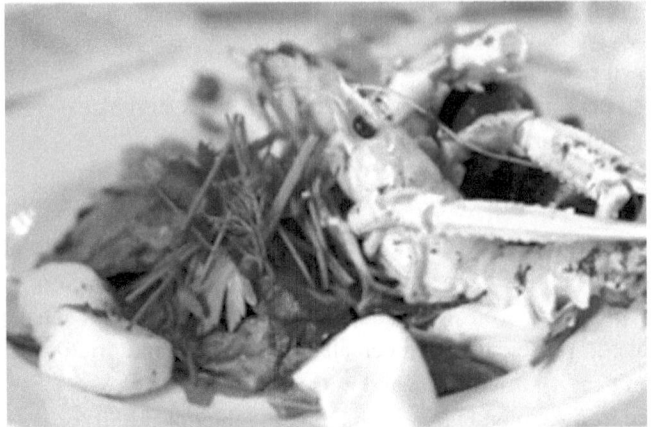

Figure 77. Avoid these foods; they interfere in the absorption of iodine

VITAMIN D

You need vitamin D during pregnancy and breastfeeding because of the following reasons:

- It regulates the amount of calcium and phosphate in the body, and these are needed to help keep bones and teeth healthy.
- For the first few months of life, your baby gets vitamin D from your breast or formula milk, so you have to take enough of the vitamin yourself. Deficiency in vitamin D can lead to softening of children's bones and consequently cause rickets (a disease that affects bone development in children).

You should take 400 units (10 µg) of vitamin D daily if you are pregnant or breastfeeding. Although there is a small amount of vitamin D in some foods namely oily fish like sardines, fortified margarines, some breakfast cereals, and taramasalata, most of the vitamin D that we get is made in the skin with the help of sunlight. It is, therefore, suggested that if you get little or no sunshine on your skin, you should be given 800 units (20 µg) daily. Just 15 minutes in the sun can produce enough vitamin D that you need. If you have dark skin or always cover your skin, you may be at particular risk of lacking vitamin D.

CALCIUM

Food rich in calcium are dairy products, fish with edible bones like sardines, breakfast cereals, dried fruit such as figs and apricots, bread, almonds, tofu (a vegetable protein made from soya beans), and green leafy vegetables like watercress, broccoli, and curly kale. Calcium is used for making your baby's bones and teeth.

VEGETARIAN (THOSE THAT DO NOT EAT ANIMAL PRODUCTS) AND SPECIAL DIETS

Iron and vitamin B12 can be hard to obtain from a vegetarian diet. If you are vegan (i.e. you do not eat any animal products) or you eat a gluten-free diet, because of food intolerance, coeliac disease, or for religions reason, talk to your doctor or midwife about it. Ask to be referred to a dietician for advice on how to make sure you are getting all the nutrients you need for you and your baby.

HEALTHY SNACKS

Between meals, you may like to have snacks. Avoid snacks that are high in fat and/or sugar; the following are recommended:
- Fresh fruit, sandwiches or pitta bread filled with grated cheese, lean ham, mashed tuna, salmon or sardines, and salad.
- Salad vegetables.
- Low-fat yoghurt or fromage frais.
- Hummus and bread or vegetable sticks.
- Ready-to-eat apricots, figs, or prunes.
- Vegetable and bean soups.
- Unsweetened breakfast cereals or porridge and milk.
- Milky drinks or unsweetened fruit juices.
- Baked beans on toast or a baked potato.

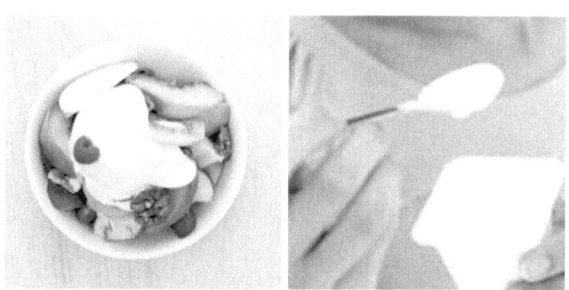

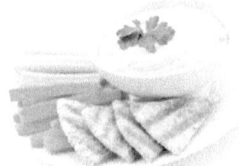

Figure 78. Healthy snacks

Sources

- Healthy Eating: Eating While You Are Pregnant. Published by Food Standards Agency UK, 2002, pre-printed with amendments August 2004 and August 2008.
- The NHS Pregnancy Book. Publish by COI for the Department of Health; 2005, 2006.
- www.eatwell.gov.uk
- www.foodgov.uk
- Labour and childbirth. The first weeks with your new baby, UK, 2009. NHS Choices.

Smoking in Pregnancy

The process behind the ill effects of smoking

Cigarette or tobacco smoke contains nicotine, which is highly addictive, and more than 4,000 different chemicals, many of which are harmful to the body. More than 60 of them cause cancer. Some of these substances are as follows:

- Nicotine
- Tar
- Carbon monoxide
- Oxidant gases
- Benzene
- Polonium

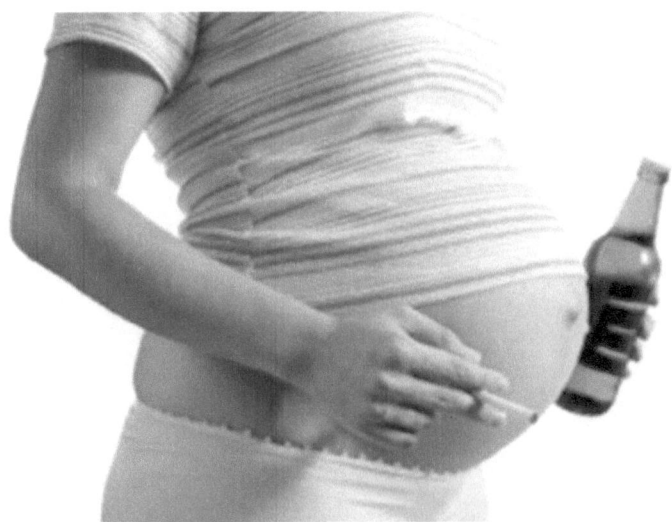

Figure 79. Smoking and drinking in pregnancy

Nicotine

- It affects your brain, within seconds of inhaling cigarette smoke, by causing a surge in the hormones in the brain called noradrenaline and dopamine. These hormones have a positive effect on your mood and your ability to concentrate. In between cigarettes, the levels of these hormones drop, leaving you feeling irritable, anxious, and in need of another cigarette (addiction). Within 24 hours, withdrawal from nicotine can cause the following side effects:
  - depressed mood
  - difficulty in sleeping
  - irritability
  - frustration or anger
  - anxiety
  - difficulty in concentrating
  - restlessness
  - decreased heart rate
  - dizziness
  - increased appetite
- It increases your heart rate.
- It increases the risk of accelerated hypertension, which is a sudden rise in already high BP; this can cause headaches, blurred vision, and vomiting.
- It also causes the small blood vessels in your skin to contract (become narrower), reducing the blood flow that is needed to ensure that your skin remains healthy.

Tar

Every breath of tobacco smoke deposits tar in your lungs. Tar contains chemicals called carcinogens, which encourages the development of cancer cells in your body.

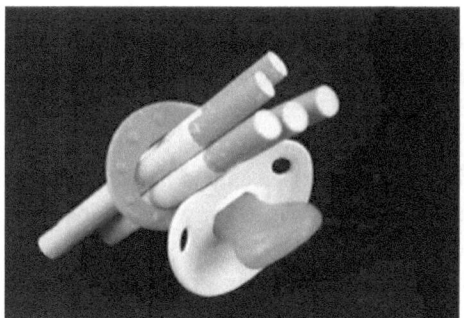 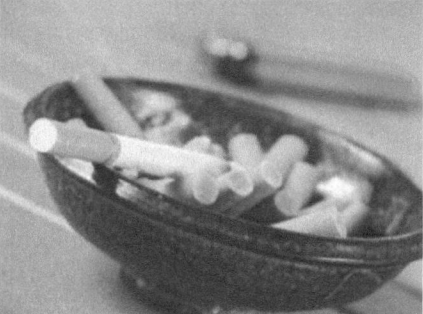

Figure 80. Smoking is dangerous to your health and that of your baby

CARBON MONOXIDE

When cigarette smoke is inhaled, the poisonous gas carbon monoxide binds itself to the haemoglobin in your bloodstream and prevents it from carrying enough oxygen around your body. This is particularly dangerous when you are pregnant because this cuts down the oxygen reaching your baby in the womb and therefore causes lack of oxygen in the unborn baby (this is known as foetal hypoxia); the end result is a growth-restricted baby.

OXIDANT GASES

Oxidant gases are gases that react with oxygen. They make your blood more likely to clot, which increases your risk of having a heart attack or stroke.

BENZENE

Exposure to benzene can cause cell damage at the genetic level and has been linked to a range of different cancers such as leukaemia and kidney cancer.

POLONIUM

Polonium is a highly radioactive substance, and even tiny amounts can cause extensive damage to human tissue.

OTHER HARMFUL SUBSTANCES

Some of these substances can cause thickening and fatty changes of your blood vessels called arteries, which then causes heart disease. Others can increase the acid content in your stomach, putting you at risk of developing ulcers in your stomach or small bowel.

RISKS OF SMOKING

RISKS TO YOURSELF
- Premature death.
- Cancer of different organs namely lungs (responsible for 90% of lung cancer), cervix, bladder, pancreas, mouth, gullet, stomach, kidney, and others.
- Respiratory diseases (conditions that affect breathing)
- Cerebrovascular diseases (conditions that affect the brain and its blood supply)
- Cardiovascular diseases (conditions that affect the heart and blood vessels)
- Other conditions that can be caused by smoking, or for which smoking is a significant risk factor, include
    - Crohn's disease (a bowel condition that causes abdominal pain and diarrhoea)
    - stomach ulcers
    - gum disease
    - asthma

- loss of sight caused by diabetes
- impotence
- breakdown of the retina (light-sensitive layer of the eye), causing gradual blindness
- Infertility, in both men and women
- skin wrinkling
- osteoporosis (weak and brittle bones)

RISKS TO YOUR PREGNANCY

- Although smoking at any stage of pregnancy can harm your baby, most of the harmful effects of smoking occur at weeks 14 - 27. Therefore, if you quit smoking during the first 3 months of pregnancy, you will have a similar risk of giving birth to a LBW baby as a non-smoker.
- A greater chance of complications occurs during pregnancy and labour, such as sickness, miscarriage, bleeding, preterm birth, stillbirth, and SGA baby.
- Increased risks of problems in your child if he or she was exposed to cigarette smoke when you were pregnant (i.e. you were smoking); the problems are as follows:
  - Developmental delay throughout childhood.
  - Poor performance at school.
  - Increased risk of developing behavioural problems and attention deficit hyperactivity disorder in older children.

RISKS TO OTHERS

When you smoke, it is not just your health that is at risk but also the health of anyone around you who breathes in cigarette smoke. A smoker only inhales about 15% of the smoke from a cigarette. The other 85% is released into the atmosphere and inhaled by other people. Breathing in this secondary smoke is known as passive smoking or secondary smoking, which predisposes to the following:

- An increased risk of smoking-related diseases, particularly lung cancer and heart disease.
- Risks to children namely
  - increased risk of developing chest infections during their first 5 years.
  - a greater risk of sudden infant death syndrome, also known as cot death.
  - more vulnerable to ear infections and asthma.

MANAGEMENT

If you want to quit smoking, initially, it is a good idea to see your GP. They can provide help and advice about quitting. If you live in the UK, they will

- refer you to a NHS 'Stop Smoking Support Service'.
- ask you about your smoking habits with a view of assessing your level of addiction and also outlining the benefits of quitting.
- help you to identify any factors that may make quitting difficult for you, such as living with others who smoke, or any stress that you experience in day-to-day life.
- prescribe a smoking cessation treatment namely nicotine replacement therapy if counselling does not help you to stop smoking. It works by releasing nicotine steadily into your bloodstream at much lower levels than in a cigarette smoke, without the tar, carbon monoxide, and other poisonous chemicals present in a tobacco smoke. This helps to control the cravings for a cigarette that occur when your body starts to miss the nicotine from smoking.

QUITTING SMOKING

Three stages to giving up smoking are
- preparing to stop
- stopping
- stopping permanently

STAGE 1: PREPARING TO STOP

Write down your reasons (benefits) for quitting smoking. The reasons can be as follows:
- You want to live longer and feel healthier.
- You wish to wear clean clothes.
- You can get more money to spend on other things.
- Your skin will be clearer, brighter, and more hydrated.
- You are no longer harming others through passive smoking.
- You limit harm to your unborn baby.
- You will eliminate or reduce the entire risks associated with smoking, generally.

Refer to the above list when you are tempted to light up. Remember that most of the pleasure you get from smoking comes from relief of your nicotine withdrawal, not the cigarette itself. Nicotine replacement therapy can provide the same effect without the need for smoking and helps you quit at the same time. Having drawn up the above list, make a plan that may include the following things:
- Select a specific date to give up or cut down on the number of cigarettes that you smoke.
- Get the support of your family and friends to help you give up smoking.
- Have a reward for the end of your first day, first week, or first month.
- Get rid of everything related to smoking, such as cigarettes, ash trays, and lighters.

STAGE 2: STOPPING

- Get through the first day without smoking.
- Engage in activities that will remove your mind from smoking.
- Chew sugar-free gum or eat something else that is healthy, such as fruit, if you need to put something in your mouth.
- Take some deep breaths and delay giving in to the urge if you feel a strong craving. The feeling will usually pass within a couple of minutes.
- Find something to fiddle with such as a pencil, a coin, or a stress-relief ball if you need to do something with your hands.

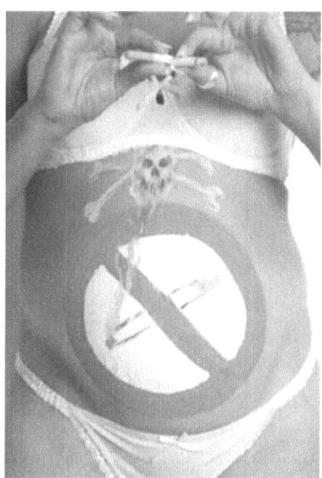

Figure 81. Quitting smoking in pregnancy

STAGE 3: STOPPING PERMANENTLY

- Keep reminding yourself of your reasons for giving up and what you are gaining by quitting smoking.
- Think positively, remain determined, and reward yourself.
- Change your normal routine to avoid situations that you would normally associate with smoking, for example avoiding alcohol for a while.
- Do not let yourself be tempted to smoke one cigarette after the first smoking-free weeks because this can easily lead to two or three cigarettes, which increase your risk of becoming a smoker again.

SOURCES

- www.givingupsmoking.co.uk
- NHS Choices, Your health, your choices. Last reviewed: 2011.
- Smoking and pregnancy. NHS information for pregnant women, partners and families. Department of Health. Order No. 50808. July 2003.

- The NHS Pregnancy Book. Your complete guide to: a healthy pregnancy, labour and childbirth. The first weeks with your new baby, UK, 2009.

ALCOHOL AND DRUGS IN PREGNANCY

DRINKING IN PREGNANCY

THE PROCESS BEHIND THE EFFECT OF ALCOHOL ON YOUR BABY

When you drink alcohol, it passes from your bloodstream to the placenta and from there to the baby's bloodstream. Alcohol taken by an adult is normally processed by the liver. A baby's liver is one of the last organs to develop fully and does not mature until the latter half of the pregnancy. Your baby cannot, therefore, process and get rid of the alcohol as fast as you can; so the baby is exposed to greater amounts of alcohol for longer time than you are, and this adversely affects him or her.

THE EFFECT OF ALCOHOL ON PREGNANCY

If you drink more than 2 units of alcohol on more than 2 occasions a week (that's above the recommended amount), then you will have an increased risk to yourself or your baby.

- Before pregnancy:
  Drinking heavily (over 6 units per day) can cause infertility (no pregnancy after trying for a baby for at least 1 year).
- During pregnancy
  Drinking can cause the following problems:
  - Miscarriage.
  - Stillbirt
  - SGA baby.
  - Preterm birth - the evidence for this is currently inconclusive.
  - Child may have physical and learning difficulties.
  - Susceptibility of the baby to illness later on in adult life.
  - The foetus may develop a combination of features called 'foetal alcohol syndrome'(Figure 82) which includes the following:
    - Abnormalities of the face
    - LBW
    - Inappropriate development of the brain in terms of structure or function
    - Learning and behavioural disorders after birth

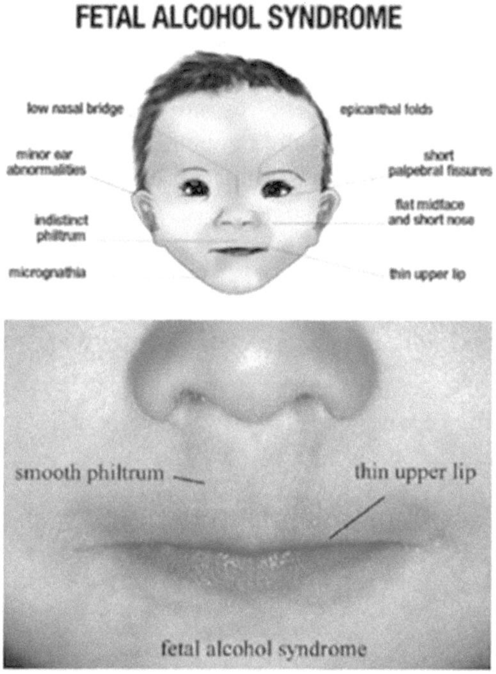

FETAL ALCOHOL SYNDROME

low nasal bridge

epicanthal folds

minor ear abnormalities

short palpebral fissures

indistinct philtrum

flat midface and short nose

micrognathia

thin upper lip

smooth philtrum

thin upper lip

fetal alcohol syndrome

Figure 82. Impact of alcohol on your baby

The features of foetal alcohol syndrome are very uncommon and do not occur unless you drink very heavily throughout pregnancy (over 6 units a day). The features can be isolated or appear in different combinations. It is also important to note that it is dangerous to drink when you are taking some medicines such as tranquillisers and sedatives that make you feel sleepy.

PREVENTION OF THE EFFECTS OF ALCOHOL IN PREGNANCY

- Do not drink during pregnancy. If you do choose to drink, then protect your baby by not drinking more than 1-2 units of alcohol once or twice a week, and don't get drunk. A unit of alcohol is equivalent to the following respectively:
  - 10 mL or 8 g of pure alcohol in the UK
  - ½ pint of beer, lager, or cider at 3.5% ABV
  - a single measure (25 mL) of spirit (whisky, gin, Bacardi, vodka, etc.) at 40% ABV
  - ½ standard (175 mL) glass of wine at 11.5% ABV

ABV or alcohol by volume is a standard measure of how much alcohol (ethanol) is present in an alcoholic beverage.

- If you are drinking with friends
  - find a non-alcoholic drink that you enjoy
  - sip any alcohol or drink slowly to make it last
  - don't let people pressure you into drinking
- Alcohol can affect your baby throughout pregnancy, but when you cut down or stop drinking at any stage in pregnancy, it can make a difference to the baby. However, in some cases, once the damage has been done, this cannot be reversed.

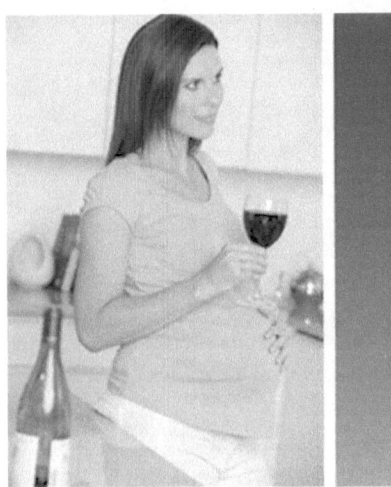

Figure 83. Quitting drinking

DEGREES OF ALCOHOL CONSUMPTION

The UK government's maximum recommended number of units of alcohol for women who are not pregnant is 14 units per week, and this can be extrapolated to African condition too. Light drinking is defined as under 2 units a day, while heavy drinking is defined as over 6 units a day.

Binge drinking is defined as drinking 5 or more units of alcohol on any one occasion; it causes intoxication. When you become drunk, the consequences are as follows:

- The possibility of unprotected sex, the consequence of which can be unplanned pregnancy and STI.
- Adverse effect on the way you think about yourself and the way you behave in social situations.
- Adverse effect on your relationships and your lifestyle.
- Adverse effect on your baby, as enumerated above, during and after pregnancy.

However, a single episode of binge drinking around the time of conception is less likely to be harmful to you or your baby. If you have had a one-off binge, unprotected sex, and don't want to get pregnant, you should ask your health care professional about the following:

- emergency contraception, which can only be used within a specific time and not used if you are already pregnant
- screening for STI
- regular contraception

If you find out you are pregnant and decide to continue with your pregnancy, then you should stop drinking or stay within the recommended amount for the rest of your pregnancy.

PREGNANCY AND STREET DRUGS - HEROIN INJECTION AND COCAINE.

They cause the following:
- Increased risk of miscarriage
- LBW
- Premature labour
- Stillbirth
- Withdrawal symptoms in baby after birth

Furthermore, apart from the above ill effects, cocaine causes the following:
- Premature separation of the placenta (placental abruption) and
- Abnormalities in the fetus

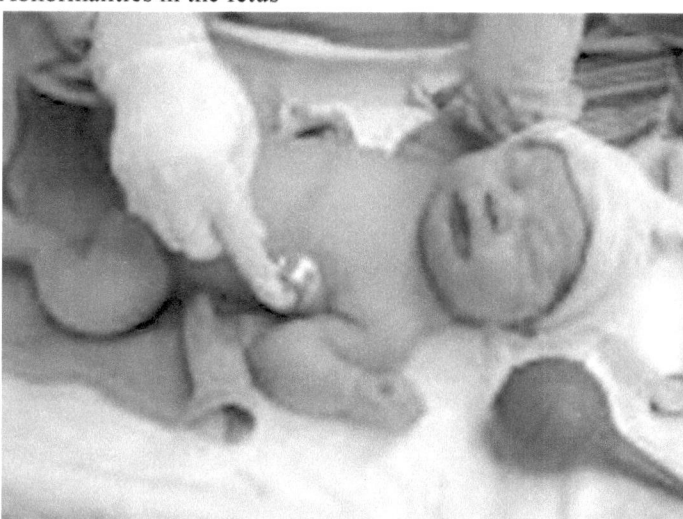

Figure 84. LBW baby as a result of drug abuse

159

So if you take street drugs orally or as injection, you are strongly advised to stop taking them before you become pregnant. Seek help from your doctor if you have difficulty in doing that.

PREGNANCY AND MEDICATION

Some drugs have been well studied in pregnant women and known to be safe (e.g. penicillin), while others are unsafe (e.g. thalidomide). However, for many drugs, we do not know for sure if they are safe or unsafe. So if you are planning a pregnancy or you are pregnant, you should minimise the use of drugs and herbal remedies that can be bought from the pharmacy. If in doubt, ask your doctor for advice.

SOME COMMONLY USED DRUGS THAT CAN BE BOUGHT OFF THE COUNTER

- Paracetamol: At normal dose, paracetamol is safe and useful for headaches, backache, and other aches and pains that may occur during pregnancy.
- Linctus: Simple linctus is safe in pregnancy.
- Diarrhoea drugs: You can use oral rehydration sachets. Do not use loperamide.
- Ibuprofen: This drug may be taken in the second trimester (weeks 14-27), but avoid taking it in the first and third trimesters unless advised by your doctor. Generally, it is better to avoid it during pregnancy.
- Laxatives: Constipation is common in pregnancy, and you may need drugs that help with that (laxatives). First, you should increase the fibre content in your diet and the amount of non-alcoholic fluids that you drink. If this fails, then fibre supplements such as bran, ispaghula, and sterculia are safe. If you need something stronger, then it is best to discuss this with a doctor. Laxatives such as docusate and lactulose may be used for a short time.
- Antihistamines: These are drugs used to treat reactions to drugs. The safest one to use in pregnancy is Piriton. However, it tends to make some people drowsy. If you require an alternative, then it is best to see a doctor for advice.
- Decongestants (drugs used for treating blocked nose): It is best to avoid these drugs in the early stages of pregnancy; speak to your doctor if concerned.

PRESCRIBED DRUGS

To be on the safe side, you should

- talk to your doctor if you take regular medication—ideally before you start trying for a baby or as soon as you find out you are pregnant.

- always check with your doctor, midwife, or pharmacist before taking any medicine.
- make sure that your doctor, dentist, or other health professional knows you are pregnant before they give you treatment.

In some cases, the risk of taking the drug has to be balanced against the risk of not taking it.

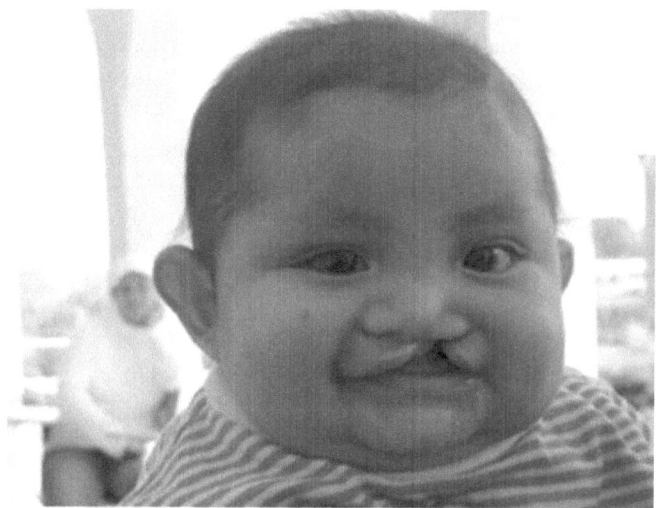

Figure 85. Anticancer drugs in pregnancy. Cleft lip and palate

HOMEOPATHIC REMEDIES AND AROMATHERAPY

We do not have much evidence for these remedies. Not all 'natural' remedies are safe in pregnancy. Confirm that that your practitioner is qualified to give the service.

X-RAYS

X-rays are generally safe during pregnancy. According to the American College of Radiology, no single diagnostic X-ray has a radiation dose significant enough to cause adverse effects in a developing embryo or foetus. However, there is quite a bit of controversy surrounding this issue. Studies have been conflicting, and therefore, X-rays should only be performed when the benefits outweigh the risks.

Not all X-rays are the same, and most pose little exposure to the uterus and developing foetus. With dental X-rays, there is hardly any exposure to any part of the body except the teeth. X-ray examinations on the arms, legs, or chest do not expose your reproductive organs to the direct beam. However, X-rays of the torso, such as the abdomen, stomach, pelvis, lower back, and kidneys, have a greater chance of exposure to the uterus. It is always important that you let the health care provider know that you are pregnant if you might need an X-ray.

Sources

- RCOG statement No.5. March 2009.
- RCOG information of patients. Alcohol and pregnancy, 2006.
- Royal College of Psychiatrist leaflet. Information for the public: alcohol and depression, help is at hand, January 2004.
- US Public Health Surgeon General's Advisory on Alcohol and Pregnancy. Food and Drink Administration Bulletin 1981;11:9-10.
- The Pregnancy Book. Your complete guide to: a healthy pregnancy, labour and childbirth. The first weeks with your new baby, UK, 2009.
- www.patient.co.uk
- Pregnancy and X-Rays: Good or Bad? American Pregnancy Association. March 2007.

Recreational Exercise in Pregnancy

Definition and Introduction

Recreational exercise is defined as any planned regular exercise that you do during pregnancy or after delivery, which involves aerobic (e.g. jogging and dancing) and/or muscle-strengthening activity (e.g. climbing stairs and walking uphill). The aim of the exercise is to keep you fit throughout the pregnancy so that you can cope with the physical changes that take place within your body and your developing baby.

You should not be training for peak fitness or for sporting events. During pregnancy, hormone changes can affect your muscles and ligaments, making your joints more lax and more mobile. Therefore, if you are not careful during exercise, you can sustain an injury.

Physical Activity that You Can Do Whilst Pregnant

Aerobic Physical Activity

This is an activity that makes your heart and lungs work harder. It causes blood to circulate more quickly around the body, and as a result, more oxygen reaches the muscles. Examples of aerobic exercise are given in the following figures:

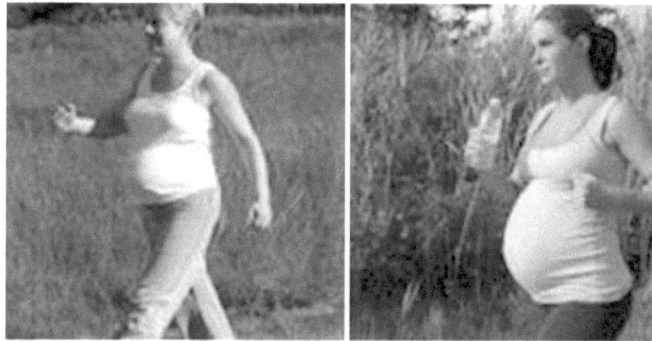

Figures 86a and b. Brisk walking

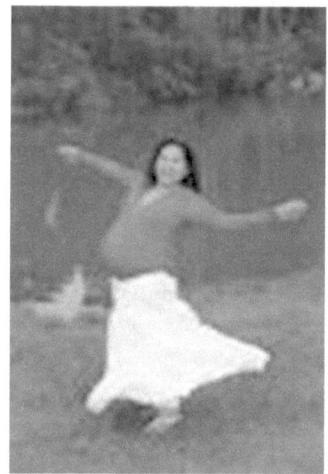

Figure 86c. Dancing

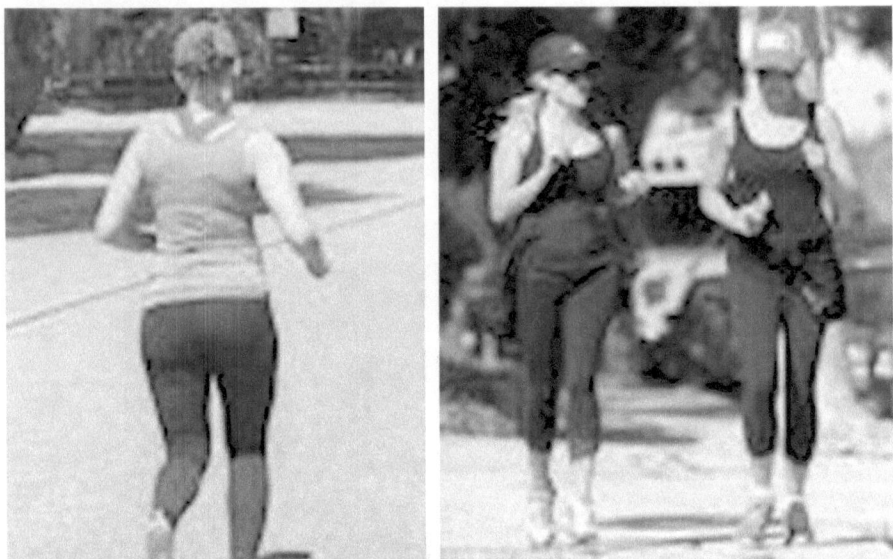

Figures 86d and e. Jogging

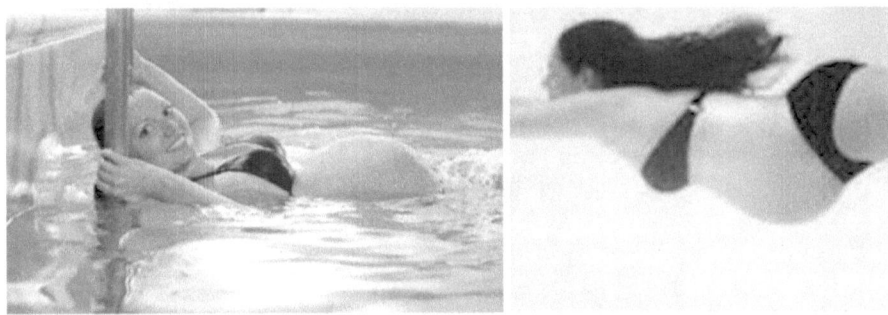

Figures 86f and g. Swimming in pregnancy

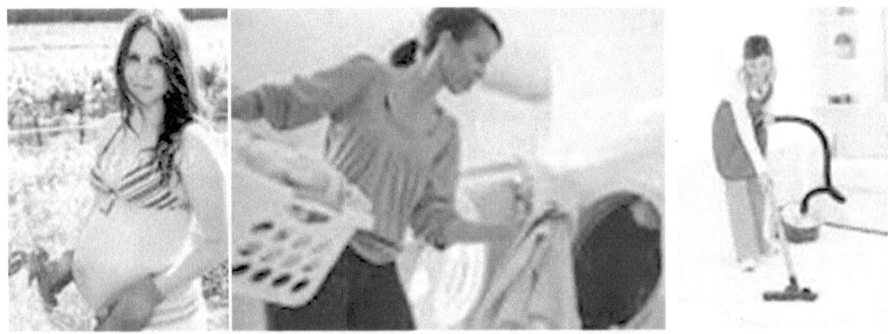

Figure 87a. Gardening   **Figures 87b and c. Homework**

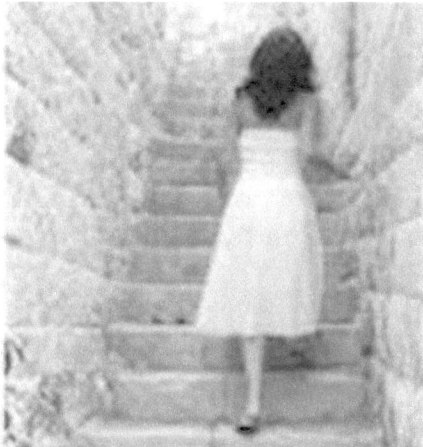

Figures 87d and e. Climbing stairs

If you do not exercise routinely before pregnancy and you are starting an aerobic activity, you should begin with no more than 15-minute continuous exercise 3 times per week, increasing gradually to a maximum of 30-minute sessions 4 times a week to daily. Other aerobic exercises that you can do are given in the following figures:

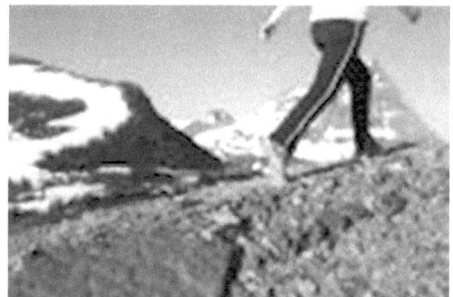

Figure 88a. Walking uphill

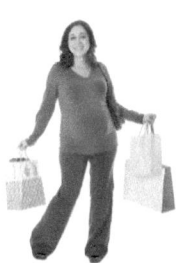

Figure 88b. Carrying shopping

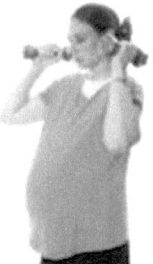

Figure 88c. Weightlifting

MUSCLE-STRENGTHENING ACTIVITY

This form of exercise helps to increase your overall fitness and involves slow, controlled movements. They are stomach-strengthening exercises, yoga, pelvic tilt exercise, pelvic floor exercise, foot exercise, and others.

STOMACH-STRENGTHENING EXERCISE

It strengthens abdominal muscles and ease backache, which can be a problem in pregnancy.

- Start in a box position (on all fours), with your knees under your hips, your hands under your shoulders, your fingers facing forward, and your stomach muscles lifted so that your back is straight.
- Pull in your stomach muscles and raise your back up towards the ceiling, curling your trunk and allowing your head to relax gently forward. Don't let your elbows lock.
- Hold for a few seconds and then slowly return to the box position.
- Take care not to hollow your back—it should always return to a straight or neutral position.
- Do this slowly and rhythmically 10 times, making your muscles work hard and moving your back carefully. Only move your back as far as you can comfortably.

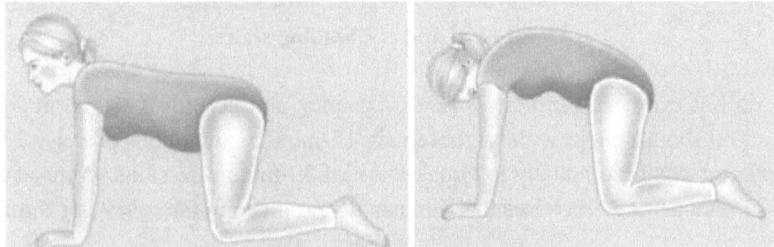

Figures 89a and b. Stomach-strengthening exercise

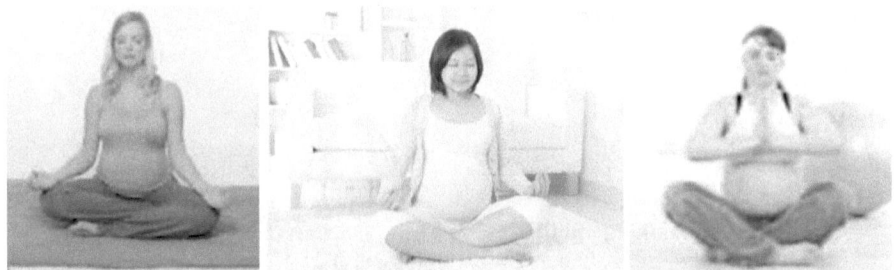

Figures 90a-c. (Please see Yoga on page 134)

PELVIC TILT EXERCISE (FIGURE 91)

- Stand with your shoulders and bottom against a wall.
- Keep your knees soft.
- Pull your belly button towards your spine so that your back flattens against the wall.
- Hold for 4 seconds and release. Repeat up to 10 times.

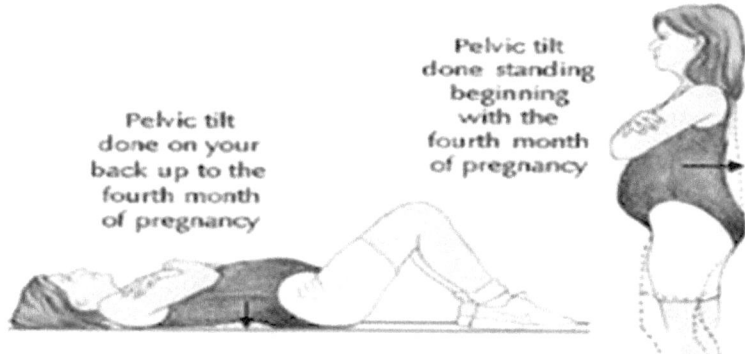

Figure 91. Pelvic tilt exercise

PELVIC FLOOR EXERCISES

It helps to strengthen the muscles of the pelvic floor, which are placed under great strain in pregnancy and childbirth. The pelvic floor consists of layers of muscles which stretch like a supportive hammock from the pubic bone (in front) to the base of the backbone. There are three openings in the muscle: the back passage, vagina (birth canal), and urethra (bladder outlet) – Fig. 92.

A specialist physiotherapist should guide you through pelvic floor exercise. It is performed as follows:

- Close up your back passage as if trying to prevent a bowel movement.
- Draw in your vagina, as if you are gripping a tampon, and your urethra, as if to stop the flow of urine, at the same time.
- Do this exercise quickly first, tightening and releasing the muscles straightaway.
- Do it slowly then, holding the contractions for as long as you can before you relax. Try to count to 10.
- Try to do 3 sets of 8 squeezes every day. To help you remember, you could do them once at each meal.

167

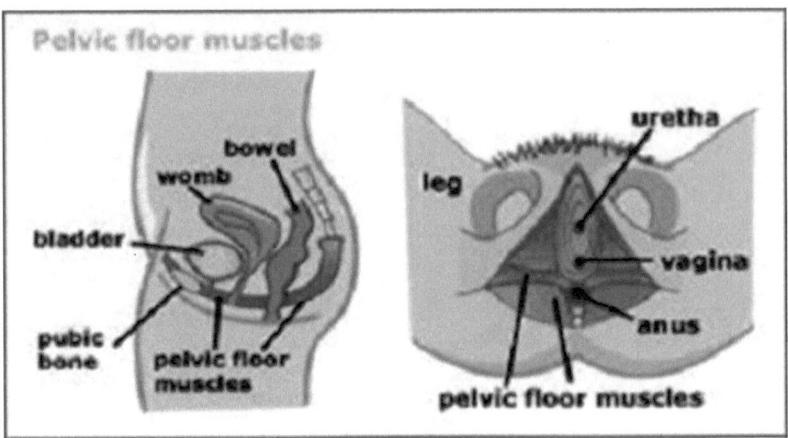

Figure 92. The female pelvic floor

FOOT EXERCISES

Foot exercises can be done by sitting or standing. They improve blood circulation, reduce swelling in the ankles, and prevent cramp in the calf muscles.

- Bend and stretch your foot vigorously up and down 30 times.
- Rotate your foot 8 times one way and 8 times the other way.
- Repeat with the other foot.

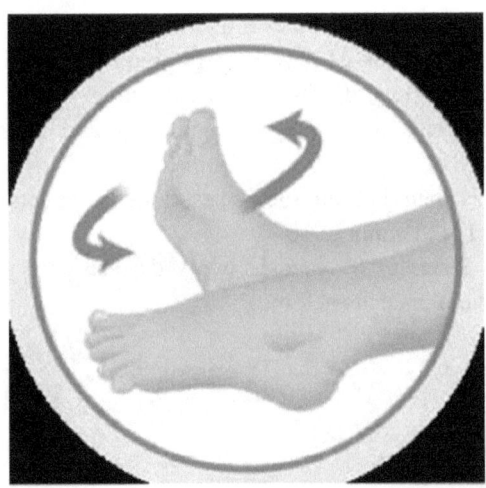

Figure 93. Foot exercises

PROTECTING YOUR BACK

- Sit up straight with your bottom against the back of your chair. Tuck a small cushion behind your waist if you wish.
- Bend your knees, not your back, when you pick something up.
- Try to stand tall.

YOUR EXERCISE PROGRAMME

Try to build physical activity into part of your everyday life. Take the stairs and not the lift at work or in the shopping centre. Take a brisk walk at lunchtime. Try not to sit for long periods in front of the television or in front of a computer. Walk, instead of driving, to the shops.

If you exercised regularly before pregnancy, you should be able to engage in the same high-intensity exercise programmes, such as running and aerobics, with no adverse effects for you or the baby. As your pregnancy progresses, you should be aiming to gradually reduce your overall activity. Speak to your doctor or midwife.

A health care professional with a specialist training in teaching exercise will weigh up the potential benefits and harms of a range of exercises. Depending upon your current exercise routine, a programme should be recommended for you during pregnancy. This will include

- appropriate types of exercise
- the length of each exercise session
- the number of exercise sessions each week
- how intensely you should exercise

Some exercises are recommended for a fitter pregnancy. They are as follows:

- Stomach-strengthening exercise
- Pelvic tilt exercise
- Pelvic floor exercise
- Foot exercise
- Protecting your back

THE BENEFITS OF RECREATIONAL EXERCISE DURING PREGNANCY

BENEFITS FOR YOU

- Makes you feel less tired and less likely to develop back pain.
- Reduces your chance of developing varicose veins and swelling of your feet, ankles, or hands.
- Improves muscles tone, strength, and endurance.
- Improves sleep.

- Reduces your chance of becoming anxious or depressed.
- Makes it easier to carry the weight you gain during pregnancy and helps prepare you for the physical challenges of labour.
- Reduces your risk of developing gestational diabetes during your pregnancy, and if you do develop it, it may help to improve the control of the diabetes by improving your sugar levels.
- Reduces your risk of developing BP during your pregnancy.
- Provides the long-term benefits of physical activity, namely protection against heart disease, osteoporosis, high BP, colon cancer, and breast cancer.
- Helps maintain a healthy weight during and after your pregnancy.

BENEFITS FOR LABOUR
- Short labour time
- Fewer delivery complications

RISKS OF RECREATIONAL EXERCISE DURING PREGNANCY AND THEIR PREVENTION

The chance of risks occurring is high when you do inappropriate exercise and when you overexert yourself. These risks can be reduced by adjusting your exercise as the pregnancy progresses. The risks include the following:

Getting too hot: Exercise during pregnancy leads to increase in body temperature; if this rises above 39.2°C during the first 12 weeks, it may affect the baby's development, leading to disability at birth. You can prevent getting too hot by

- drinking plenty of water before and during exercise.
- avoiding overexertion, particularly in the first 12 weeks of pregnancy.
- avoiding exercising in a very hot and humid climate until you have acclimatised.

Exercise in water: If you are exercising in water, as in aquanatal classes, or you are using a hydrotherapy pool, the water temperature should not exceed 32°C in a swimming pool and 35°C in a hydrotherapy (water treatment) pool. Swimming can make it more difficult for you to notice your body heating up because the water makes you feel cooler.

Low blood pressure: After 16 weeks, pressure on a blood vessel called vena cava, which lies in your back when you lie on the back during exercise, can lead to low BP. This can make you feel light-headed and faint.

Physical injury due to too much movement (hypermobility): During pregnancy, your joints and ligaments are loose and less stable because of the effects of hormones; you can flex and extend particular parts of your body more than usual, such as your elbows, wrists, fingers, and knees. This is called hypermobility, and it happens in preparation for birth. You are, therefore, at increased risk of injuring yourself. To reduce the risk of physical injury, you should

- make sure that you do warm-up and cool-down exercises.
- avoid sudden changes of direction if you are doing aerobic exercise.
- consider wearing pelvic support belts during exercise.

Insufficient oxygen in the baby (hypoxia): At high altitudes, for example in aeroplane, the flow of blood to the womb is decreased and so the baby receives less oxygen. If a woman exercises at high altitudes, the amount of blood flowing to the womb is decreased even further. This leads to insufficient oxygen for the baby. To avoid this happening, avoid exercise at altitudes over 2,500 metres until you have acclimatised; this may take a few days.

Significant reduction in blood sugar levels during exercise: Blood glucose is a source of energy for both you and the baby. It is, therefore, important that you eat well during pregnancy and exercise for no more than 45 minutes at a time. If you have pre-existing or gestational diabetes mellitus (GDM), then you should have your blood glucose monitored after exercise, eat at regular times, take rest at specific times, and ensure that your baby is carefully monitored. Discuss with your midwife or doctor.

EXERCISES TO BE AVOIDED DURING PREGNANCY

- You should not exercise while you are lying on your back after 16 weeks of pregnancy, for the reason given above.
- You should not scuba-dive during pregnancy. When you return to the surface of water after diving, bubbles of a special gas called nitrogen gas can form in your baby's bloodstream and block the blood circulation in small blood vessels in his or her brain and elsewhere, causing decompression sickness.
- You should avoid contact sports where there is a risk of being hit in the abdomen, such as kick-boxing, judo, or squash.

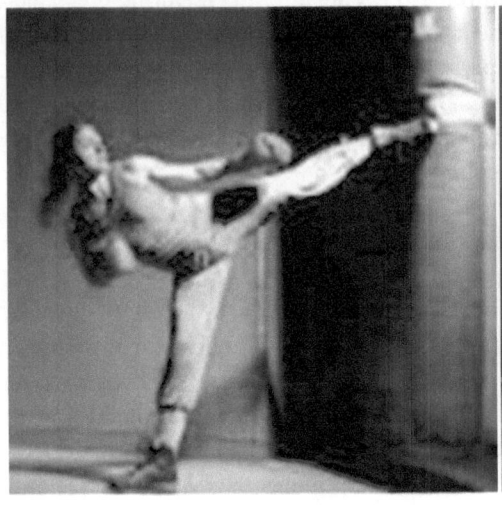
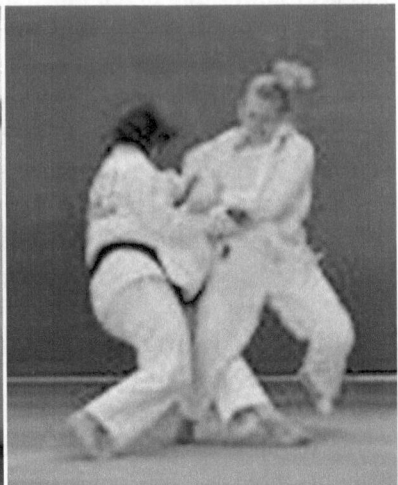

Figure 94. Kick-boxing   **Figure 95. Judo**

- You should be careful when engaging in exercise where you are likely to lose your balance (because of hypermobility in pregnancy) and fall injuring your abdomen, and possibly injuring your developing baby. Such activities include horse riding, downhill skiing, ice hockey, gymnastics, and cycling. It might be best to avoid these exercises unless you do them regularly and you generally take extra care.
- You should avoid exercising at heights over 2,500 metres until you have acclimatised. This is because you and your baby are at risk of acute mountain sickness (decrease in oxygen).

SELF-ASSESSMENT FOR OVEREXERTION DURING PHYSICAL EXERCISE

You should aim to do moderate-intensity physical activity. This means that you get warm, mildly out of breath, and mildly sweaty. You should always have a warm-up and a cool-down period. There are also various techniques to assess whether you are overexerting yourself or not.

- The 'talk test': You should aim to be able to talk and hold a conversation whilst you are doing physical activity. If you become too breathless to talk, it probably means that you are doing too much.
- Monitoring your heart rate: When doing aerobic exercises, you should have a target zone for your heart rate. The target zone will depend upon your age and your exercise routine (as below). If you had a sedentary lifestyle prior to pregnancy, you will probably be advised of a maximum heart rate of 60-70% above your normal rate. If you are aiming to

maintain fitness during pregnancy, then the upper limit of 60-90% of maximum heart rate will be advised.

Maternal age	Heart rate target zone (beats/minute)
Less than 20 years	140-155
20-29 years	135-150
30-39 years	130-145
Over 40 years	125-140

Normal age-related heart rate during recreational exercise in pregnancy.

WHEN TO STOP EXERCISING

If you have any unusual symptoms, you should not continue to exercise. If your symptoms began during aerobic exercise, it is important that you do not bring your exercises to an end abruptly as this can make you feel very faint. Instead, you should either walk around slowly for a short while or continue transferring your weight from one foot to the other by lifting one heel and then the other. You should contact your health care professional immediately afterwards. Unusual symptoms may include any of the following:

- Dizziness or feeling faint
- Excessive tiredness
- Feelings of muscle weakness
- Headache
- Excessive shortness of breath
- Difficulty getting your breath whilst exercising
- Chest pain and palpitation
- Pain in your abdomen, back, or pubic area
- Pain in your pelvic girdle
- Calf pain or swelling
- Weakness in your muscles
- Abdominal, pelvic, or back pain
- Painful uterine contractions, signs of labour, or any leakage of amniotic fluid
- Vaginal bleeding
- Concerns that your baby is moving less

CONTRAINDICATION TO PHYSICAL ACTIVITY DURING PREGNANCY

Physical activity during pregnancy is safe for most women. However, if you have a medical condition or you develop it during pregnancy, then you should talk with your doctor before doing any recreational exercise. He or she will be able to advise you whether it is safe for you to take part in physical activity.

If you have any of the following, you should not do recreational exercise during pregnancy:
- Diseases of different organs and systems, for example the heart, lungs.
- Obstetric problems like vaginal bleeding, a history of preterm labour in the past, any signs of preterm labour, premature rupture of membranes, SGA baby, multiple pregnancy, placenta praevia, known weakness of the cervix, cervical stitch, and so on.
- Poorly controlled diabetes, epilepsy, thyroid disease, severe anaemia, and bone or joint problems that may affect ability to exercise.
- Eating disorder such as anorexia.

You should speak with your doctor or midwife before you start doing any physical activity during pregnancy if you
- smoke more than 20 cigarettes a day.
- are someone who normally does not do much physical activity at all.
- are very overweight (have a BMI of more than 40).

TRAINING FOR ATHLETIC COMPETITIONS
If you are an athlete, you can continue to train for competitions, but do not expect to retain peak fitness. You will need supervision by an obstetrician. You will need to talk with your trainer about your requirements for additional hydration and nutrition.

SOURCES
- Exercise in Pregnancy. RCOG, January 2006. http://www.rcog.org.uk/resources/
- Exercise during pregnancy. Frequently asked questions. ACOG. 2011
- Recreational exercise and pregnancy: information for you. Published September 2006 by the RCOG.
- Tobacco, Alcohol, drugs and pregnancy. Frequently asked questions. ACOG. 2013
- Back to normal. Post natal advice and exercises. Published by the Obstetric Physiotherapy team, Norfolk & Norwich Health Care NHS Trust, March 2001.
- Nutrition during pregnancy.
- Weight management before, during and after pregnancy. NICE Public Health Guidance, July 2010. Dietary interventions and physical activity interventions for weight management before, during and after pregnancy.

Air Travel in Pregnancy

RISKS ASSOCIATED WITH AIR TRAVEL
IN PREGNANCY AND PREVENTION INFORMATION

RISKS TO YOU
Formation of blood clot in your leg (DVT)—Sitting still for a long time increases the risk of DVT (page xx). This is particularly so if your flight lasts more than 8 hours and worse if you already have risk factors (such as a previous DVT or obesity) for DVT. No special preventive measure is needed if you are on a short-haul flight (under 4 hours). For a medium or a long-haul flight (over 4 hours) you should

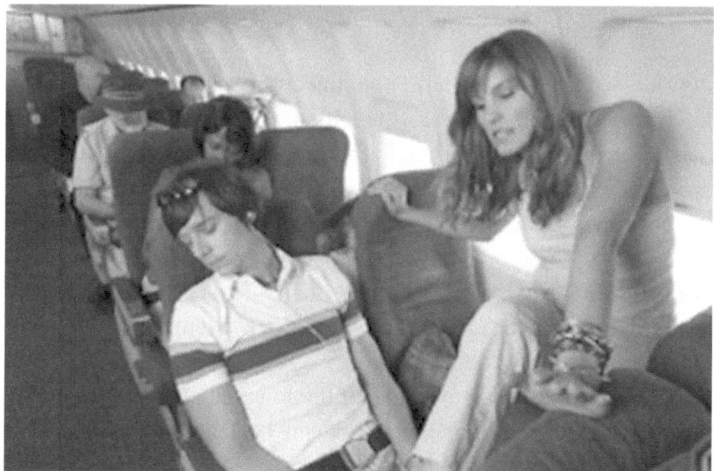

Figure 96. Aisle seat in an aeroplane

- get an aisle seat and take regular walks around the plane every 30 minutes.
- have cups of water at regular intervals throughout your journey.
- cut down on drinks which contain caffeine (coffee, fizzy drinks).
- wear graduated elastic compression stockings.

175

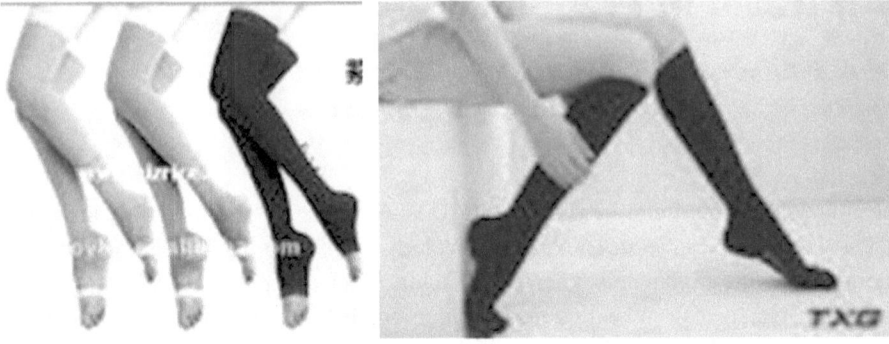

a. above knee   b. below knee

Figure 97. Graduated compression elastic stockings

- **be** advised to take heparin (an injection which reduces the likelihood of forming blood clots in your blood vessels) on the day of the flight, whatever the length of your flight, and for several days afterwards if you have additional risk factors for DVT. For security purposes, you will need a letter from your doctor to enable you to carry this medicine on to the plane.

Increased discomfort due to
- swelling of your legs from fluid retention (oedema).
- nasal congestion (blocked nose).
- problems with the ears because of the lowered air pressure in the plane.
- motion sickness during the flight can occur, and this can worsen your pregnancy sickness if you have it already.

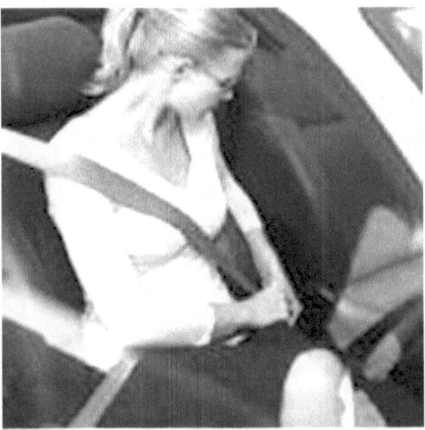 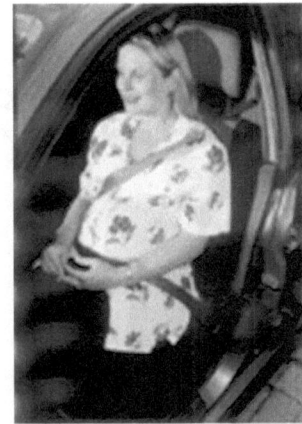

a. Non-pregnant   b. Pregnant.

Figure 98: Seat belt

High risk of injury to you—You should, therefore, wear a seat belt. The strap of your seat belt should be reasonably tightly fastened under your tummy and across the top of your thighs as in figure 98b.

RISKS TO YOUR BABY

If you are healthy, have a low-risk pregnancy and engage in occasional flights, there is no evidence that

- the condition in the aeroplane (drop in air pressure and/or decrease in humidity) will have a harmful effect on your baby.
- early labour will occur or your waters will break.
- you will have an increased risk of miscarriage.

SAFE TIME TO FLY IN PREGNANCY

The safest time to fly is

- before 37 weeks if you are carrying one baby. The chance of going into labour increases significantly after this time, and therefore, many airlines do not allow women to fly after this week.
- before 34 weeks if you are carrying an uncomplicated twin pregnancy.

Generally, if you are over 28 weeks pregnant, your airline will demand a letter from your midwife or doctor stating when your baby is due and confirming that you are not at an increased risk of any complications.

CONTRAINDICATIONS TO FLYING

You may be advised not to fly if you have the following:

- Increased risk of going into labour before your due date.
- Severe anaemia, that is when the level of red blood cells in your blood is lower than normal.
- Sickle-cell anaemia (a condition which affects red blood cells) and you have recently had a sickling crisis.
- Recent significant vaginal bleeding.
- A serious condition affecting the lungs or heart, and it is difficult to breathe.
- Unmended fractured bone in the leg, or you have a cast in place, and your leg is swollen.
- Recent bowel surgery, for example removal of appendix.
- Ear infection (otitis media) or infection of the air space in the bone of the nose.

It is important you discuss any health issues or pregnancy complications with your doctor or midwife before you fly.

MANAGEMENT OF SUDDEN OBSTETRIC PROBLEM WHILE ON A FLIGHT

If you develop any obstetric or medical problem on a flight, there is no guarantee that a medical specialist will be on board the flight. Therefore, the pilot may have to divert the flight.

OTHER ISSUES TO BE CONSIDERED BEFORE TRAVELLING

- The availability of specialised medical treatment in the country you are going to in case of an unexpected complication with your pregnancy necessitating emergency treatment.
- Specific medical risks in the country you are visiting and how to prevent it, for example malaria in Africa and Asia.
- Necessary immunisations and recommended medication for the country you are travelling to.
- Travel insurance cover for you and your unborn baby in case you give birth unexpectedly.
- Consultation with your doctor and/or midwife for advice and preparation for the journey.

SOURCES

- Royal College of Obstetricians and Gynaecologists (RCOG). Information for patients. Air travel and pregnancy. Information for you. Published January 2011 by the RCOG.
- Travel during pregnancy. Frequently asked questions. ACOG. 2011.
- Air travel during pregnancy. ACOG Committee Opinion. Number 443, October 2009.
- Royal College of Obstetricians and Gynaecologists (RCOG). Scientific Advisory Committee (SAC) Opinion Paper. Air travel and pregnancy, 2008.
- www.patient.co.uk. NHS Choices, Your health, your choices. Last reviewed: 2011.

Management of Common Symptoms of Pregnancy

INTRODUCTION

This chapter deals with minor and common symptoms of pregnancy, which in most cases are considered as normal adaptation to the growing pregnancy. We have analyzed the views of women on how they cope with such symptoms and given scientific interpretation to them. Most importantly, we have highlighted, in almost all the cases, when women must inform their health care professional about their symptoms. We have grouped the symptoms and conditions according to the organs and systems that they affect.

NAUSEA AND VOMITING

Please see page 43.

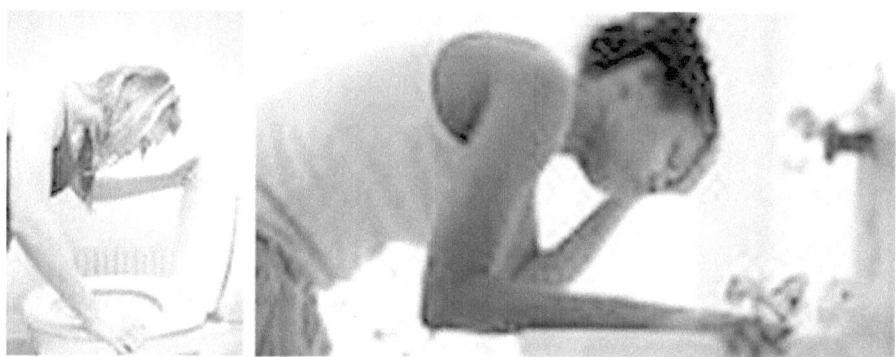

Figure 99a and b. Vomiting in pregnancy

INDIGESTION AND HEARTBURN

Indigestion is a vague feeling of discomfort and pain in the upper abdomen and chest, including feeling of fullness and bloating, belching and nausea, and occasionally heartburn. Symptoms can be triggered by eating fatty or spicy or too much high-fibre foods, eating too fast or too much, and drinking too much caffeine, alcoholic, or carbonated beverages. Symptoms have also been shown to be worsened by anxiety and depression.

Heartburn is a burning feeling or discomfort felt behind the middle of the chest and/or the throat. It may be accompanied by acid backflow from the stomach reaching the throat and/or the mouth, causing a bitter or sour taste. About 22 out of 100 women report heartburn in the first trimester, 39 out of 100 in the second, and 72 out of 100 in the third trimester of pregnancy.

Organs of the Digestive System

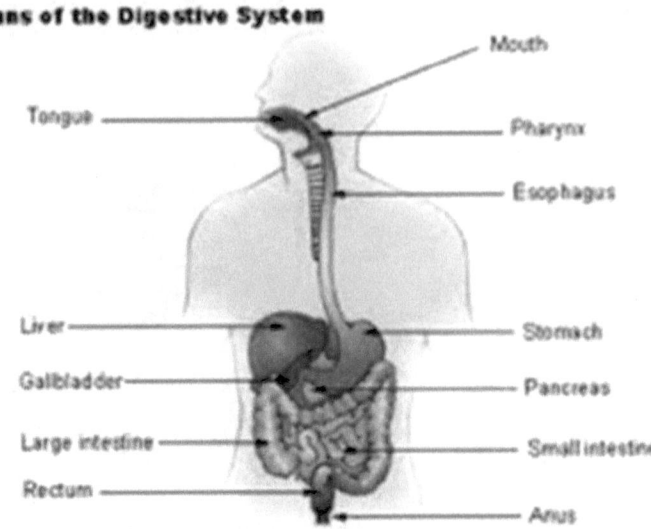

Figure 100. Digestive organs

We do not know exactly why heartburn occurs, but during pregnancy, the hormonal changes in your body may cause relaxation of the valve between your stomach and the food pipe (oesophagus) and also interfere with the movement of the stomach, resulting into backflow of acid from the stomach into the food pipe. In later pregnancy, your growing uterus presses on your stomach and may also predispose to heartburn. Heartburn is not associated with adverse outcomes of pregnancy, and therefore, its treatment is intended to provide relief of symptoms.

MANAGEMENT
You should see your obstetrician who will ask you certain question and perform investigations in order to exclude serious conditions that may be associated with indigestion and heartburn, namely PE, liver and other bowel problems. If those conditions are ruled out, you will be reassured, and the treatment of only heartburn will be initiated.

HOW TO AVOID HEARTBURN AND INDIGESTION
- Dietary modification
  - Eat smaller meals more often.
  - Avoid the food which triggers the problem, for example high-fat, fried, or highly spiced food and stomach irritant caffeine.
  - Drink a glass of milk. Have one glass of milk by your bed in case you wake with heartburn in the night.
  - Avoid eating and drinking for a few hours before going to bed.

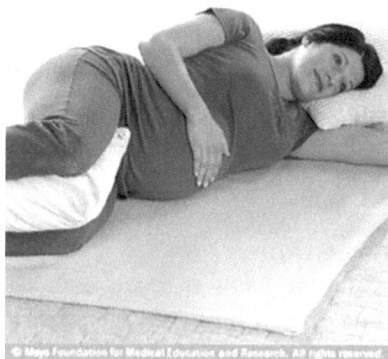

Figure 101. Lying propped up

- Awareness of posture
    - Sit up straight when you are eating as this takes the pressure off your stomach.
    - Heartburn is often brought on by lying flat. Sleep well propped up with plenty of pillows.

TREATMENT (HOW TO EASE HEARTBURN/INDIGESTION)

You have to see you doctor who will prescribe the necessary medication for you. Some of the drugs that are normally used are listed below.

- Drugs that neutralise and bind the acid that is produced in the stomach, for example antacids and alkali mixtures.
- Drugs that reduce acid secretion by the stomach, for example ranitidine and cimetidine.
- Drugs that alleviate symptoms by reducing the acid reflux, for example omeprazole and Gaviscon.

CONSTIPATION

This means delay in the passage of food residue through the bowel, associated with pain when opening bowel and abdominal discomfort. About 39 out of 100 pregnant women report symptoms of constipation at 14 weeks of gestation, 30 at 28 weeks, and 20 at 36 weeks. Possible causes or associations are as follows:

- Poor dietary fibre intake.
- Rising levels of the hormone progesterone, which is produced by the placenta; it causes a reduction in stomach movement and therefore increases the time that food takes to leave the stomach (gastric transit time).

181

MANAGEMENT

You should inform your doctor or obstetrician who will ask you certain questions and conduct investigations aimed at ruling out serious conditions that may be associated with constipation, for example inflammatory bowel disease, mass or swellings in the abdomen. If the sinister signs and symptoms are absent and the investigations give normal results, you will be reassured, and the treatment of constipation will be initiated.

HOW TO AVOID CONSTIPATION

- Modify your diet—eat foods that are high in fibre, like wholemeal breads, wholegrain cereals, fruit and vegetables, and pulses such as beans and lentils.
- Exercise regularly to keep your muscles toned.
- Drink plenty of water.
- Avoid iron supplements; ask your doctor whether you can manage without them or change to a different type of medication.

TREATMENT

When the constipation is not relieved by the measures above, drugs called laxatives (drugs that help to open bowel) can be used, for example lactulose.

PILES (HAEMORRHOIDS)

Piles, also known as haemorrhoids, are swollen veins around the back passage (anus), which may itch, bleed, ache, and also cause soreness when opening bowel. You can usually feel the lumpiness of the piles around the anus. About 8 out of 100 pregnant women experience piles in the last 3 months of pregnancy, but they usually resolve within weeks after birth. They occur more in pregnancy because of the following reasons:

- Pregnancy hormones relax the walls of blood vessels called veins.
- Eating low-fibre diet.

MANAGEMENT

Your doctor or obstetrician will examine you to confirm the diagnosis. Treatment includes the following:

- Diet modification as under 'Constipation'.
- Helpful advices are as follows:
  - Avoid standing for long periods.
  - Take regular exercise to improve your blood circulation.
  - Apply to the pile a cloth wrung out in ice water; you may find it helpful.

– Push any piles that stick out gently back inside using a lubricating jelly.
- Creams (such as Anusol) can be applied. Your midwife or doctor may suggest other types of cream or ointment for you.
- Surgical removal of the piles can be carried out in the third trimester when the vein has been blocked by blood clot or the pile has rotten. Surgery is, however, rarely considered an appropriate intervention for the pregnant woman since piles may resolve after delivery.

BACKACHE

As your baby grows, the hollow in your lower back may become more pronounced due to the increasing weight in the womb and increased laxity of supporting muscles caused by a placental hormone called relaxin. This leads to backache. Furthermore, the structures holding the womb in its place become softer and stretch to prepare you for labour. This can put a strain on the joints of your lower back and pelvis, which can also cause backache.

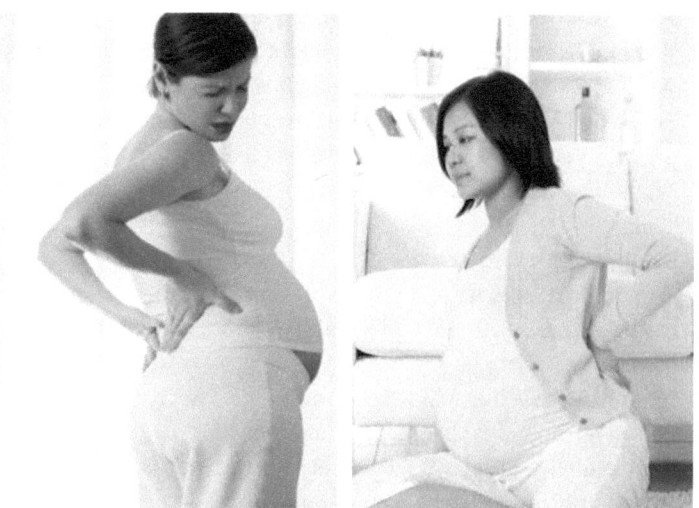

Figure 102a and b. Backache

It affects 35-61 out of 100 pregnant women, especially at 20-28 weeks. Symptoms are worse in the evenings, and it can interfere with your daily activities and sleep patterns. The reassurance is that it is rare for the symptoms not to resolve completely after pregnancy.

Management

You should always report backache to your midwife or doctor. The presence of the following may indicate that the backache is caused by other conditions unrelated to pregnancy:

- Loss of sensation in your back or extremities
- Muscle weakness
- Bladder or bowel symptoms
- Abdominal tenderness
- Severe disability related to the pain

If none of the above symptoms is present, you should be reassured, and the advice and treatment, as outlined below, may be offered. If after such measures your symptoms worsen, you will need to see your doctor again.

How to Avoid Backache

- Avoid lifting heavy objects.
- Bend your knees and keep your back straight when lifting or picking something up from the floor.
- Move your feet when turning round to avoid twisting your spine.
- Wear flat shoes that allow your weight to be evenly distributed.
- Work at a surface that is high enough so that you don't stoop.
- Try to balance the weight between two bags when carrying shopping.
- Sit with your back straight and well supported.
- Make sure you get enough rest, particularly later in pregnancy.

How to Ease Backache

- A firm mattress can help to prevent and relieve backache. If your mattress is too soft, put a piece of hardboard under it to make it firmer.
- Massage can help.
- Exercising in water will help to reduce backache.
- Group or individual back-care classes can help.
- Simple analgesia (paracetamol) is safe and may be helpful.
- A physiotherapy referral should be offered.

Pelvic Joint or Girdle Pain (Symphysis Pubis Dysfunction)

This condition is caused by a slight misalignment or stiffness of your pelvic joints. The diagnosis is based on the following:

- Feeling pain in your pelvic joints, especially in front when walking, climbing stairs, or turning in bed.
- Clicking in the joint at the back when walking or changing position.

184

- Having problems with moving the leg away from the midline (abduction) and moving it back (adduction) when standing.

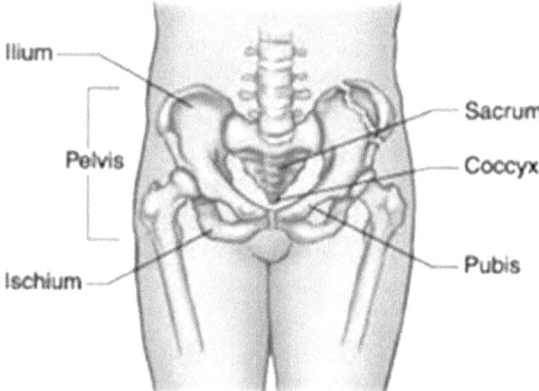

Figure 103. Pelvic bones

It affects 1 out of 4 pregnant women. Some women have minor discomfort, while others may have much greater immobility; 7 out of 100 sufferers continue to experience serious symptoms after birth.

MANAGEMENT

A thorough examination and investigation to rule out other serious backache problems as stated under 'Backache' above and also urinary tract infection will be carried out by your doctor.

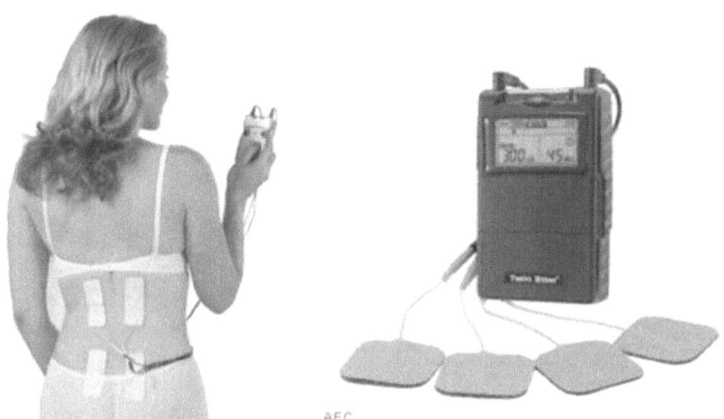

Figure 104a and b. TENS machine

The diagnosis, however, is based on the symptoms alone, although after pregnancy, imaging procedures, for example X-ray, ultrasound, and others, may be needed.

TREATMENT

- Physiotherapy: everyday living advices are
    - Avoid doing strenuous exercise, prolonged standing, vacuum-cleaning, stretching exercises, and squatting.
    - Brace the pelvic floor muscles before performing any activity, which might cause pain.
    - Rest the pelvis.
    - Sit down for tasks where possible (e.g. preparing food, ironing, and dressing).
    - Avoid lifting and carrying.
    - Avoid stepping over things.
    - Avoid straddle movements especially when weight bearing.
    - Bend the knees and keep the legs 'glued together' when turning in bed and getting in and out of bed.
    - Place a pillow between the legs when in bed or resting.
    - Avoid twisting movements of the body.

- Pain relief: If oral painkillers are not effective, you will be admitted and injections will be given. TENS machine (see above) can be used too.
- Referral to pain management team if pain is not controlled.
- Pelvic support devices such as elbow crutches, which will help take the weight off the pelvis and assist with movement, wheelchair, or pelvic brace can be used if the pain is very severe.
- Acupuncture is suggested.

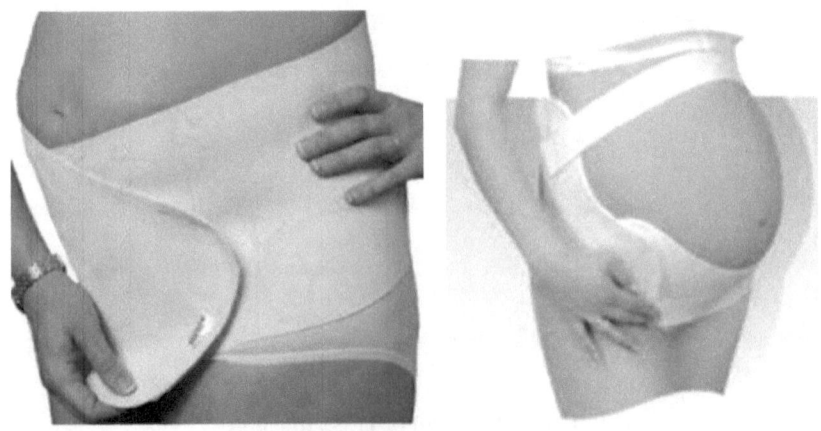

Figure 105a and b. Pelvic brace

- Surgery is considered after pregnancy to stabilise the pelvis in very extreme cases, but success rates are very poor.

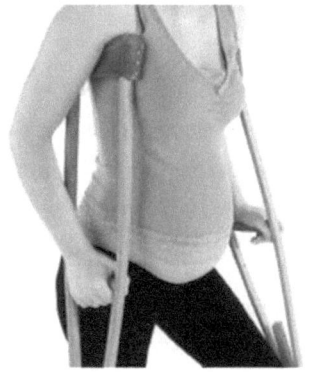

Figure 106. Crutches in pregnancy

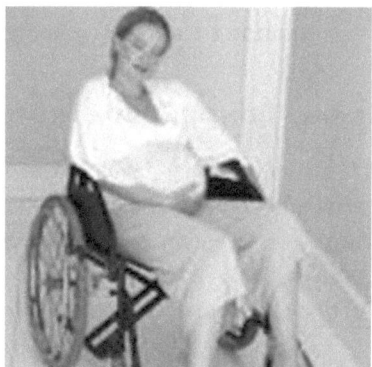

Figure 107. Wheelchairs in pregnancy

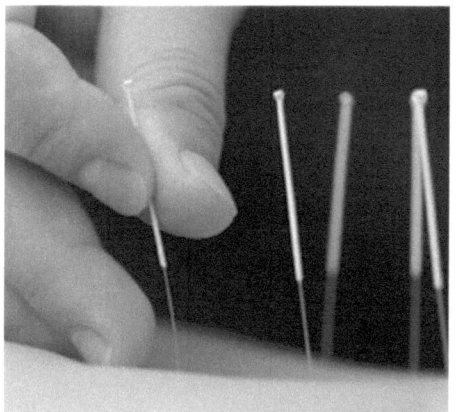

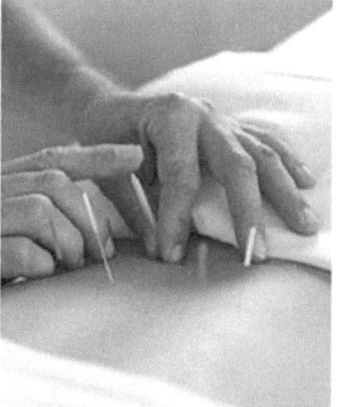

Figure 108a and b. Acupuncture

BIRTH PLANNING

- Caesarean section is not offered, except in the most extreme cases when movement is severely restricted.
- Birthing pool is recommended as the water supports the joints and assists with pain relief. The lithotomy position will not be used because of the pain it causes and the potential damage which can occur as the pelvis is misaligned.
- The use of epidural anaesthesia in labour runs the risk of masking pain and causing women to overextend their legs without realising it, and this may cause more damage to the joint.

- Birth in an upright position, with knees slightly apart, not exceeding maximum comfort zone.
- The midwife or doctor will be careful not to cause more damage to pelvic joints, for example when moving the legs in preparation for suturing a tear or episiotomy.

CARPAL TUNNEL SYNDROME

This is a condition that develops due to pressure on the 'carpal tunnel', which is in the wrist and contains the median nerve (see figure below). Any swelling around the carpal tunnel can press on the nerve, causing the syndrome.

You're more likely to develop the condition if any of the following is applicable to you:
- pregnancy
- overweight
- a job that involves repeated forceful movements, for example using a screwdriver
- rheumatoid arthritis in the wrist joint
- thyroid problems
- acromegaly, a condition caused by too much growth hormone in the blood
- diabetes
- cysts in the carpal tunnel

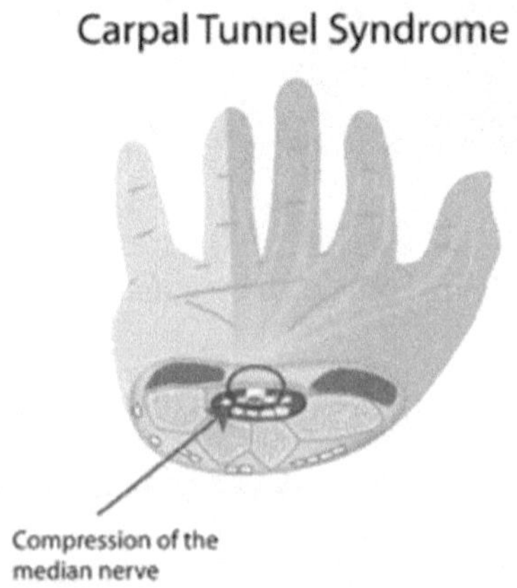

Carpal Tunnel Syndrome

Compression of the
median nerve

Figure 109. Involved fingers and palm

About 3 in 100 men and 5 in 100 women develop carpal tunnel syndrome at some point in their life. It occurs in 21-62 out of 100 pregnant women.

SYMPTOMS

- Feeling of numbness, tingling and burning in the thumb, index finger, middle finger, and at the side of the ring finger, nearest to the middle one as shown above.
- Pain in the forearm, shoulder, and neck.
- Symptoms may be mild, lasting for only short periods of time, may tend to worse at night or first thing in the morning, may get better after you have used your hand for a while, but may then get worse afterwards.
- If the symptoms occur all the time, hand muscles may become so weak that it may be difficult to grip objects or perform manual tasks.

DIAGNOSIS

This is based on the following:

- The symptoms of carpal tunnel syndrome as enumerated above
- If there are no symptoms at the time of visit, your doctor may tap on your wrist and ask you to bend the palm of your hand; if you start having the symptoms, it means it's likely that you have carpal tunnel syndrome.
- If it is still doubtful, you may be referred to an neurologist (a doctor who specialises in conditions that affect the nervous system) who may do a special test called 'nerve conduction test' to check for damage to your median nerve. This test is unfortunately not available in every country, especially in the developing countries.

TREATMENT

Sometimes, carpal tunnel syndrome improves without any treatment, especially if you're pregnant or under the age 30. Treatment helps to relieve your symptoms by reducing the pressure on the median nerve. Combination of the various forms of treatment may give a good result in some severe cases. The treatment options include the following:

- Self-help
  - Limit any activity that makes your symptoms worse, for instance repetitive movements.
  - Rest your hands and wrists regularly.
  - Shake your hands when they are numb or tingling.
  - Apply cold compress on the wrist, such as an ice pack or ice wrapped in a towel. You shouldn't apply ice directly to your skin as it can damage it.
- Steroids in the form of prednisolone tablets to swallow or injection to inject into the carpal tunnel in your wrist.

- Wrist splints help to keep your wrist straight and reduce pressure on the compressed nerve.
- Carpal tunnel brace can be used.
- Ultrasound sound waves to the wrist. The wave does the following:
  - breaks down scar tissue caused by many healing cycles
  - relieves pain
  - enhances healing of injured tissue in the wrist

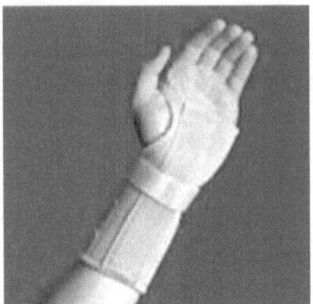

Figure 110. Carpal tunnel brace

  - increases blood flow to the wrist
  - reduces carpal tunnel inflammation
  - drives medicated gel deep into your wrist

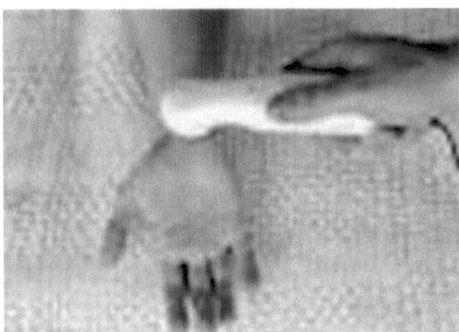

Figure 111. Ultrasound wave treatment

- Surgery in severe cases to release the nerve.
- Physiotherapy may be helpful.
- Performing yoga may help to reduce pain.

VARICOSE VEINS

They are veins which have become swollen. They are caused by the pooling of blood in the surface veins as a result of inefficient valves that would normally prevent blood draining back down the leg. They occur as blue swollen veins on the calves, on the inside of the legs, and cause itching and general discomfort. They also occur in the vulva, around the vagina. Feet and ankles can also become swollen. They are a common complaint in pregnancy and usually get better after delivery.

MANAGEMENT

You should report to your doctor who will exclude a more serious problem called DVT (page 348.)

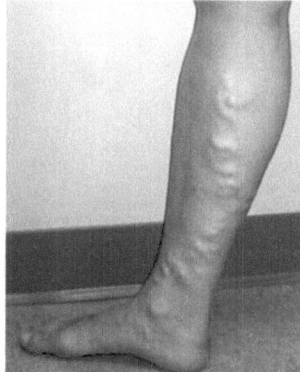

Figure 112. Varicose veins of the leg

TREATMENT

If DVT is ruled out, treatment is as follows:
- Important advice
  - Avoid standing for a long period of time.
  - Try not to sit with your legs crossed.
  - Sit with your legs up as often as you can to ease the discomfort.
  - Do foot exercises and other antenatal exercises such as walking and swimming, which will help your blood circulation.
  - Wear support tights called thromboembolic deterrent TED stockings on your legs. The stockings can improve the symptoms but will not prevent varicose veins from emerging.

Swollen Ankles, Feet, and Fingers (Oedema)

Ankles, feet, and fingers often swell in pregnancy and that is normal. The reasons for the swelling are as follows:

- Changes in your blood cause fluid to shift into your tissue, and therefore, your body is holding more water than usual.
- Your growing uterus puts pressure on your pelvic veins and your vena cava (the larger vein on the right side of the body and at the back of the uterus that carries blood from your lower limbs back to the heart). The pressure slows the return of blood from your legs, causing it to pool, and this forces fluid from your veins into the tissues of your feet and ankles.
- Towards the end of the day, especially if the weather is hot or if you have been standing a lot, the extra water tends to gather in the lowest parts of your body.

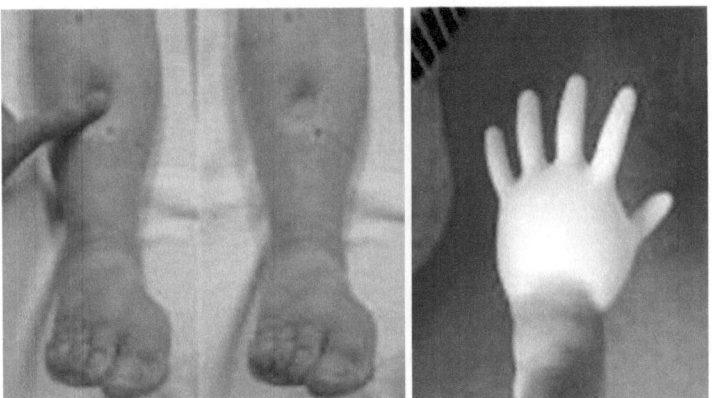

Figure 113. Swelling in pregnancy

Some Tips on How to Minimise the Swelling

- Relieve the increased pressure on your veins by lying on your side with a pillow under your tummy and another between your knees. Since the vena cava is on the right side of your body, left-sided rest works better.

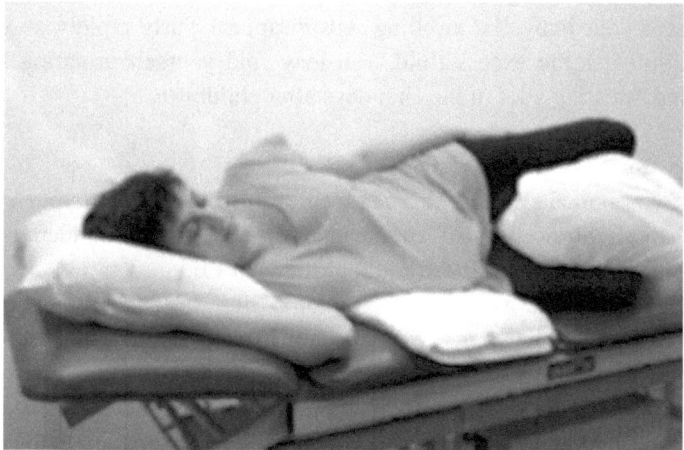

Figure 114. Posture taken to reduce oedema

- Put your feet up as much as you can. Try to rest for an hour a day with your feet higher than your heart.
- Don't cross your legs or ankles while sitting but stretch them.

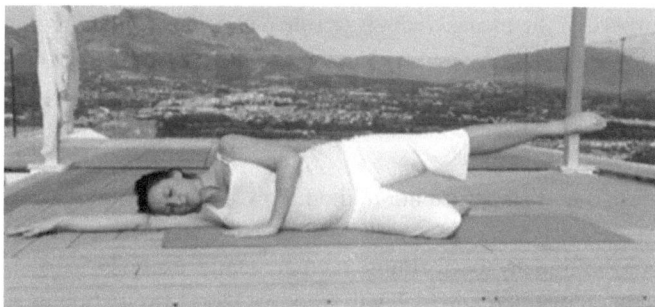

Figure 115. Putting the feet up

- Avoid standing or sitting for long time. A short walk will enhance blood circulation in your blood vessels.
- Wear comfortable shoes that stretch to accommodate the swelling.
- Don't wear socks or stockings that have tight bands around the ankles or calves.
- Try waist-high maternity support stockings. Put them on before you get out of bed in the morning so blood doesn't have a chance to pool around your ankles.
- Drink plenty of water since it surprisingly helps your body retain less water.
- Exercise regularly, especially foot exercise.

- Do not let pregnancy swelling get you down. Remember, after you have your baby, the swelling will disappear fairly rapidly as your body eliminates the excess fluid. You may find yourself urinating frequently and sweating a lot in the first days after childbirth.

WHEN TO GET HELP

- If you notice swelling in your face or puffiness around your eyes, more than slight swelling of your hands, or excessive or sudden swelling of your feet or ankles, these could be signs of PE.
- If you notice associated symptoms like headache, blurring vision, speckles before your eyes, and pain in your upper abdomen, these are also signs of PE.
- If one leg is significantly more swollen than the other, especially if associated with pain, this can be a sign of clots formation in the calf veins.

CRAMP

Cramp is a sudden sharp pain, usually in your calf muscles or feet, common at night, and we do not really know what causes it.

MANAGEMENT

The main purpose of the management is to rule out serious conditions that may cause cramps, for instance clots in the calf veins (DVT) and associated blood clots in the lung veins. So see your doctor or obstetrician when you have cramps in the leg.

TREATMENT

After ruling out blood clots formation, the following simple measures would help:

- Avoid cramp by performing regular gentle exercise, particularly ankle and leg movements, which will improve blood circulation in your leg.
- Ease cramps by pulling your toes up towards your ankle or rub the muscle hard.

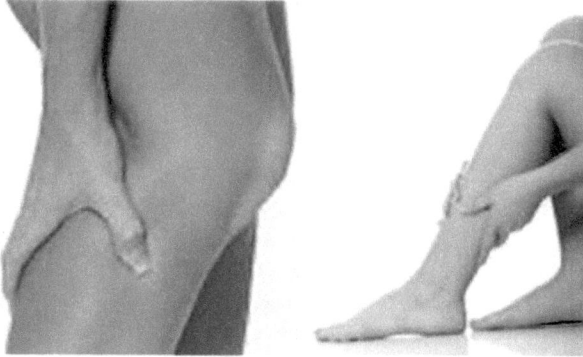

Figure 116a and b. Rubbing the muscle

TEETH AND GUMS

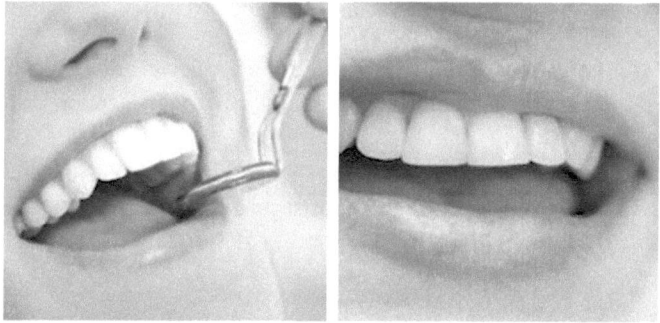

Figure 117a and b. Teeth decay in pregnancy

Dental health problems during pregnancy are as follows:

- Tooth decay: Increased acid in the mouth during pregnancy can lead to tooth decay. Furthermore, when you vomit during pregnancy, the acid content of the stomach reaches the mouth, and this worsens the problem.
- Loose teeth: Hormones which are produced during pregnancy can relax the structures holding the teeth in place and therefore loosen them, even without gum infection.
- Gum disease: The hormonal changes in pregnancy can cause inflammation of the gum (gingivitis), making it bleed; if untreated, it may lead to adverse pregnancy outcome like preterm birth and LBW. Pregnancy can cause enlargement of the gum.

Teeth and Gum Care

- Use a soft toothbrush and clean your teeth and gums carefully.
- Ask your dentist to show you a good brushing method to remove all the plaque.
- Avoid having sugary drinks and foods too often.
- Floss regularly. Rinse with a fluoride mouthwash.

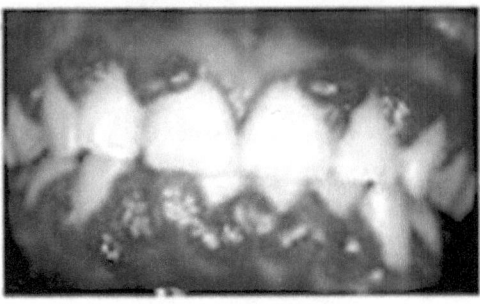

Figure 118. Inflammation of the gum

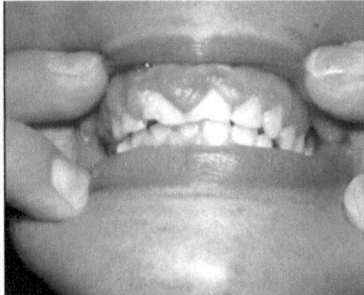

Figure 119. Enlargement of the gum

- Rinse your mouth with a solution of baking soda and water after vomiting if you have morning sickness. Mix one teaspoon baking soda in one cup of water.
- Schedule a dental check-up before pregnancy to treat any dental problems ahead of time. Also visit your dentist regularly during pregnancy.

Itching and Rashes

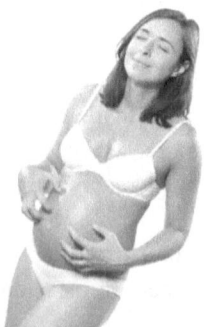

Figure 120. Itching in pregnancy

Mild itching is common in pregnancy because of the increased blood supply to the skin. In late pregnancy, the skin of the abdomen is stretched as the baby grows, and this may also cause itching. You may also find that things that normally make you itchy, for example dry skin, eczema, food allergies make you even itchier when you're pregnant.

How to Avoid Itching

- Wear loose clothes.
- Try to avoid synthetic materials.
- Avoid hot showers and baths, which can dry out your skin and make the itching worse. Use mild soap and be sure to rinse it off well. Use an unscented moisturiser.
- Avoid going out in the heat of the day since heat can intensify the itching.

Specific Skin Conditions Causing Itching in Pregnancy

They occur in about 1% of pregnancy and present with different types of rashes (small red bumps, small fluid-containing rash, spots, and others) on different part of the body, including over stretch marks. Most of the conditions start around the beginning of the third trimester and may last for few weeks to 3 months after delivery. A bland ointment, drugs for itching, and oral steroids are all used. You should always report a rash or itching to your doctor.

The most important rashes are as follows:

- Eczema in pregnancy
- Pemphigoid gestationis

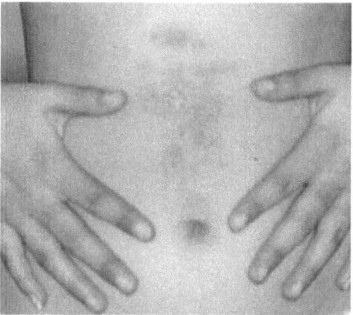

Figure 121. Eczema in pregnancy

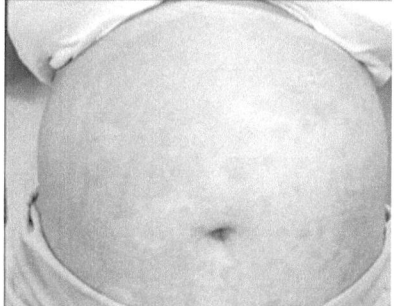

Figure 122. Pemphigoid gestationis

Skin and Hair Changes

These changes may be noticeable from about 20 weeks onwards. The darker your skin, the more likely you are to see changes. If you're very fair or have red hair, you may not notice any at all. The changes are as follows:

- Your nipples and the area around them may become darker due to hormonal changes taking place in pregnancy.

197

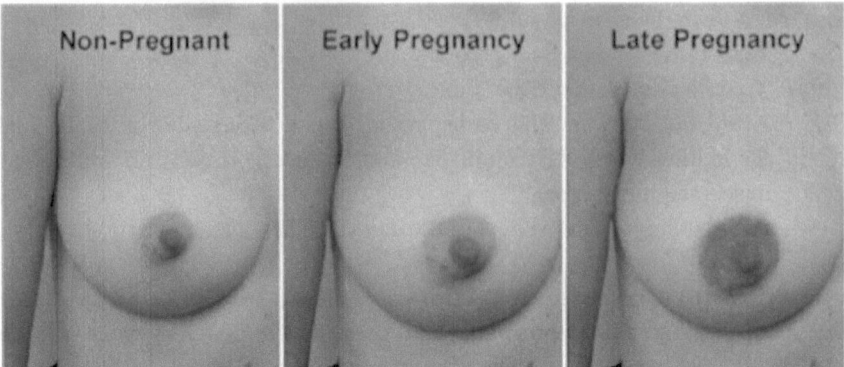

Figure 123a-c. Areola (nipple and area around it)

- You may have a mask-like colouration on the face, which can be irregular and blotchy.
- Your birthmarks, moles, and freckles may also darken.
- You may have a dark line called linea nigra, which appears from the belly buttons down to the top of the pubic hair.

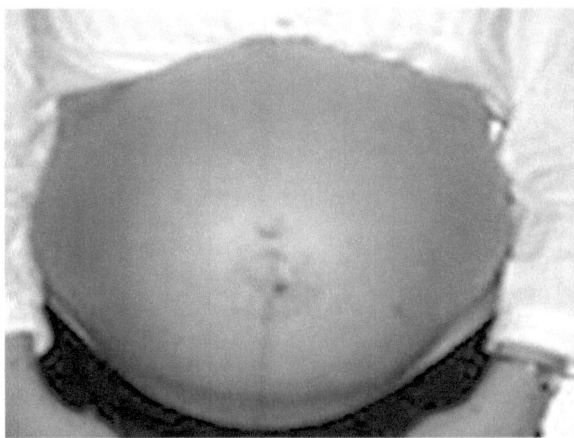

Figure 124a and b. Linea nigra

- You may get tanned easily and unevenly when in the sun or using sunbed. While there's no evidence that sunbathing or sunbeds are harmful to your baby, it is advised not to stay in the sun for very long.
- Your hair may grow more and be greasier, but hair loss also increases. It's okay to use hair colourants and perm lotions on your hair, although you may find the results are different from what you have been used to. This may be because hair can be more porous in pregnancy, affecting the way it reacts to a product.

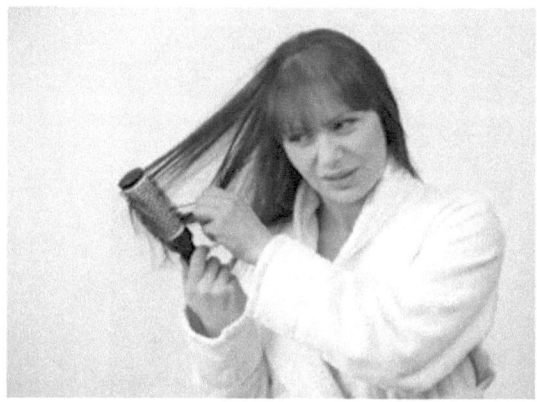 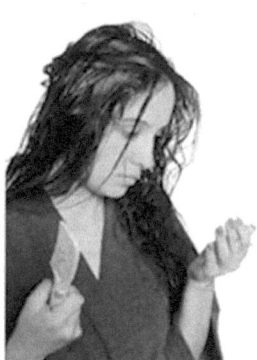

Figure 125a and b. Hair loss

- It may seem as if you are losing a lot of hair after birth. In fact, you are simply losing the extra hair that you grew during pregnancy. The skin changes will gradually fade away, although your nipples may remain a little darker.

STRETCH MARKS

Stretch marks are small depressed streaks in the skin, which usually occur on the abdomen and sometimes on the upper thighs, buttock, or breasts in the later stages of pregnancy when the womb is rapidly expanding to accommodate your growing baby. At least half of pregnant women get stretch marks. They start out pink, reddish brown, purple, or dark brown, depending on your skin colour.

RISK FACTORS FOR DEVELOPING STRETCH MARKS IN PREGNANCY
- It can run in a family. If your mother or sister got stretch marks during pregnancy, you're more likely to get them too.
- You are more likely to get the marks if you are a young mother.
- The more your skin has to expand during pregnancy and the more quickly it happens, the more likely you will develop stretch marks. For this reason, you're more likely to get stretch marks if
  - you gain a lot of weight rapidly.
  - you're carrying multiple pregnancy.
  - you're carrying a big baby.
  - you have excess amniotic fluid.

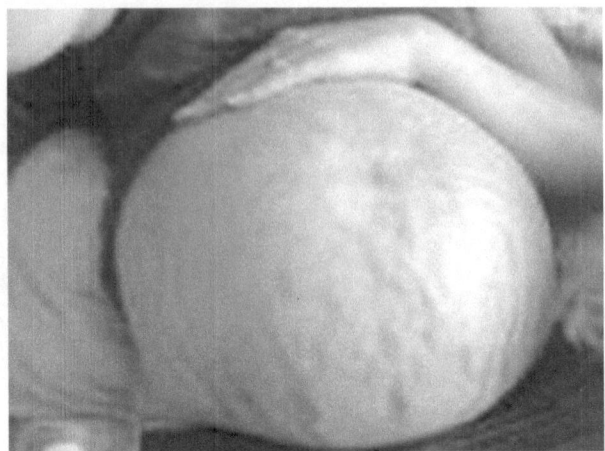

Figure 126. Stretch marks

PREVENTION OF STRETCH MARKS IN PREGNANCY

- It is good to gain not more than the recommended weight in pregnancy, in most cases, 25-35 pounds (11.3-15.9 Kg), and gain it slowly.
- It is very doubtful whether oil or cream help to prevent stretch marks. However, keeping your belly well moisturised as it grows may reduce itching.

THE FATE OF STRETCH MARKS AFTER DELIVERY

The good news is that after childbirth, the marks should gradually pale and become less noticeable. You won't be able to banish them altogether, but if your stretch marks still bother you after your pregnancy, talk to a dermatologist. The marks can be minimised by using the following treatment options:

- Topical medications such as tretinoin (Retin-A) and glycolic acid can be used, but not to be used in pregnancy and during breastfeeding.
- Laser treatments can help to restore the skin's elasticity and also change the pigmentation so that the stretch marks better match the rest of your skin.

NOSEBLEEDS

The blood vessels in your nose expand under the influence of pregnancy hormones; this coupled with the increased blood volume during pregnancy puts more pressure on those delicate vessels, causing them to rupture easily. Nosebleeds don't usually last long but can be quite heavy. As long as you don't lose a lot of blood, there is nothing to worry about. You may also find that your nose gets more blocked up than usual.

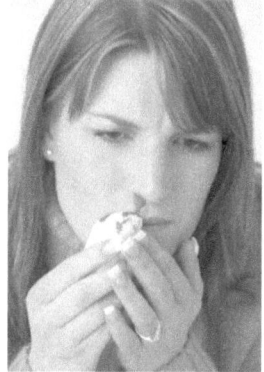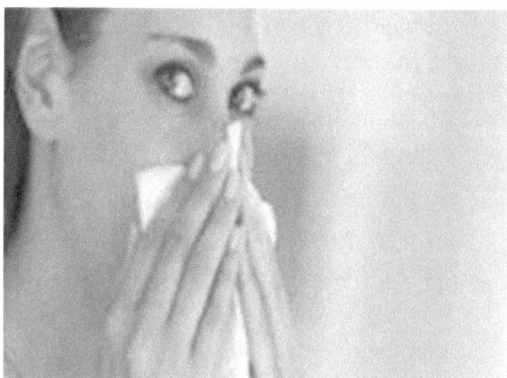

Figure 127a and b. Nosebleeding

You're especially likely to get a nosebleed in the following conditions:
- When you have a cold, sinus infection, or allergies.
- When the membranes inside your nose dry out, as they do in cold weather, air-conditioned rooms, airline cabins, and other dry environments.
- When you have trauma and certain medical conditions such as high BP or a clotting disorder.

How to Prevent Nosebleed
- Drink extra fluids to help keep all of your mucous membranes well hydrated.
- Blow your nose gently. Aggressive blowing can lead to nosebleeds.
- Try to keep your mouth open when you sneeze.
- Avoid dry air, especially in winter or in dry climates, by running a humidifier inside your house and not overheating your bedroom.
- Prevent irritation of the nose in the following ways:
  - Stay away from nasal irritants like smoke.
  - Don't overuse medicated nasal sprays or decongestants because they can dry out and further irritate your nose.
- Use a lubricant to prevent nasal dryness.
  - Some experts recommend petroleum jelly.
  - Others suggest a special water-based nasal lubricant that is available over the counter at pharmacies.
  - Saline nasal sprays or drops can help, too.

How to Stop Nosebleeds
- Always sit down with your head higher than your heart. Press the sides of your nose together between your thumb and forefinger, just below the bony part, for 5-10 minutes and try not to swallow the blood. Repeat for

a further 10 minutes if this is unsuccessful. If the bleeding continues, seek medical advice as a matter of urgency.

- Generally, always report nosebleed to your doctor.

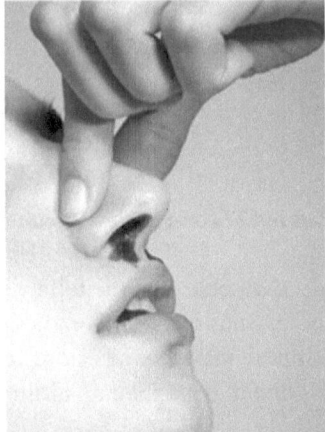

Figure 128. Stopping nosebleeding

LEAKING NIPPLES

In pregnancy, the breasts may start to produce milk around weeks 14-26. The substance that is produced is called colostrum. Leaking is normal and nothing to worry about.

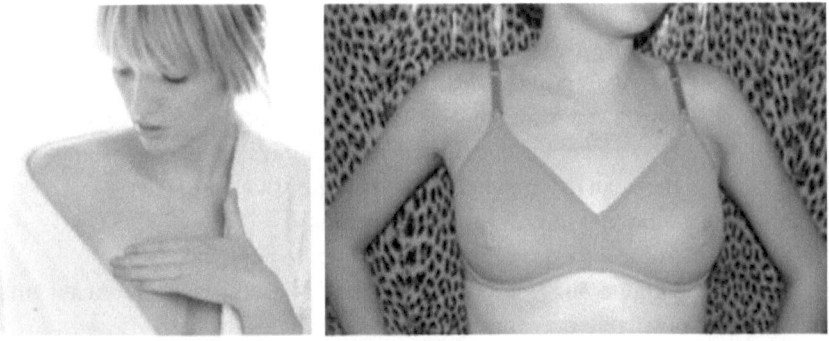

Figure 129a and b. Leaking nipples

If it bothers you, you can try putting a tissue or an absorbent breast pad sometimes called nursing pads in your bra to absorb the milk. Please see your midwife or doctor if the milk becomes bloodstained.

VAGINAL DISCHARGE

Vaginal discharge, which is clear and white and with no unpleasant smell, is more common in pregnant women than in non-pregnant women. If the discharge
- has a strong or unpleasant odour
- is associated with itch or soreness
- is associated with pain on passing urine

you should see a medical staff (your doctor or midwife) because you may have vaginal infection namely
- BV
- vaginal trichomoniasis
- thrush

However, vaginal discharge may also be caused by a range of other conditions such as skin problem of the vulva and allergic reaction.

CANDIDIASIS (THRUSH)
It is very common. It presents with vulval itching and white thick discharge. The presence of the following sinister findings may indicate the presence of other problems unrelated to thrush:
- vaginal bleeding
- offensive vaginal discharge

High vaginal swab may clarify the diagnosis.

TREATMENT
If the above sinister findings are absent, you will be reassured and given canesten pessary and cream while waiting for the swab result. You should see your doctor again if this treatment does not relieve your symptoms. If any of the sinister findings above is present, your doctor should review you. You can prevent thrush by wearing loose cotton underwear.

TRICHOMONIASIS
This is a sexually transmitted infection caused by a parasite called 'Trichomonas vaginalis'. It is characterised by the following:
- green-yellow frothy discharge from the vagina.
- pain when passing urine.
- associated with preterm labour and LBW.

A drug called metronidazole or Flagyl is used for its treatment.

URINARY INCONTINENCE IN PREGNANCY

The main causes of urinary incontinence in pregnancy are water infection, stress incontinence, and overactive bladder. For water infection, please see page xxx.

STRESS INCONTINENCE

The muscles in the bladder neck (sphincter) and in the pelvic floor are overwhelmed by the extra pressure on the bladder induced by the growing womb. Urine may, therefore, leak out of the bladder when there is an additional increase in the pressure in the abdomen, for example when coughing, sneezing, laughing, moving suddenly, or just getting up from a sitting position. The incontinence may be mild, but it can be severe for some people. The treatment of choice in pregnancy is pelvic floor exercise.

OVERACTIVE BLADDER

You will need to urinate more often than usual because the bladder has uncontrollable spasms. When you have to go, you must do that quickly or else, you will pass urine on yourself. The treatment is as follows:

- Behavioural methods.
  - Timed voiding: You use a chart or diary to record the times that you urinate and when you leak urine. This will give you an idea of your leakage 'patterns' so that you can avoid leaking in the future by going to the bathroom at those times.
  - Bladder training: You 'stretch out' the intervals at which you go to the bathroom by waiting a little longer before you go. For instance, you can go once an hour, then every 90 minutes, and so on.
- Some drugs can help to relax an overactive bladder, but they are not used in pregnancy.

PASSING URINE OFTEN

Needing to pass urine often may start in early pregnancy. Sometimes, it continues right throughout the pregnancy. In later pregnancy, it is the result of baby's head pressing on the bladder. Some tips to help with the problem are as follows:

- If you find that you have to get up in the night, try cutting out drinks in the late evening, but make sure you keep drinking plenty during the day.
- Later in pregnancy, some women find it helpful to rock backwards and forwards while they are on the toilet. This lessens the pressure of the uterus on the bladder so that you can empty it properly. Then you may not need to pass water again quite so soon.

You will need to ask for help in the following situation:
- If you have any pain while passing water or you pass any blood, you may have a urinary infection, which will need treatment. Drink plenty of water to dilute your urine, and contact your doctor within 24 hours.

HEADACHES

If you get headaches, try and get more regular rest and relaxation. Paracetamol in the recommended dose is safe in pregnancy, but there are some painkillers that you should avoid. Speak to your nurse, midwife, or doctor about it. You should always report headaches to your midwife or doctor, especially if they are frequent. They may be associated with preeclampsia or swelling in the brain.

FEELING FAINT

You may feel faint when you are pregnant. This is because of hormonal changes

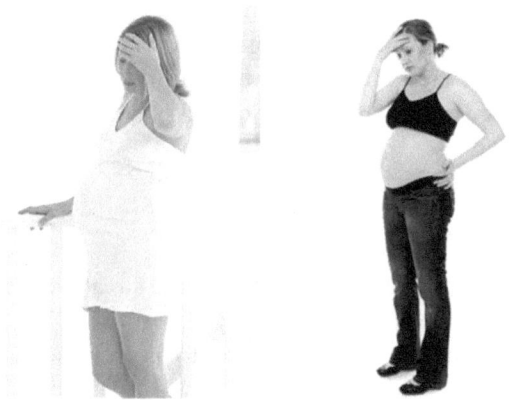

Figure 130a and b. Headaches

taking place in your body and happens if your brain is not getting enough blood and therefore enough oxygen. You are most likely to feel faint if you
- stand still for too long.
- get up too quickly from a chair or out of a hot bath.
- lie on your back.

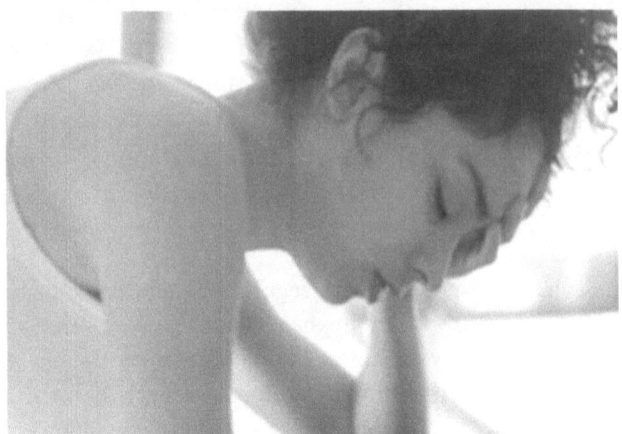

Figure 131. Feeling faint

How to Avoid Fainting
- Try to get up slowly after sitting or lying down.
- Find a seat quickly if you feel faint when standing still, and the feeling should pass; if it doesn't, lie down on your side.
- Turn on your side if you feel faint while lying on your back. It is advisable not to lie flat on your back at any time in later pregnancy or during labour.

Feeling Hot

During pregnancy you are likely to feel warmer and sweat more than normal. This is due to the following reasons:
- Hormonal changes in your body lead to an increase in the blood supply to your skin.
- The amount of blood in your body increases by as much as 50% during pregnancy. To better handle all that extra blood, your blood vessels dilate slightly, allowing the blood to come off the surface, which can make you feel hot.
- The rate at which your body uses up energy when it is at rest increases by about 20% in the third trimester. This can also add to the overheated feeling. You may sweat more too.

The good news is that everything will return to normal after delivery. Until then, you'll have to find ways to deal with feeling hot, which are as follows:
- Wear loose clothes made of natural fibres, which are more absorbent and trap less heat than synthetic fibres.

- Drink plenty of water; this prevents dehydration and makes you feel more comfortable, especially when it's hot outside.
- Consider using electric fans.
- Lock yourself in your room and go bare or topless especially when you are alone at home.
- Take several baths a day.

Tiredness

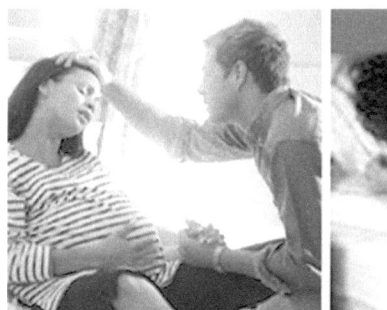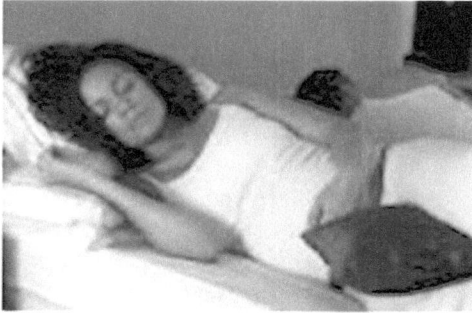

Figure 132a and b. Feeling tired

Tiredness occurs throughout pregnancy. At first, it might be morning sickness keeping you awake, or it could just be anxiety and worry about impending motherhood, while in third trimester, discomfort and frequent trips to the toilet can all interrupt your good night's sleep, and all these can lead to tiredness. Tiredness can be reduced in the following ways:

- Try to accept that some tiredness is a normal part of the pregnancy experience rather than let yourself get stressed by pregnancy tiredness.
- Try and get as much rest as possible.

When to Get Help

If there is associated headache or the tiredness is getting worse, you should see your midwife or doctor who will do a blood test to rule out anaemia.

Sleep

You may sleep more than usual during the first trimester of your pregnancy because your body has just started adapting to the pregnancy. Late in pregnancy, sleeping becomes difficult especially during the night because of the following reasons:

- Increasing size of the foetus, which can make it hard to find a comfortable sleeping position. If you've always been a back or stomach sleeper, you might have trouble getting used to sleeping on your side as recommended by doctors.

- Frequent urge to urinate and urge incontinence.
- Increased heart rate—as more of your blood supply goes to the uterus, your heart will be working harder to send sufficient blood to the rest of your body.
- Shortness of breath—at first, you will breathe in more deeply under the influence of hormones. Later in pregnancy, your enlarging uterus presses against your diaphragm (the muscle just below your lungs) and thereby making it more difficult to breathe.
- Leg cramps and backaches.
- Heartburn and constipation.
- Vivid dreams and nightmares.
- Stress—you may be worried about your baby's health and delivery and anxious about your abilities as a parent. These feelings are normal, but they might keep you up at night.

MEASURES TO HELP YOU ACHIEVE GOOD SLEEP

- Lie on your side; left better than right. This will take pressure off your back and improve blood circulation.
- Place a pillow under your abdomen and/or between your legs.
- Cut out caffeinated drinks like soda, coffee, and tea from your diet as much as possible or restrict any intake of them to the morning or early afternoon. At bedtime, have a warm caffeine-free drink such as milk with honey.

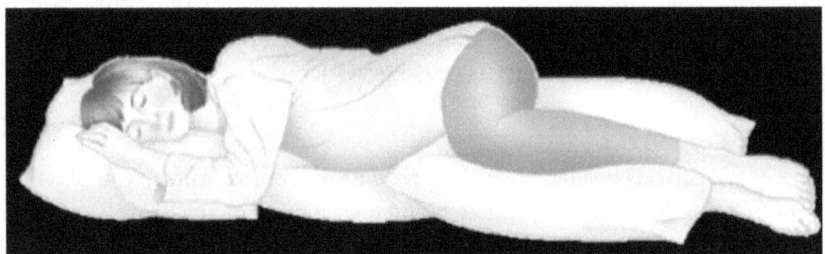

Figure 133. The best sleeping position in pregnancy
(from UK NHS Pregnancy Book, 2009)

- Avoid drinking a lot of fluids or eating a full meal before going to bed at night. Eat more at breakfast and lunch and then have a smaller dinner.
- Prevent nausea with measures outline on page 45 if it is keeping you up.
- Avoid rigorous exercise right before you go to bed. Instead, do something relaxing, like soaking in a warm bath for 15 minutes.

- Press your feet hard against the wall or stand on the leg if a leg cramp awakens you. Also, make sure that you're getting enough calcium in your diet, which can help to reduce leg cramps.
- Take a class in yoga or learn other relaxation techniques to help you unwind after a busy day.
- Consider enrolling in a childbirth or parenting class if fear and anxiety are keeping you awake.
- Get up and do something, for example read a book, listen to music, watch TV, when you can't sleep, instead of tossing and turning and worrying that you're not asleep. Eventually, you'll probably feel tired enough to get back to sleep. If possible, take short naps (30-60 minutes) during the day to make up for lost sleep.

SOURCES

- The NHS Pregnancy Book. Your complete guide to: a healthy pregnancy, labour and childbirth. The first weeks with your new baby, UK, 2009.
- Antenatal Protocol. King's College Hospital, London, 2009.
- Murry MM. Dental health during pregnancy. www.mayoclinic.com. June 2, 2009.
- Tiredness in pregnancy. www.kidspot.com.au/Pregnancy-Third-trimester-Pregnancy-tiredness+1487+114+article.htm
- Chang L. Incontinence during pregnancy and after childbirth.
- www.webmd.com/urinary-incontinence-oab/america-asks-11/pregnancywww.webmd.com/urinary-incontinence-oab/america-asks-11/pregnancy
- Swollen extremities (edema) during pregnancy. Reviewed by the BabyCenter Medical Advisory Board En Español.

Obstetric Problems in Pregnancy

INTRODUCTION

Obstetric problems in pregnancy have been defined, for the purpose of better understanding of the book, as those conditions and situations that are specific to pregnancy. We have included in this chapter those cases that are met often. They are as follows:

- Problems of foetal size
    - SGA foetuses and FGR
    - LGA foetuses
- Problems associated with amniotic fluids
    - Polyhydramnios (too much amniotic fluids around the baby)
    - Oligohydramnios (too little amniotic fluids around the baby)

- Timing of birth
  - Preterm labour
  - Post-term pregnancy (when you are overdue by 2 weeks and more)
- Bleeding in pregnancy
- Electronic foetal monitoring (EFM) and decreased foetal movements

PROBLEMS OF FOETAL SIZE

For assessment of fetal size, please see page 116.

ABNORMAL FOETAL GROWTH INCLUDING SGA/FGR

SGA foetus refers to a foetus that has failed to achieve the tenth centile for AC and/or estimated birth weight threshold at a specific GA. It is severe when these parameters are less than the fifth centile (Please see Figure 54 for centile chart and also the ''glossary '' for the meaning of centile chart.)

SGA foetuses are classified into two different groups:
- Foetuses that have failed to achieve their genetically determined growth potential (FGR).
- Foetuses that are constitutionally small, that is small normal foetuses. Approximately 50-70 in 100 of foetuses with a birth weight below tenth centile for GA are constitutionally normal.

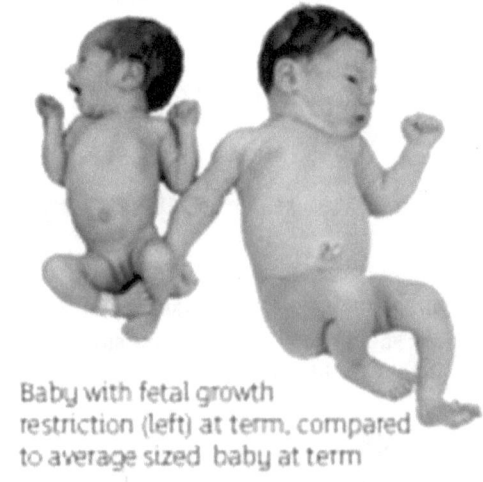

Baby with fetal growth restriction (left) at term, compared to average sized baby at term

Figure 134. Foetal growth restriction

Abnormal growth is further subdivided into the asymmetric and symmetric types based on the following ultrasound findings:

- Head to abdominal circumference ratio (HC/AC)
- Head circumference to femur length ratio (HC/FL)
- Abdominal circumference to femur length ratio (AC/FL)

ASYMMETRIC TYPE OF GROWTH

There are different categories of asymmetric growth.

- FGR (due to impaired placental function)
    - This occurs when the foetus has grown normally for the first two trimesters but encounters difficulties in the third, in most cases, secondary to PE.
    - AC is the single best measure of foetal nutrient status. A small AC suggests FGR, which can be asymmetrical if the HC is normal or symmetrical if the HC is also small (see below).
    - The AC is smaller than what it is suppose to be, but the HC is of normal size; therefore, the HC/AC ratio is high.
    - EFW is low
- Abnormal skeletal development called dysplasia (dwarfism or short stature)
    - Short limbs but the head and abdomen circumferences are in the normal range.
    - HC/FL and AC/FL ratios are high.
    - This occurs in about 1 in 4,000 children.
- Microcephaly (small head)
    - HC is significantly smaller than normal for age and sex, but the AC and FL are normal.
    - HC/AC and HC/FL ratios are low.
    - This occurs because the brain fails to grow at a normal rate, and therefore, the skull is also small.
    - Causes are viral infections, genetic disorders, and severe malnutrition.
- LFD baby (macrosomia) due to maternal diabetes
    - AC is high, and HC and FL are normal.
    - HC/AC and FL/AC ration are low.

SYMMETRIC TYPE (NORMAL HC/AC)

- The foetus has developed slowly throughout the duration of the pregnancy and was thus affected from a very early stage.
- The HC of such a newborn is in proportion to the rest of the body, including AC.
- The expected birth weight is small.
- It is normally a severe FGR due to
    - impaired placental formation
    - chromosomal abnormalities

211

- genetic problems
- viral infection (e.g. rubella, toxoplasmosis) of the baby early in pregnancy
- anaemic conditions
- drug abuse (e.g. drinking too much alcohol)

RISKS ASSOCIATED WITH FGR

Babies having FGR are at greater risk of the following:

- Not getting enough oxygen through the umbilical cord during pregnancy and childbirth
- More chance of having intervention (e.g. Caesarean section in the antenatal period and in labour because of abnormal trace of baby's heart, taking blood from the baby's head in labour to confirm that it is receiving enough oxygen, instrumental deliveries, etc.)

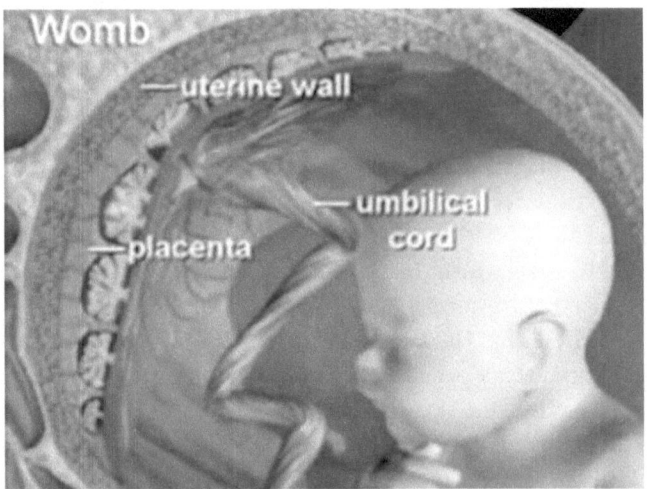

Figure 135. Less oxygen to the baby

- Stillbirth
- Complications in the newborn—dry peeling skin, thin umbilical cord, low sugar levels, and others
- Impaired neurodevelopment
- Possibly type 2 (non-insulin-dependent) diabetes and hypertension in adult life

BIRTH WEIGHT

Birth weight classification is shown in the table below.

Classification	Birth weight (g)
Normal birth weight at term delivery	2,500-4,200
LBW	1,500-2,500
Very LBW	1,000-1,500
Extremely LBW	Less than 1,000

Table 8. Classification of birth weight

The most important cause of LBW is preterm labour. About 6-30 out of 100 pregnant women develop LBW in developing countries; the corresponding figure in the developed countries is 8.1 out of 100. SGA is not a synonym of LBW; for a 2,250-g baby delivered at 35 weeks, the weight is appropriate for GA but is a LBW.

CAUSES OF SGA BABIES

These are already pointed out under abnormal growth above. Others are as follows:
- Foetal
  - Heart disease
  - Malformations
  - Multiple pregnancy and others
- Maternal
  - Diseases of different organs and systems
  - Sickle-cell disease
  - Fever
  - Smoking and others
- Placental factors
  - Separation of the placenta, low-lying placenta
  - Sticky blood (thrombophilia)
  - Post-term pregnancy

MANAGEMENT

PREDICTION OF FGR AT THE BOOKING CLINIC (11-13+6 WEEKS OF PREGNANCY)
- Blood test to check for the level of an ingredient in the blood called PAPP-A, which is produced by the placenta.
- Ultrasound scan to check the number of blood vessels in the umbilical cord.

213

Low levels of Papp-A and one artery in the umbilical cord are risk factors for FGR. High-risk patients are monitored in a specialised unit called foetal medicine unit.

PREDICTION OF **FGR** AT **20-23 WEEKS**

At ultrasound scan, the blood flow to the womb through an artery called uterine artery will be assessed. High resistance to the blood flow is a risk factor for FGR (page 112), and such patients are best monitored in a fetal medicine unit.

ABDOMINAL PALPATION AND MEASUREMENT OF **SFH**

Normally at each visit to your midwife or doctor, you will be screened for SGA baby by abdominal palpation and measurement of the SFH from about 26 weeks of pregnancy. If SGA is suspected, you will be referred for ultrasound scan.

DIAGNOSTIC PROCEDURES

- Ultrasound scan is used to assess baby's growth, AFV, and blood flow (page 116.) This will determine further management of the pregnancy.
- Assessment for chromosomal defects: When a small foetus is diagnosed, assessment for risk of chromosomal defects on ultrasound is indicated at any stage in pregnancy. Up to 19% of foetuses with AC and EFW less than the fifth centile may have chromosomal defects. The risk is higher when growth restriction is associated with structural abnormalities, a normal liquor volume, or a normal blood flow in baby's umbilical artery and uterine artery. Where indicated, invasive investigation (amniocentesis) may be performed.
- EFM (page 136) is also used in monitoring the well-being of the baby.
- TORCH (toxoplasmosis, rubella, CMV, herpes) screen (page 289) to rule out viral cause of FGR may be indicated.

FURTHER MANAGEMENT

Steroid is administered if GA is below 36 weeks, and decision has been made to deliver the baby. Antenatal steroids significantly reduce the incidence of breathing problems in the baby after birth.

DELIVERY

Generally, the decision to deliver the baby is based on the following:

- How far you have gone in your pregnancy.
- Ultrasound findings of whether baby is growing or not, AFV, and blood flow in baby's blood vessels.
- Findings on EFM CTG.
- Your own opinion.

A trace of the baby's heart will be performed in labour. Delivery will be either by Caesarean section or vaginal route, based on the severity of the problem. It should be in a unit where there are baby specialists, and also, facilities for resuscitation should be available.

MACROSOMIA (LARGE-FOR-DATE BABY)

DEFINITION
The average weight of a newborn is 3.4 kg (7 lb 8 oz). Babies weighing more than 4.5 kg (9 lb 15 oz) are considered to be LFD babies.

DIAGNOSIS
- Screening for SGA by abdominal palpation and measurement of the SFH at each antenatal visit from 26 weeks will reveal those babies that are likely to be macrosomic. If a macrosomic baby is suspected, you will be referred for ultrasound scan.
- There can be a 10% discrepancy between your baby's weight predicted by ultrasound during pregnancy and the actual weight at birth.
- Baby's weight is confirmed at birth.

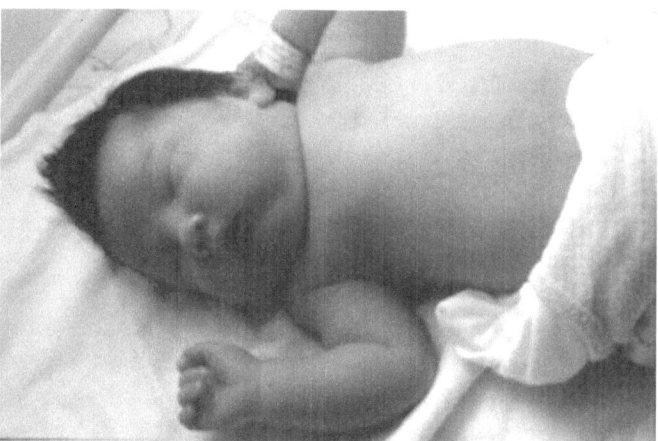

Figure 136. Large-for-date baby

PREDISPOSING FACTORS/CAUSES OF MACROSOMIA
- Genetics—for example, if you were a big baby at birth, you are more likely to have a big baby.
- Gestational diabetes or pre-existing diabetes.
- High BMI at the start of your pregnancy.
- Gaining a lot of weight during pregnancy.
- Post-term pregnancy—more than 2 weeks past your due date.
- Gaining a lot of weight between pregnancies.

- Baby's sex—boys are more often larger than girls.
- Previous baby's weight—if you had a big baby in the past, you are more likely to have big babies in future pregnancies.

The good thing is that even if any of the above factors applied to you, you are still more likely to have a normal size baby than a macrosomic baby. Most macrosomic newborns are born to women with a low risk of having a big baby.

RISKS ASSOCIATED WITH MACROSOMIC PREGNANCY

- Gestation or pre-existing diabetes
- Increased chance of incurring a complication during childbirth; examples are as follows:
  - Perineal tear
  - Injury to your tail bone (coccyx)
  - Shoulder dystocia (shoulder stuck after delivery of the head) with the associated injury to you and your baby (page xxx)
  - Increased blood loss
  - Increased risk of having Caesarean section

MANAGEMENT

- Glucose tolerance test to rule out diabetes.
- Ultrasound scan to monitor your baby throughout the pregnancy.
- Inducing labour earlier than term doesn't have any proven benefit for you nor your baby. The only exception to this rule is if you have diabetes. So induction of labour is normally conducted at term if you do not go into spontaneous labour just as in any normal pregnancy.
- You will have an intravenous access set up on your arm; this will enhance quick intravenous infusion if you bleed (a complication that is associated with macrosomia) after delivery.
- A doctor will be present at delivery so that if baby's shoulder becomes stuck after delivering the head(a problem which is also associated with macrosomia), the problem can be dealt with quickly.

SOURCES

- The NHS Pregnancy Book. Your complete guide to: a healthy pregnancy, labour and childbirth. The first weeks with your new baby, UK, 2009.
- RCOG Green-top Guideline No. 31. The investigation and management of the small-for-gestational-age foetus. Februray 2013.
- Snijders RJ, Sherrod C, Gosden CM, Nicolaides KH. Foetal growth retardation: associated malformations and chromosomal abnormalities. Am J Obstet Gynecol. 1993;168:547-55. RCOG Guideline No. 31, p. 11 of 16.

- Soothill PW, Ajayi RA, Campbell S, Nicolaides KH. Prediction of morbidity in small and normally grown foetuses by FHR variability, biophysical profile score and umbilical artery Doppler studies. Br J Obstet Gynaecol. 1993;100:742-45.
- FMF website.
- BabyCentre Medical. Last reviewed: August 2011.

AMNIOTIC FLUID

In the first 16 weeks of pregnancy, amniotic fluid (liquor) is produced by the following organs:
- developing placenta
- the water bag surrounding baby
- umbilical cord
- foetal skin

After 16 weeks, it is made up of foetal urine and the fluid secreted by the foetal respiratory tract (breathing pipe and the lung) and removed by foetal swallowing.

Adequacy of amniotic fluid around baby is normally assessed with ultrasound scan.

DECREASED AMNIOTIC FLUID LEVELS (OLIGOHYDRAMNIOS)

DEFINITION
The diagnosis is made if the deepest pool of amniotic fluid is less than 3 cm.

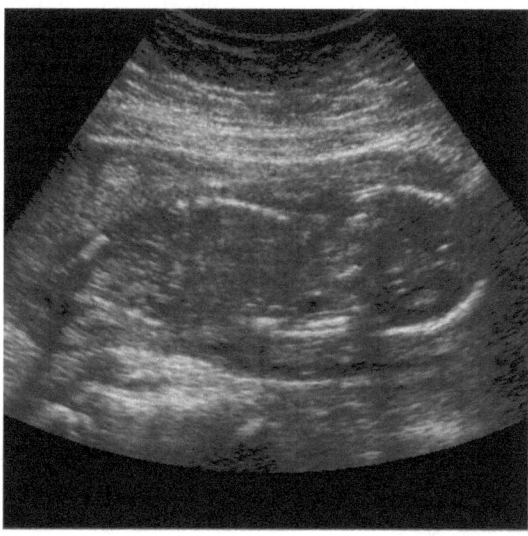

Fig. 137. Oligohydramnios (Small amount of fluids around baby.)

PREVALENCE

Oligohydramnios complicates approximately 45 out of 1,000 pregnancies generally and 12 out of pregnancies that last beyond 41 weeks. Severe oligohydramnios where there is almost no amniotic fluid around baby occurs in 7 out of 100 pregnancies.

CAUSES AND ASSOCIATIONS

They are as follows:

- The waters break (page 232).
- The placenta is not functioning well, and therefore, the baby is also small.
- A decrease in foetal urine production or excretion due to abnormalities of his or her urinary tracts.
- Blood supply to kidney is decreased, leading to reduced urine production.
  - Less blood going to the kidneys and more going to more vital organs like the heart and the brain if the baby is lacking in oxygen.
  - Foetal kidney failure leading to less or no urine production.
- Post-term pregnancy
  - The cause of decreased AFV in post-term pregnancies is unknown.
  - The decreased efficiency of placental function has been proposed as a cause.
- The donor foetus in twin-to-twin transfusion syndrome (TTTS).
- Chromosomal factor.
- Foetal death.
- Drug-induced causes include indometacin and drugs that belong to a group called angiotensin-converting enzyme (ACE) inhibitors.
- A smaller SFH measurement than expected during a routine antenatal assessment.
- Unknown causes.

COMPLICATIONS

- The risk of foetal infection is increased (by the presence of prolonged rupture of the membranes).
- There is a high risk of the following complications in the foetus if oligohydramnios occurs as early as the second trimester and the pregnancy progresses:
  - The lungs will fail to expand.
  - Contractures of the limbs.
  - Amniotic band on foetal limbs in early pregnancy causing
    - ➢ constriction rings around the fingers and toes, arms, and legs
    - ➢ swelling of the extremities distal to the point of constriction
    - ➢ amputation of digits, arms, and legs

INVESTIGATION

- Speculum examination will be performed to look for a pool of liquor in the vagina; you may be asked to cough to see if there is any leakage of liquor from the womb.
- Ultrasound scan is done to check for liquor volume, blood flow to the baby and abnormalities.
- Any condition that can affect the function of the placenta, e.g. preeclampsia will be looked for.

MANAGEMENT

Management of oligohydramnios is based on the GA at diagnosis and the possible cause of the problem. Transfer to a tertiary referral centre may be appropriate if oligohydramnios is severe.

- If you are dehydrated, treatment with oral or intravenous fluids has been shown to increase the liquor.
- Before term:
  - Expectant management is often the most appropriate course of action, depending on your condition and that of your baby.
  - Ongoing foetal well-being assessment with ultrasound and trace of the baby's heart.
- At term:
  - Delivery is often the most appropriate management, taking into consideration foetal well-being, the severity of the oligohydramnios, GA, and the favourability of the cervix.
- In labour, if the trace of the baby's heart is abnormal, normal saline can be transfused into the womb through a catheter that is introduced into amniotic fluid—amniotransfusion.

INCREASED AMNIOTIC FLUID LEVELS (POLYHYDRAMNIOS)

DEFINITION AND PREVALENCE

Polyhydramnios is defined as increased liquor volume with the deepest at least 8 cm. It is classified into the following categories of severity:

- Mild, when the deepest pool of the fluid is 8-11 cm
- Moderate, when the deepest pool of the fluid is 12-15 cm
- Severe, when the deepest pool of the fluid is 16 cm or more

In the second and early third trimester, it occurs in about 1 in every 200 pregnancies.

CAUSES AND ASSOCIATIONS

They are as follows:

- Baby cannot swallow the amniotic fluid as much as he or she should do due to
  - abnormalities of the head and spine
  - tumours of the face or neck
  - bowel obstruction
  - tumours compressing the lung and/or chest
  - others
- Baby passes lot of urine; this occurs in the following situations:
  - you have diabetes
  - baby's heart works more because of
    - ➢ anaemia in the baby
    - ➢ foetal and/or placental tumours
- The recipient foetus in TTTS
- Placental tumours
- Others

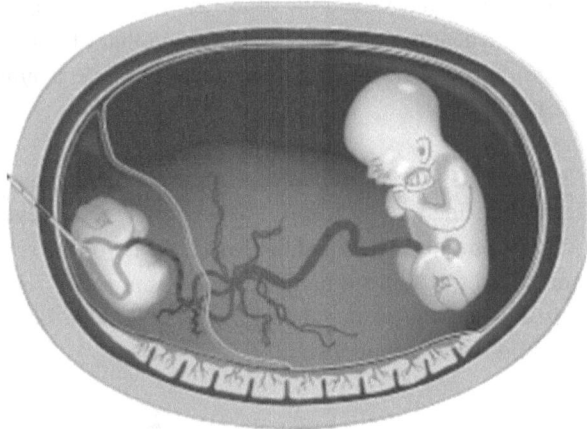

Figure 138. Twin-to-twin transfusion syndrome (Transverse section.)

PRESENTATION
- The SFH will be bigger than you have actually gone in your pregnancy, that is LFD baby.
- Abdominal discomfort or pain when it is severe.
- It may be difficult to feel for foetal parts, for example the head.

COMPLICATIONS
- High incidence of preterm labour and delivery
- Premature rupture of the membranes
- Premature separation of the placenta

- Malpresentation
- Bleeding after childbirth
- Cord prolapse
- High incidence of Caesarean section

INVESTIGATION

- Ultrasound scanning to check liquor volume, rule out foetal abnormalities, and assess the risk of preterm birth by measuring cervical length.

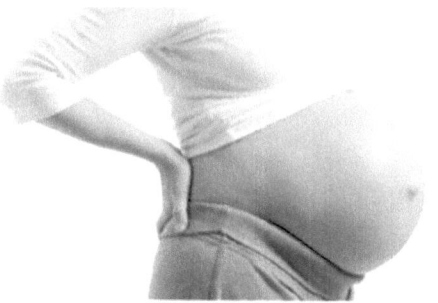

Figure 139a. Tummy larger than expected due to polyhydramnios

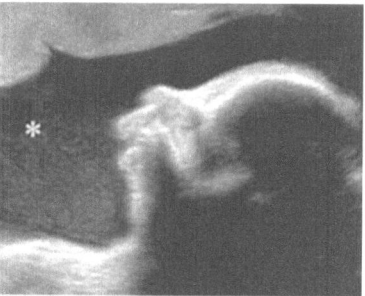

Figure 139b. Polyhydramnios on scan

- Glucose tolerance test to rule out gestational or undiagnosed pre-existing diabetes.
- TORCH screen to rule out viral infection is sometimes offered.
- Other tests may be indicated depending on the suspected cause of the problem.

MANAGEMENT

- The first step is to identify the possible cause and deal with it.
- Mild polyhydramnios can be simply monitored at different intervals.
- If your waters break at any stage of the pregnancy, it is important that you call your midwife or doctor and go to the labour ward immediately so that cord prolapse can be ruled out and management can be planned.
- Reduction of pain and the risk of delivering your baby early. This is done in two ways:
    - Repeated tap and drainage of large volumes of amniotic fluid.
    - Alternatively, a drug called indomethacin should be taken orally; it is meant to reduce the amount of urine produced by your foetus. It is effective in cases where the condition is related to increasing

foetal urine production. It is contraindicated in twin-to-twin syndrome or after 35 weeks, as adverse effects outweigh the benefits in these cases.

- Injection of steroids into your muscle is indicated since the risk of PTD is significantly high. This helps to improve lung maturity of your baby.
- Treatment of TTTS, which complicates multiple pregnancy (page xxx), may improve polyhydramnios that is associated with it.
- Mode of delivery—IOL with drugs and controlled rupture of the amniotic membranes is indicated.

Sources

- Amnioinfusion for oligohydramnios during pregnancy, NICE Interventional procedure guidance, 2006.
- Baxter JK, et al. Oligohydramnios imaging, Medscape, April 2011.
- Information for doctors 'Oligohydramnious', www.patient.co.uk, 14 December 2011.
- Information for doctors 'Polyhydramnious', www.patient.co.uk, 14 December 2011.
- Carter BS, et al. Polyhydramnios and oligohydramnios, Medscape, February 2008.
- FMF website UK, 2013.
- Mathew M, Saquib S, Rizvi SG. Polyhydramnios. Risk factors and outcome. Saudi Med J. 2008;29(2):256-60 [abstract].
- Management of diabetes, Scottish Intercollegiate Guidelines Network—SIGN, March 2010.

Reduced Foetal Movements

Characteristics of Normal Foetal Movements

- Foetal movements are defined as any discrete kick, flutter, swish, or roll.
- They are first perceived between 18 and 20 weeks of pregnancy and rapidly acquire a regular pattern.
- Foetal movements peak in the afternoon and evening periods from as early as 20 weeks of pregnancy. They are usually absent during foetal 'sleep' cycles, which occur regularly throughout the day and night and usually last for 20-40 minutes but rarely exceed 90 minutes in the normal foetus.

The Significance of Foetal Movements

- Foetal movements provide an indication of the integrity of the central nervous and musculoskeletal systems of your baby.

- It is believed that a significant reduction or sudden alteration or absent of foetal movements is a warning sign of a possible impending poor perinatal outcome. About 55 out of 100 women who experience a stillbirth perceive a reduction in foetal movements prior to diagnosis.

FACTORS THAT AFFECT FOETAL MOVEMENTS

You should perceive most foetal movements when lying down, fewer when sitting, and fewest while standing. It is, therefore, not surprising that if you are busy and not concentrating on foetal activity, you may not feel it. The following factors decrease foetal movements:

- A placenta that is located on the front wall of the womb prior to 28^{+0} weeks of pregnancy.
- Drugs that make people sleep and cross the placenta, such as alcohol, benzodiazepines, methadone, and others.
- Cigarette smoking.
- The administration of corticosteroids, which enhances foetal lung maturation.
- Major foetal malformations.
- High blood glucose levels, but some scientists refute this.
- Foetal position, when foetal spine lies in front.

ASSESSMENT OF FOETAL MOVEMENTS

- Foetal movements are assessed by your own subjective perception of it. The mean time to perceive 10 movements varies between 21 minutes for focused counting to 162 minutes for unfocused perception of foetal movements.
- You should be aware of your baby's individual pattern of movements. If they are reduced or absent after 28^{+0} weeks, you should contact your maternity unit immediately.
- You should lie on your left side and focus on foetal movements for 2 hours if you are unsure whether foetal movements are reduced or not after 28^{+0} weeks of gestation. If you do not feel 10 or more discrete movements, you should contact your midwife or maternity unit immediately.
- Ultrasound is better than maternal perception in assessing foetal movements.

MANAGEMENT OF RFMs

- You should always attend the maternity day unit or labour ward when you are concerned about foetal movements.
- The goal of assessment and possible antenatal foetal surveillance are as follows:

- – to exclude foetal death
- – to exclude foetal compromise
- – to identify pregnancies at risk of adverse outcome while avoiding unnecessary interventions
- Your hand-held note will be assessed to find out your risk assessment at booking. A relevant history will be taken to assess your risk factors for stillbirth, such as multiple consultations for RFM, known FGR, hypertension, diabetes, extremes of maternal age, first time pregnant, smoking, placental insufficiency, and so on.
- It is prudent to measure BP and test urine for proteinuria as PE is also associated with placental dysfunction.
- CTG, to exclude foetal compromise, will be carried out for 20 minutes if the pregnancy is over 28^{+0} weeks. Some units will do it from 26 weeks. The presence of a normal FHR pattern is indicative of a healthy foetus.
- RFM between 24^{+0} and 28^{+0} weeks of gestation—The presence of a foetal heartbeat will be confirmed with a hand-held device. There is no evidence for routine use of CTG surveillance in this group. If there is clinical suspicion of FGR, consideration will be given to ultrasound assessment.
- RFM prior to 24^{+0} weeks of gestation—Foetal heartbeat will be confirmed with a hand-held device. Placental insufficiency is very unlikely at this stage of pregnancy. If foetal movements have never been felt by 24 weeks of gestation, referral to a specialist foetal medicine centre will be considered to look for evidence of foetal neuromuscular conditions (i.e. condition affecting foetal brain, spinal cord, and muscles).
- Ultrasound scan within 24 hours of RFM for growth, liquor volume, blood flow studies and to rule out abnormalities will be conducted after 28^{+0} weeks of pregnancy in the following situations:
  - – Perception of RFM persists despite a normal CTG.
  - – There are additional risk factors for FGR/stillbirth.
  - – Presentation with the same problem more than once (recurrent RFM).
  - – No foetal heart activity on EFM.
- You should be reassured that 70 out of 100 pregnancies with a single episode of RFM are uncomplicated.
- There is no evidence to support formal foetal movement counting (kick charts) if investigations are normal. However, if you have normal investigations after one presentation with RFM, you should contact your maternity unit if you have another episode.
- The decision on whether or not to induce labour at term, if you present with recurrent RFM when the growth, liquor volume, blood flow studies,

and CTG appear normal, will be made after careful consultant-led counselling of the pros and cons of induction on an individualised basis.

Sources
- RCOG Green-top Guideline No. 57. Reduced fetal movements, February 2011.
- The Pregnancy Book. Your complete guide to: a healthy pregnancy, labour and childbirth. The first weeks with your new baby, UK, 2009.

Threatened Preterm Labour

This presents with regular or irregular contractions of the womb about 3 or less in 10 minutes not giving rise to changes in the cervix. More than 80% of women who present to the labour ward with painful and regular uterine contractions at 24-36 weeks of pregnancy are not in true labour and do not deliver within the subsequent 7 days. Prediction of the risk of progression of threatened preterm labour to actual preterm labour is achieved by using either of the two methods given below.
- Transvaginal ultrasound: If the cervical length is more than 15 mm in singletons or more than 25 mm in twins, the risk of delivery within the subsequent 7 days is less than 1%. If the cervix is less than the above figures (positive test), the risk of PTD increases significantly.
- Foetal fibronectin test: Delivery occurs in about 25% of those with a positive foetal fibronectin result and in 1.0% of those with a negative result.

If your test is positive in either of the above two methods, the following will be done:
- You will be admitted into the hospital.
- You will be offered painkillers.
- You will be screened for possible infection with blood, urine, and vaginal swab tests.
- Your baby will be monitored with CTG, and scan will be done to check his or her growth, liquor volume, and blood flow.
- You will be given steroid to accelerate the maturation of your baby's lungs so that he or she can adapt adequately to life outside the womb if you deliver.
- You will be given treatment to stop the contractions for 48 hours; this period is needed for the steroid to act on your baby's lung.
- You will be transferred to another hospital, where your baby can be taken care of adequately if you deliver, if your primary hospital is full or it is not equipped enough to take care of premature babies at your age of pregnancy. During transfer, you will be on treatment to stop contractions.

225

You will be in the hospital for at least 24 hours; if everything is all right, you will be discharged home, and your pregnancy will be reclassified to the high risk category if you are not already in that group. If you screen negative with any of the tests above, you will be reassured and discharged home unless the contraction pain is so severe that you need much painkillers; your situation will then be reassessed a few hours later.

PRETERM DELIVERY

INTRODUCTION
Preterm delivery is defined as birth between age of viability and 37 completed weeks of pregnancy. Age of foetal viability is the age at which the baby can survive if delivered. It depends on the level of care given when the baby is born. In most countries of the world, this age is 24 completed weeks of pregnancy, but in developing countries, for example Sub-Saharan Africa, it is likely to be 28 weeks of pregnancy.

The overall prevalence of spontaneous delivery before 34 weeks is about 1 in 100 pregnant women when cases due to foetal abnormalities are excluded. However, some believe that the incidence is 7 out of every 100 deliveries before the thirty-seventh week of pregnancy. If you have any reason to think that your labour may be starting early, get in touch with your doctor or midwife straightaway.

CLASSIFICATION OF PRETERM DELIVERY
Preterm deliveries are classified according to the age at delivery into the following:
- Extreme PTD (<28 weeks)
- Early PTD (28 to <31 weeks)
- Moderate PTD (31 to <34 weeks)
- Mild PTD (34 to <37 weeks) which constitutes the majority of preterm birth

CAUSES
- Medical reasons, mainly PE and FGR in 1/3 of cases.
- Spontaneous PTD due to premature onset of labour or preterm pre-labour rupture of the membranes (PPROM). This accounts for 2/3 of the cases of preterm deliveries.
- Multiple pregnancy.
- Others.

IMPACT OF PRETERM DELIVERY
- LBW.
- Greater risk for a serious lung condition, known as respiratory distress syndrome (RDS).

- Underdeveloped organs or systems.
- Greater risk for life-threatening infections.
- Problem with feeding.
- Need for admission and sometimes transfer of the baby to another hospital after birth.
- Increased incidence of stillbirths and neonatal death (during the first 4 weeks of life) mainly in the extreme, early, and moderate subgroups.
- Heart problems (patent ductus arteriosus PDA and low blood pressure). PDA affects babies born before 30 weeks. It is a persistent opening between two major blood vessels in the heart. It can close on its own but if it doesn't and is left untreated it can cause heart failure.
- Bleeding in the brain in labour for babies born before 28 weeks. Most bleeding resolve with little short-term impact. But some babies may have larger brain bleeding which causes permanent brain injury leading to accumulation of fluids in the brain over several weeks and requiring surgery.
- Poor temperature control in babies. Babies can lose body heat rapidly because they don't have the stored body fat of a full-term infant and they can't generate enough heat to counteract what's lost through the surface of their bodies.
- The earlier a baby is born, the greater his or her risk is of developing bowel problem called necrotizing enterocolitis (NEC). The cells lining the bowel wall are injured premature baby starts feeding. Breast milk reduces the incidence of the condition.
- Anaemia in the newborn
- Low level of blood sugar (hypoglycaemia) because preterm babies have smaller stores of glycogen (stored glucose) than do full-term babies and also their immature livers have trouble producing glucose.

LONG-TERM IMPACTS
- Cerebral palsy which is a disorder of the brain
- Impaired developmental milestones.
- Behavioural and psychological problems such as attention deficit hyperactivity disorder, depression or generalized anxiety, and difficulties interacting with kids of their own age.
- Eye problem called retinopathy of prematurity in those born before 30 weeks – vision may be impaired.
- Increased risk of hearing loss
- High risk of chronic health issues in the future and sudden infant death syndrome (SIDS).

SCREENING FOR PRETERM BIRTH

Screening is necessary to predict the 2/3 cases that contribute to spontaneous PTD before 34 weeks. As far as screening for PTD is concerned, pregnant women are classified into two categories.

- Those with previous late miscarriage or spontaneous PTD, that is high-risk group for PTD; they contribute 15 out of 100 cases of PTD and constitute 3 out of 100 pregnancy population.
- Those in their first pregnancy or had previous pregnancies which resulted in deliveries at term, that is low-risk group; they contribute 85 out of 100 cases of PTD and constitute 97 out of 100 pregnancy population.

Consequently, any strategy at reducing the rate of PTD that is focused only on the high-risk group would have a very small impact on the overall rate of PTD. The best recommended strategy, therefore, is that every pregnant woman should be screened for the risk of preterm delivery PTD, starting from $11-13^{+6}$ weeks(when nuchal screen is normally carried out). Methods that are used for the screening are as follows:

- Maternal factors and obstetric history
- Cervical length at 11-13 and 22-24 weeks or 22-24 weeks alone
- Cervicovaginal foetal fibronectin at 22-24 weeks
- Combined screening strategy (cervical length and maternal and obstetric history)

MATERNAL FACTORS AND OBSTETRIC HISTORY

The risk of a pregnancy ending in PTD is increased in the following circumstances:

- Low maternal height.
- Older women.
- African racial origin.
- Cigarette smoking in pregnancy.
- Getting pregnant after using ovulation-induction drugs.
- Previous miscarriage between 16 and 23 weeks and 6 days.
- Previous spontaneous preterm deliveries. The lower the age of pregnancy at which the previous PTD occurred and the more the number of previous PTD, the more the chance of having preterm birth in the index pregnancy. Previous term delivery confers some protection against preterm birth.
- Maternal blood levels of PAPP-A, which is a substance produced by the placenta, is reduced at $11-13^{+6}$ weeks in those who end up with preterm labour.

CERVICAL LENGTH AT 11-13 AND 22-24 WEEKS OR 22-24 WEEKS ALONE

Cervical length is measured by transvaginal ultrasound. The normal value is 32.4 mm. The smaller the cervical length, the more the risk of spontaneous PTD. Specifically, the risk of PTD is significantly increased in the following situations:

- You are carrying one baby and the length of the cervix is 15 mm or less.
- You are carrying more than one baby and the length of the cervix is **25 mm or less.**

Generally, it is better measuring cervical length at 11-13 weeks for the following reasons:

- Early detection of cervical incompetence or short cervix
- Early treatment in detected cases

COMBINED SCREENING STRATEGY
(CERVICAL LENGTH, MATERNAL, AND OBSTETRIC HISTORY)

This strategy provides a better prediction of spontaneous preterm birth than either factor alone. This screening strategy is not offered in every hospital. Discuss with your GP or midwife; they should be able to refer you to a hospital or clinic where the service is offered. The screening is important because if you are found to be at risk of PTD, something can be done to at least reduce that risk.

CERVICOVAGINAL FOETAL FIBRONECTIN AT 22-24 WEEKS

Foetal fibronectin is a substance produced by the cells in the amniotic fluid and is also produced by your baby in the early stages of development. It acts as a glue that binds the foetal sac to the uterine lining. Level is assessed by taking a swab from the vagina. A positive test (higher than what the normal level should be) is applied as follows:

- The test is performed at 22-24 weeks in other to predict those women who are likely to deliver before 34 weeks of pregnancy. It is positive in 4% of pregnant women population but also in 25% of those who deliver before 34 weeks.
- Prediction of the likelihood of threatened preterm labour or early preterm labour progressing into fully established preterm labour.

PREVENTION OF PRETERM BIRTH

Management varies in different countries and units. A more flexible approach is as follows:

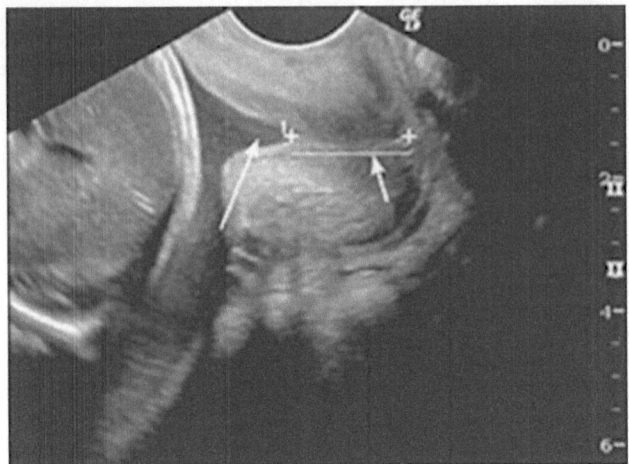

Figure 140. Cervical length measurement

CERVICAL LENGTH OF 15 MM OR LESS IN A LOW-RISK POPULATION

If the length of the cervix is less than 15 mm at the mid-trimester scan of 20-23 weeks, you would be offered prophylactic progesterone (vaginal pessary of 200 mg per night) from 20 to 34 weeks of pregnancy. You will be followed up with cervical scan at 26, 28, 32, and 34 weeks apart from your regular scans. At any stage if the cervix is 10 mm long or less, you would be given steroid to accelerate the maturity of the baby's lungs in case you go into labour early. This management should reduce the risk of extreme and early PTD by about 25%. Some obstetrician will offer minor operation—cervical stitch instead of progesterone if the scan is offered at 11-13[+6] weeks.

PREVIOUS HISTORY OF SPONTANEOUS SECOND-TRIMESTER (14-24 WEEKS) MISCARRIAGE OR PRETERM DELIVERY

If you have a history of one of such events in the past, your risk of recurrence is 5-10% before 34 weeks of pregnancy. The risk is reduced by

- giving you vaginal progesterone pessary every night from 22 to 34 weeks of pregnancy.
- having serial scans (16, 18, 20, and 22 weeks) to measure cervical length, and if the length is reduced to less than 25 mm, then cervical stitch will be inserted.

If you have a history of two or more of such events, your risk of recurrence is about 20%. The risk is reduced by

- giving you vaginal progesterone every night from 20 to 34 weeks.
- inserting cervical stitch after the twelfth-week scan has excluded major foetal defects.

MULTIPLE PREGNANCY

It is important to note that although multiple pregnancy is associated with a high risk of PTD, cervical stitch is not used at all to prevent it. It can actually increase the risk of PTD. Progesterone vaginal pessary can be used.

MANAGEMENT OF ACTUAL PRETERM LABOUR

Management depends on the GA, and as already stated, you will have your baby in a unit that is well equipped to deal with the problems of preterm babies.

34-36^{+6} WEEKS

Labour can be induced if necessary. Management as in term pregnancy except the following:
- Epidural anaesthesia is the preferred method of pain relief in labour.
- Forceps is preferred to ventouse if instrumental delivery is indicated.
- It is preferable that your baby is delivered in his or her water bags.

LESS THAN 34 WEEKS

We do not know the most appropriate mode of delivery at this GA—vaginal or Caesarean section. However, recent evidence suggests that Caesarean section cannot be recommended unless there are other obstetric indications to justify it. You are, therefore, more likely to be offered vaginal birth instead of Caesarean section.

IOL is rarely offered. During labour, the following will happen:
- Baby's heart is traced continuously.
- Obstetrician may proceed straight to Caesarean section, without taking blood from the baby's head to confirm whether it is in distress or not, if there is any abnormality on the CTG tracing.
- Forceps delivery is allowed but ventouse is contraindicated because it can cause significant problem in your baby.
- A drip to contract the womb will be offered if you are not progressing adequately in labour.
- Epidural anaesthesia is the preferred method of pain relief in labour.
- It is preferable that your baby is delivered in his or her water bags.
- A paediatrician must be there at delivery, and depending on the gestation, a special baby cot should be present, too.

CERVICAL LENGTH AND ITS CLINICAL APPLICATIONS IN OBSTETRIC PRACTICE

Measurement of cervical length with ultrasound is clinically useful in the following situations:
- Prediction of PTD in both low and high-risk patients.

- Prediction of the likelihood of delivery within subsequent 7 days if you present with threatened preterm labour.
- Polyhydramnios: If you have too much fluid around your baby during the second or early third trimester of pregnancy, measurement of cervical length will determine the risk of PTD and therefore the need to tap out some of the fluids (amniodrainage).
- Planned elective Caesarean section: Measurement of cervical length at 37 weeks can help in deciding whether to carry out the delivery at 38-39 weeks and therefore prevent emergency surgery if you go into labour or delay the operation until after 39 weeks.
- IOL: The pre-induction cervical length gives useful prediction of the induction-to-delivery interval and the likelihood of vaginal delivery and Caesarean section.
- Prolonged pregnancies: Measurement of cervical length at 40-41 weeks can predict the likelihood of spontaneous onset of labour and vaginal delivery over the subsequent 10 days.

WHEN YOUR WATERS BREAK EARLY (24-37 WEEKS) BEFORE LABOUR

Normally, your waters break just before labour starts, once labour has started, or during labour. If it happens before labour starts between 24 and 37 weeks, it means that your waters have broken earlier than normal and is called PPROM. The amount of amniotic fluid you lose may vary from a trickle, making you feel damp, to a gush; it is clear or slightly pink. About 2 out of every 100 women experience PPROM during pregnancy, but it is associated with 40 out of 100 preterm deliveries.

CAUSES
In most cases, the cause is not known. There is a link between PPROM and the growth of certain bugs called BV in the vagina. These bacteria produce a substance called enzyme which can weaken the amniotic membranes and cause the waters to break. It is unlikely that anything that you have done caused your waters to break early, neither is there anything that could have been done to prevent it happening.

RISK TO YOUR BABY
- There can be preterm delivery.
- There can be infection in the womb called chorioamnionitis, which can trigger a preterm birth and infection of your baby.
- The lungs may fail to expand (pulmonary hypoplasia). The amniotic fluid is needed for the baby's lungs to develop. If the waters break very early

in the second trimester, there may not be enough fluid for your baby's lungs to develop normally, and therefore, the lungs will be small.

- There is also a small risk of foetal death, and also baby can die during the first month after birth. It is worse if your waters have broken before 24 weeks and you give birth; in this situation, sadly, it is unlikely that your baby will survive. Babies who do survive are likely to have serious health problems.

Risks to You

Infection of the fluid surrounding the baby (clinical chorioamnionitis) presents as following:

- Temperature increases.
- Heart rate increases.
- Pain when feeling the womb.
- Offensive vaginal discharge.
- Blood test showing high levels of inflammatory markers, for example white cells.
- Bugs can be cultured from the amniotic fluid; the bugs increase the risks of PTD, neonatal sepsis, and cerebral palsy.
- CTG showing increased heart rate of your baby.

Diagnosis

If you think that you are leaking fluid from the vagina, it is advisable to wear a sanitary pad (not a tampon) and monitor the colour and smell of the fluid, as well as how much is leaking. Sometimes, the leaking fluid may be urine. Amniotic fluid smells different from the smell of urine. If you think the fluid is amniotic fluid, contact your local hospital or midwife immediately.

The diagnosis is based on the following:

- A history suggestive of spontaneous rupture of membranes.
- A speculum examination demonstrating pooling of fluid in the vagina.
- Internal examination with the fingers will not be performed unless there is a strong suspicion that you may be in labour. This is because bugs may be transported from the vagina into the cervix leading to infection inside the womb, and also, your body may release natural prostaglandin, which may cause preterm labour.
- A swab test called AmniSure or Actim PROM has been shown to be very accurate in the diagnosis of PPROM.
- CTG is useful, and indeed, increased FHR is used in the diagnosis of water infection.
- Ultrasound scan to check liquor volume, growth, blood flow, foetal movements, and tone can be carried out, but it is of limited value in

predicting foetal infection. It can demonstrate less fluid around your baby and may help with the diagnosis.

If it is confirmed by various tests that your waters have not broken down, you will be discharged home. If a very small amount of amniotic fluid leaks out, it may not be easy to confirm that your waters have broken down. If you go home and continue to leak fluid, you should return to the hospital for a further check-up.

INVESTIGATION

The tests are meant to rule out infection. They are as follows:
- Blood test
- Vaginal swab
- Urine test
- Ultrasound, as above

FURTHER MANAGEMENT

On presentation to the hospital, if the diagnosis of PPROM is confirmed, you will be admitted into the hospital for about 48 hours; within that time, if you have a subclinical infection and you are to go into labour, it will happen. If you do not go into labour within this time interval, you will be managed at home. The primary aim of further management is to timely identify infection of the placenta and the water bag (chorioamnionitis). It can be prevented by the following recommendations:
- Avoidance of vaginal sex.
- Regular monitoring for signs of labour, mainly contractions.
- Checking your temperature, pulse, and heart rate every 8-12 hours. A normal temperature is 37 or less, and your pulse should be less than 90 bpm.
- Checking the colour of the amniotic fluid that is coming out. You should wear a sanitary pad rather than a tampon.
- Regular trace of baby's heart; if you are being managed at home, you may need to go to the hospital 2-3 times a week for foetal monitoring.
- Weekly ultrasound scan to measure the amount of amniotic fluid around your baby and his or her blood flow and 2 weekly scan for growth.
- Procedures that do not have sufficient evidence to support their application include
  - Weekly blood tests and vaginal swab for sign of infection.
  - Infusing fluids into the amniotic space (amnioinfusion) when PPROM occurs very early in the second trimester to enhance the development of the lungs.
  - Sealing the hole in the amniotic membrane with fibrin sealants when PPROM occurs in the second trimester.

WHEN TO CALL FOR HELP IF MANAGED AT HOME

Contact your doctor and/or return to the hospital immediately if you experience any of the following:
- raised temperature (more than 37°C)
- foetal movements are not normal
- flu-like symptoms (feeling hot and shivery and achy)
- vaginal bleeding
- leaking fluid becomes greenish or smelly
- abdominal pain
- contractions

TREATMENT

There is no treatment that can replace the fluid, but the baby's kidneys will continue to produce amniotic fluid. You may continue to leak fluids for the rest of the pregnancy. The purpose of the treatment is to prevent infection and help get ready for birth.

The following treatment will be offered:
- A 10-day course of antibiotic erythromycin is administered since it is associated with significant reduction of the following:
  - infection of the placenta and the water bags
  - neonatal infection
  - numbers of babies born within 48 hours
  - number of babies with an abnormal brain scan prior to discharge from hospital
  - reduction of foetal death and baby's death within 1 month of birth
- Erythromycin will still be given if GBS has been isolated in the past or at presentation from the vagina or urine, but many obstetricians will give intravenous benzylpenicillin instead, and if within 24-48 hours you do not go into labour, they will change to erythromycin.
- Steroid should be given to you. It does not increase the risk of infection in you nor in your baby. It reduces the chance of the following occurring in your baby if you deliver prematurely:
  - breathing problems
  - bleeding in the brain
  - bowel destruction (necrotising enterocolitis)
  - death in the first month of life (neonatal death)
- Drug to stop contraction can be given if you are to be transferred to a hospital with better facilities. It may also be used if more time is needed for the steroids to work.

DELIVERY

The recommendation is that delivery should be considered from 34 weeks of pregnancy. If you are delivered at 34 weeks or less, baby is likely to suffer from prematurity more than if you were delivered at 36 and more weeks. However, the presentation of the prematurity at 34 weeks is not severe, mainly in the form of high bilirubin levels and transient breathing problems. All other problems of prematurity are the same from 34 to 37 weeks. Where expectant management is considered beyond 34 weeks, the risk of chorioamnionitis increases.

SOURCES

- Beta J, Akolekar R, Ventura W, Syngelaki A, Nicolaides KH. Prediction of spontaneous preterm delivery from maternal factors, obstetric history and placental perfusion and function at 11-13 weeks. Prenatal Diag. 2011;31:75-83. doi: 10.1002/pd.2662.
- Guideline for Practice. Harris Birthright Research Centre for Fetal Medicine, King's College Hospital, London, 2011, 2012.
- Greco E, Lange A, Ushakov F, Calvo JR, Nicolaides KH. Prediction of spontaneous preterm delivery from endocervical length at 11 to 13 weeks. Prenatal Diag. 2011;31:84-89. Published online 28 December 2010.
- Royal College of Obstetricians and Gynaecologists (RCOG) Green-top Guideline No. 44. Preterm prelabour rupture of membranes, November 2006, October 2010.
- When your waters break early (preterm prelabour rupture of membranes). Information for you. RCOG, March 2008.

TWIN/MULTIPLE PREGNANCY

Generally, twins account for about 2% of all pregnancies. In developed countries e.g. the UK, about one in every 65 pregnancies is a twin. Triplets occur naturally in 1 in 10,000 pregnancies and quads are even rarer. The highest incidence of twin pregnancy in the whole world is in Nigeria but unfortunately, there is no valuable statistics from the country.

TYPES OF TWIN PREGNANCY AND THEIR CHARACTERISTICS

There are two types of twin pregnancy:
- Identical or monozygotic
- Non-identical or dizygotic

IDENTICAL OR MONOZYGOTIC TWINS

- They occur when a single egg is fertilised, and this fertilised egg splits into two to form two babies.

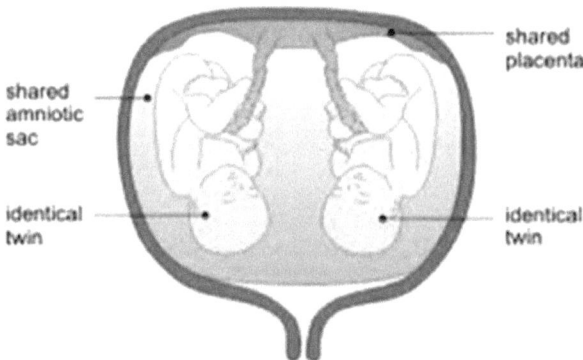

Figure 141. Twins with single placenta and single fluid sac—MCMA

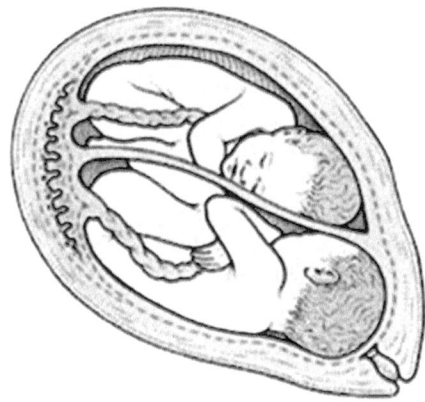

Figure 142. Single placenta but two fluid sacs—MCDA twins

- Each baby will have the same genes and therefore the same sex and look very alike.
- There may be sharing between the two babies of
  - the same placenta (MC pregnancy)
  - the same amniotic sac or inner membrane (monoamniotic pregnancy)
  - the same foetal organs (conjoined or Siamese twins)
- One-third of the monozygotic twin pregnancies have 2 placentae and two amniotic sacs and therefore called dichorionic diamniotic DCDA twins – one placenta and one sac for each baby. This happens when the fertilized egg splits into two during the 3rd – 4th day after conception.
- Two-thirds have only one placenta and one sac and therefore called monochorionic monoamniotic MCMA twins (1% of all twin pregnancies)

Prevalence of identical twins
- It may be similar in all ethnic groups (1 in 350-400 pregnancies).
- It does not run in a family.
- It does not vary with maternal age.
- It may be 2-3 times higher following assisted conception.

NON-IDENTICAL (DIZYGOTIC) TWINS
- They occur when two separate eggs are fertilised by two separate sperm at the same time and then implant into the uterus.
- Both babies will look no more alike than any other two brothers and sisters and may be of the same or different sexes.
- Each foetus or baby has its own placenta and amniotic sac (DCDA pregnancy)

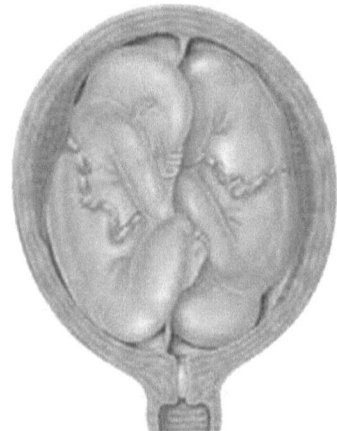

Figure 143. Two placenta and two fluid sacs—DCDA twins

Prevalence of non-identical twins
- It is more prevalent in blacks than in white women.
- It runs in the mother's side of the family.
- It increases with maternal age.
- The chance of having twins is higher, the more children you have already.
- It increases with assisted conception.

DETERMINATION OF THE TYPE OF TWINS
(NUMBER OF PLACENTAE AND NUMBER OF AMNIOTIC SACS)
The best way to do that is by ultrasound scan at 11-13^{+6} weeks, in which case the chance of confirming the number of placentae and amniotic sacs is about 100%. The diagnosis on ultrasound is as follows:

- One placenta and one amniotic sac for both babies i.e. monochorionic monoamniotic twins MCMA
- One placenta but two sacs i.e. monochorionic diamniotic twins MCDA.
- Two placentae and two sacs i.e. dichorionic diamniotic twins DCDA
- Triplets
- And so on.

The older the pregnancy, the more difficult it is to confirm the type of twins pregnancy. Thus, by 20 weeks, only 85% of DC pregnancies can be confirmed.

COMPLICATIONS OF TWIN PREGNANCY

Chorionicity (number of placentae) is the main factor that determines pregnancy outcome as seen in the table below.

Pregnancy complication	Singleton pregnancy	DC twin	MC twin
Miscarriage after live baby at 11-13 weeks ultrasound or foetal death before 24 weeks	1%	2%	10% Due to severe early onset of TTTS or selective FGR
Perinatal mortality (death of baby from 24 weeks to 1 week after birth)	0.5%	2% Due to preterm birth in most cases	4% Due to preterm birth in most cases, TTTS and selective FGR
TTTS			15%
Selective FGR	5%	10%	15%
Risk of preterm birth between 24 and 32 weeks	1%	10%	10%
Prevalence of major structural defects	1%	1% in each of DC twins	4% in each of the twins

Table 9. Complications of multiple pregnancy

Other complications of twin pregnancy are as follows:
- Increased risk of
  - Early pregnancy symptoms, for example vomiting
  - Anaemia
  - Gestational diabetes
  - Pregnancy-induced hypertension (PIH)

- – Pre-eclampsia
- – Post-partum haemorrhage (PPH)
- – Instrumental delivery
- – Caesarean section
- Cord entanglement, for MCMA twins
- Twins reversed arterial perfusion sequence (the highest degree of TTTS) occurring in 1% of MCMA twins
- Foetal death of one of the twins
- One of the twins having birth defect.
- Conjoined twins occurring in around one in 90,000-100,000 pregnancies worldwide.

The last four complications including higher order multiple pregnancies are not treated in this edition of this book because of the technicalities involved. Such cases just like many other cases of twin pregnancy are managed in tertiary centres by foetal medicine consultants.

TTTS and Selective FGR
These two conditions occur when there is only one placenta (MC pregnancy).

Selective FGR
- It occurs in about 15% of MC twins, with poor growth of one of the twins and poor blood flow in the umbilical arteries of any of them.

Twin-to-Twin Transfusion Syndrome

Twin Pregnancy: Twin to Twin Transfusion

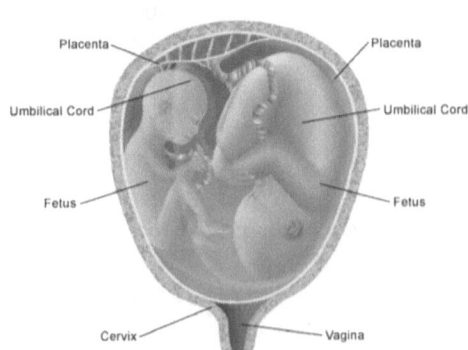

Figure 144. Twin-to-twin transfusion syndrome (Longitudinal section)

- In all MC twin pregnancies, there are blood vessels connections in the placenta which allow communication of blood circulation between the two babies.
- Imbalance in the net flow of blood across these blood vessels communications from one baby, the donor, to the other, the recipient, results in TTTS.
- In about 10% of MC twins, severe TTTS develops by 16-24 weeks with too much fluid (polyhydramnios) in the sac of the recipient foetus and no fluids (anhydramnios) in the sac of the donor twin. It means the first is producing too much urine, while the latter is not producing at all.

These conditions can be predicted or diagnosed at the $11\text{-}13^{+6}$ weeks scan with the following findings:
- More than 20% difference in the size CRL of the two babies.
- More than 20% difference in the NT of the two babies, of which the bigger baby has the bigger NT.
- More than 20% difference in the amniotic fluid of the two babies, of which the bigger baby has the bigger volume. Discrepancy in AFV is not found in selective FGR.
- Abnormal blood flow in the liver of one or both babies.

So if any of these findings is present at your dating scan, you should be referred to a specialised unit called 'foetal medicine unit' or at least to a doctor who has special interest in foetal medicine. Effective treatment for both severe TTTS and selective FGR is provided by doing keyhole surgery and separating the blood vessels in the placenta that join the blood flow between the two twins at less than 30 weeks; this is done using laser surgery. If the pregnancy has advanced more than 30 weeks, Caesarean section will be offered after giving you steroid to enhance the maturation of the baby's lungs.

The laser surgery is offered only in specialised centres in developed countries. It is not offered at all in developing countries. So if you are pregnant with twin pregnancy and you develop TTTS or selective FGR, discuss with your obstetrician about referral to a centre where the operation can be performed.

MANAGEMENT OF MC TWIN PREGNANCY
The management may be different in different centres, but the principle remains the same. We have illustrated here the practice at King's College Hospital, London, where a lot of research has been done in multiple pregnancy and other areas of foetal medicine.

The clinical schedules and appointments are as follows:
- $11\text{-}13^{+6}$ weeks: Dating scan as in singleton pregnancy.

- 16, 18, 20, 22, and 24 weeks: Ultrasound and review by a specialist in foetal medicine. Ultrasound examinations between 16 and 24 weeks focus primarily on detection of TTTS, selective FGR, and assessment of cervical length to predict the risk of preterm birth. At 22 weeks, ultrasound for foetal abnormalities and a specialised heart scan will also be performed.
- 28, 32, 34, and 36 weeks: Ultrasound and review is performed mainly for growth, liquor volume, and blood flow studies. TTTS is uncommon from 24 weeks, so the main focus is on the growth of the baby.

If there is no complication, delivery will be considered at 36 weeks. Many units deliver MC twins by elective Caesarean section because of 10% risk of acute TTTS in labour. Others go for vaginal delivery, provided the first baby is presenting by the head. Continuous foetal heartbeat monitoring will be in place.

MANAGEMENT OF DC TWINS

This pregnancy is associated with an increased risk of preterm birth and poor foetal growth; therefore, the clinic schedules and scan are as follows:

- 11-13^{+6} weeks: Dating scan as in singleton pregnancy.
- 18, 20, 22, and 24 weeks: To assess cervical length and growth. Ultrasound for observing foetal abnormalities is also performed at 22 weeks.
- 28, 32, and 36 weeks: Growth scan and review by doctor.

If poor foetal growth is identified in one of the foetuses, delivery will be considered if there is gross change in the blood flow in the umbilical artery after 32 weeks or gross change in the special vein in the liver called ductus venosus at 28-32 weeks. If all is well, delivery is carried out at 37-38 weeks, and vaginal birth if the first baby or both babies are presenting with the head, but Caesarean section will be offered if the first twin is breech. Many obstetricians will perform Caesarean section for all types of presentation except when both twins are presenting with the head.

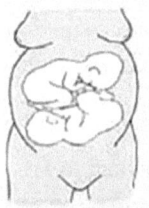 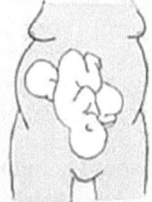 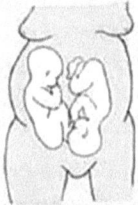 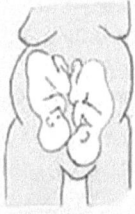 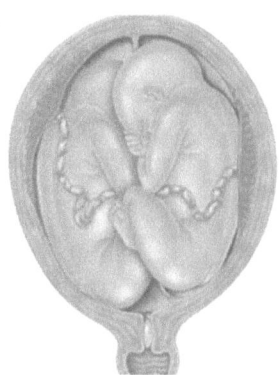

When both babies are sideways, they cannot be born through the vagina. It is very dangerous to try to deliver them at home.

When one head is down, it is a little less dangerous to deliver at home. If the head-down baby is born first, the other baby may turn.

It is even better if both babies are up and down. But a breech twin will have the same dangers as all breech babies.

It is best if both babies are head down, but it is still more dangerous than a single birth.

Figure 145. Presentation in twins

SCREENING FOR CHROMOSOMAL ABNORMALITIES

DIZYGOTIC TWINS

- The maternal age-related risk for chromosomal abnormalities for each foetus is the same as in singleton pregnancies. Therefore, the chance that at least one foetus is affected by a chromosomal defect is twice as high as in singleton pregnancies.
- Screening for Down's syndrome is by combined ultrasound and biochemical tests at 11-13 weeks as in singleton pregnancy. If the risk is more than 1 in 150 in either of the two foetuses, CVS will be offered.
- In DC twins, the detection rate DR (about 90%) and false positive rate FPR (3% per foetus or 6% per pregnancy) are similar to those in singleton pregnancies.
- If one foetus is dead and the GA is less than 9 weeks, the combined screening test as in singleton pregnancy will be used to calculate the risk of chromosomal abnormalities. However, the fact that it is a twin pregnancy with one dead foetus should be noted. If the death is after 9 weeks, then the biochemical tests will not be included; only ultrasound and maternal age will be used to assess the risk of chromosomal abnormality.

MONOZYGOTIC TWINS

- The risk for a chromosomal abnormality affecting both foetuses is the same as in singleton pregnancies.
- MC twins are monozygotic, and they are invariably concordant for foetal karyotype. However, in chromosomal abnormal foetuses, there is often discordancy in NT.

- The risk for trisomy 21 is calculated for each foetus, based on maternal age, ultrasound findings, and maternal biochemical tests, and then the average risk between the two foetuses is considered to be the risk for the pregnancy as a whole. If the risk is more than 1 in 150 for any of the babies, CVS will be offered.
- False-positive rate of screening (8% per pregnancy) is higher than in DC twins, because increased NT in at least one of the foetuses may be an early manifestation of TTTS.

AMNIOCENTESIS AND CVS IN TWINS

- In the case of amniocentesis, the procedure-related foetal loss rate is 1-2%. The amniocentesis in twins is effective in providing a reliable karyotype for both foetuses.
- In the case of CVS, the procedure-related foetal loss rate is also 1-2%, but in about 1% of cases, there may be a diagnostic error, either due to sampling the same placenta twice or due to cross-contamination.
- In pregnancies where one of the foetuses has chromosomal abnormality, the main options available are either selective foeticide, that is killing the foetus by injecting a substance called potassium chloride into its heart, or expectant management. Selective foeticide after 16 weeks of gestation is associated with three-fold increase in the risk of spontaneous abortion compared to the same procedure before 16 weeks. Therefore, CVS is better than amniocentesis.

LABOUR AND DELIVERY OF TWINS

If you are expecting twins, labour may start early because of the increased size of the uterus. It is unusual for multiple pregnancy to go beyond 38 weeks. Many health professionals will usually be present at the birth. For example, there should be two midwives, an obstetrician, and two paediatricians (one for each baby). Babies will be closely monitored with EFM, and a scalp clip might be fitted on the first baby once the waters have broken.

You will be given a drip in case it is needed later, and an epidural is usually recommended. Once the first baby has been born, the midwife or doctor will check the position of the second by feeling your abdomen and doing a vaginal examination. If the second baby is in a good position to be born, the waters surrounding the baby will be broken, and the second baby should be born very soon after the first because the cervix is already fully dilated. If contractions stop, a hormones drip will be started, or if it is already ongoing, its rate will be increased to enhance contractions. Triplets and higher order multiple pregnancies are always delivered by elective Caesarean section.

Sources

- RCOG Green-top Guideline No. 51. Management of monochorionic twin pregnancy, December 2008.
- Kagan KO, Gazzoni A, Sepulveda G, Sotiriadis A, Nicolaides KH. Discordance in nuchal translucency thickness in the prediction of severe twin-to-twin transfusion syndrome. Ultrasound Obstet Gynecol. 2007;29:527-32.
- Vandecruys H, Avgidou K, Surerus E, Flack N, Nicolaides KH. Dilemmas in the management of twins discordant for anencephaly diagnosed at 11+0 to 13+6 weeks of gestation. Ultrasound Obstet Gynecol. 2006;28:653-58. doi: 10.1002/uog.2836.
- Sebire NJ, D'Ercole C, Soares W, Nayar R, Nicolaides KH. Intertwin disparity in foetal size in monochorionic and dichorionic pregnancies. Obstet Gynecol. 1998;91:82-5.
- Ville Y. Twin-to-twin transfusion syndrome: time to forget the Quintero staging system? Ultrasound Obstet Gynecol 2007; 30: 924-927. DOI: 10.1002/uog.5221

Post-Date Pregnancy

Normal length of pregnancy is between 37 and 42 weeks. Post-date pregnancy is when the pregnancy lasts more than 42 weeks, and it occurs in 5-10% of pregnancies. Most women will go into labour within 39-41 weeks. If your labour does not start by 41 weeks, your midwife or doctor will offer you a 'membrane sweep'. This involves having a vaginal examination, which stimulates the neck of your uterus to produce hormones which may trigger natural labour. They will also suggest a date to have your labour induced (started off) before 42 weeks.

If you don't want labour to be induced and your pregnancy continues to 42 weeks or beyond, you and your baby will be monitored. Your midwife or doctor will check that both you and your baby are healthy by doing ultrasound scan for you and checking your baby's movement and heartbeat. If your baby is showing signs of distress, your doctor or midwife will again suggest that labour needs to be induced or you have a Caesarean section.

Risks of Post-Date Pregnancy
- There can be birth trauma.
- The chance of delivering a dead baby (stillbirth), baby dying within 1 week of birth (neonatal death), and further death after that (post-neonatal death) is 2.8 per 1,000 pregnancies over 41 weeks, but 4.8 per 1,000 pregnancies over 42 weeks gestation.

- There is no significant increase in admissions of newborns to a neonatal unit, baby aspirating his or her own poo (meconium aspiration) or low Apgar scores with expectant management beyond 42 weeks compared with induction of labour between 41 and 42 weeks.
- The placenta may not work well, and therefore, the foetus may show signs of distress in labour.
- The amount of fluid around the baby may decrease. This may cause the umbilical cord to become compressed before or during labour.
- The foetus grows larger, which may cause some problems during birth.
- The foetus or newborn may have post-maturity syndrome. Babies with this syndrome can have loss of fat, wrinkled and peeling skin, long nails, low blood sugar, and are at risk of stillbirth.
- There may be a greater chance of Caesarean birth compared with delivering the baby before 42 weeks.

We strongly believe that prevention and management of post-date pregnancy should be carried out in a specialised clinic called 'post-date clinic', as practised at the University College London Hospital (UCLH).

POST-DATE CLINIC

All women attending for routine maternity care should be referred to this pregnancy clinic at 40^{+4}-41^{+3} weeks of gestation. Exclusions are as follows:
- if you require delivery prior to 40^{+4} weeks
- if you request 'social' IOL prior to 40^{+4} weeks
- if you have multiple pregnancy

AIM OF THE CLINIC

- To provide a standardised assessment of all women at risk of post-date pregnancy, giving them consistent advice and booking IOL through one central point within a maternity unit.
- To predict the likelihood of delivery in the following 7-10 days.
- To ascertain factors that may necessitate early delivery or close monitoring.
- To manage women who are planning vaginal birth after Caesarean (VBAC) section, where induction should be avoided.
- To diagnose other associated obstetric conditions namely breech presentation, which should benefit from elective Caesarean section, oligohydramnios, and FGR for which immediate IOL with close monitoring should be applied.

THE PROCEDURE AT THE CLINIC

- Assessment of your height and weight and Calculation of your BMI and BP.
- Urine test.
- Abdominal ultrasound scan for foetal presentation, placental position, growth, liquor volume, and blood flow in your baby's blood vessels.
- Transvaginal scan to measure cervical length and exclude low-lying placenta or blood vessels under the presenting part PP (vasa praevia). Cervical length is the best predictor of the likelihood of spontaneous delivery in the next 7-10 days.
- Review by a midwife or by a doctor, which can complement the ultrasound findings.
  - Enquire about general health, including foetal movements.
  - Assess the SFH, lie, presentation, and engagement of your baby by feeling your tummy.
  - Discuss your chance of going into spontaneous labour within the following 7-10 days.
  - Offer you a membrane sweep.
  - Discuss process of IOL.
  - Agree on a management plan as outlined below.

HIGH-RISK PREGNANCY

Immediate induction if

- the BP is 140/90 mmHg or more.
- the estimated foetal weight is below the fifth centile.
- the deepest pool of amniotic fluid is less than 1.5 cm.

Immediate elective Caesarean section if

- the head is not presenting.
- the placenta is low or a blood vessel is in front of the PP.
- there is abnormal blood flow in the umbilical artery.

LOW-RISK PREGNANCY—NONE OF THE ABOVE
RISK FACTOR IS PRESENT

- You will be counselled by your doctor on your chance of going into spontaneous labour within the following 7-10 days on the basis of your cervical length, whether you have had a baby in the past or not (parity), and your BMI. The chance is higher if you have had a baby in the past (parous woman) than those who never had (nulliparous women). The lower your BMI and cervical length, the higher the chance of going into labour spontaneously. This principle is not yet universally adapted into clinical practice. However, it is the practice at the UCLH, where a special algorithm is used, and the outcome so far is encouraging.

- IOL will be booked for 41-41^{+6} weeks due to the gradual but significant increase in the stillbirth rate from 40 to 43 weeks and longer. About 80% of women go into spontaneous labour within 7-10 days after 40 weeks, and in this group, the Caesarean section rate is about 15%, whereas in those who do not go into spontaneous labour and require induction, the Caesarean section rate is about 35%.

- If you refuse IOL at 41^{+6} weeks, you will be offered a sweep and stretch of the cervix, but you should know that the chance of stillbirth increases. You will, therefore, be offered monitoring in maternity day unit beyond 42 weeks with twice weekly trace of baby's and one ultrasound clinic to assess amniotic fluid volume AFV. If any of the high risk criteria is identified, you will be offered again either IOL or Caesarean section.

TIMING FOR ELECTIVE CAESAREAN SECTION

Normally, elective Caesarean section at term is planned from 39 weeks. This is because the risk of breathing problems in newly born babies is halved with each completed week of pregnancy between 37 and 41 weeks. Unfortunately, delaying the operation beyond 38 weeks will result in many women going into spontaneous labour, and consequently, an elective procedure will be converted into an emergency one with increased risk to you.

Therefore, if you have been planned for elective Caesarean section from 39 weeks, there may be the need to predict if you will go into labour before the planned date. This is done by doing a transvaginal scan at 37 weeks and measuring cervical length, which can predict spontaneous onset of labour and delivery at term. If your cervical length is less than 20 mm, there is a 95% chance of you going into labour spontaneously before 40 weeks. In such situation, it may be reasonable to do your Caesarean section at 38-39 weeks (after giving you steroid for baby's lungs) to avoid the increased risk associated with possible emergency as compared with elective surgery.

If your cervical length is more than 30 mm, there is a 95% chance that spontaneous onset of labour will not occur before 40 weeks. In such situation, elective Caesarean section could be delayed until 40 weeks (provided there is no other risk to you or your baby) to reduce neonatal breathing problems.

SOURCES

- Nicolaides K. Protocol for the Prolonged Pregnancy Clinic. London: UCLH; 2009.
- Induction of Labour. NICE Clinical Guideline, 2008.

- Sanchez-Ramos L, Felicia O, Delke I, Kaunitz AM. Labour induction versus expectant management for post term pregnancies: a systematic review with meta-analysis. Obstetrics Gynaecol. 2003;101(6):1312-18.
- Hilder L, Costeloe K, Thilaganathan B. Prospective risk of stillbirth. BMJ. 2000;320:444. doi: 10.1136/bmj.320.7232.444/a (published 12 February 2000).

VAGINAL BLEEDING IN PREGNANCY

INTRODUCTION

It is classified into the following categories:
- Vaginal bleeding in early and mid-pregnancy (up to 23^{+6} weeks)
- Vaginal bleeding from 24 weeks till delivery (antepartum haemorrhage, APH)
- Vaginal bleeding after delivery (PPH)

Vaginal bleeding in early pregnancy has been discussed in the Chapters on "Early Pregnancy Problems." In this chapter, we will concentrate on antepartum bleeding APH, while vaginal bleeding after childbirth is discussed in one of the 'Pregnancy series' called *"All you need to know about labour and childbirth."* The two books complement each other, and it would be appropriate to go through them.

VAGINAL BLEEDING FROM 24 WEEKS TILL DELIVERY (ANTEPARTUM HAEMORRHAGE APH)

Antepartum haemorrhage is defined as bleeding from or into the genital tract, occurring at any time from 24 weeks of pregnancy till delivery of the baby. It occurs in 3-5 out of 100 pregnancies. The most important causes are as follows:
- Low-lying placenta—placenta praevia
- Separation of the placenta from the womb—placental abruption
- Severe adherence of the placenta to the womb—placenta accreta
- Blood vessel in the amniotic membrane lying below the PP of the baby—vasa praevia

Other causes are

- Cervical ectropion: The outlet of the cervix is turned inside out so that the inner lining of the cervix is seen when doing a speculum examination.

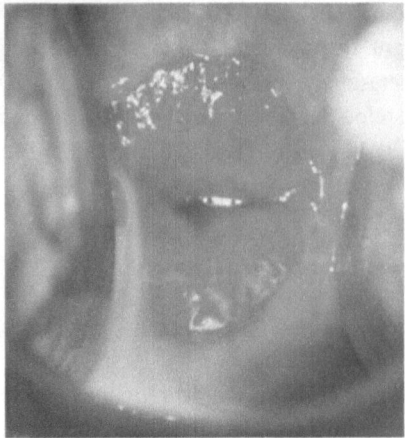

Figure 146. Cervical ectropion

- Cervical or endometrial poly: Small outgrowth from the lining of the womb or cervix.
- Cervical cancer.
- Vaginal infections.
- Small amount of blood mixed with mucus that is known as a 'show'. This is a sign that the cervix is changing and becoming ready for labour to start. You may see a "show" a few days before contractions start or during labour itself. A heavy show will be regarded as APH.

PLACENTA PRAEVIA

This is a low-lying placenta—the placenta is inserted wholly or in part into the lower part of the uterus. It is classified into the following types by ultrasound imaging (page):
- major placenta praevia, if the placenta lies over the internal cervical os, as shown.
- minor or partial placenta praevia, if the leading edge of the placenta is in the lower uterine segment but not covering the cervical os, that is within 6 cm of the internal os.

RISK FACTORS FOR PLACENTA PRAEVIA

The following are the factors that can predispose you to developing placenta praevia:
- Previous placenta praevia
- Multiparity (means you have at least 1 child and you are now pregnant)
- You are 40 or more years old
- Multiple pregnancy
- Smoking

- Deficient inner lining of the womb (endometrium) due to the presence or history of
    - uterine scar, for example from previous Caesarean section (the more the number of Caesarean section, the more the risk), previous operation on the womb like removing a fibroid
    - inflammation of the inner lining of the womb called endometritis
    - manual removal of placenta after delivery
    - previous surgical TOP
    - fibroid under the inner lining of the womb
- Assisted conception

Unfortunately, using the above risk factors, APH cannot reliably be predicted, and there is limited evidence to support interventions to prevent it. The risk can be reduced by modifying the risk factors, for example smoking.

SCREENING AND DIAGNOSIS OF PLACENTA PRAEVIA
The following are suggestive of a low-lying placenta:
- Suspected vaginal bleeding after 20 weeks of gestation
- A high PP, an abnormal lie of your baby
- Painless or provoked bleeding, irrespective of previous imaging results

The definitive diagnosis usually relies on ultrasound imaging. Placenta that is low-lying at 22 weeks may not be so at 32 weeks. For 9 out of 10 women, the placenta has moved into the upper part of the uterus by 32 weeks of pregnancy.

PLACENTA ABRUPTION
This is a complication of pregnancy, whereby the placental lining separates from the womb; it occurs from 20 weeks of pregnancy till the time prior to birth. It is the most common cause of late pregnancy bleeding and occurs in 1% of pregnancies worldwide.

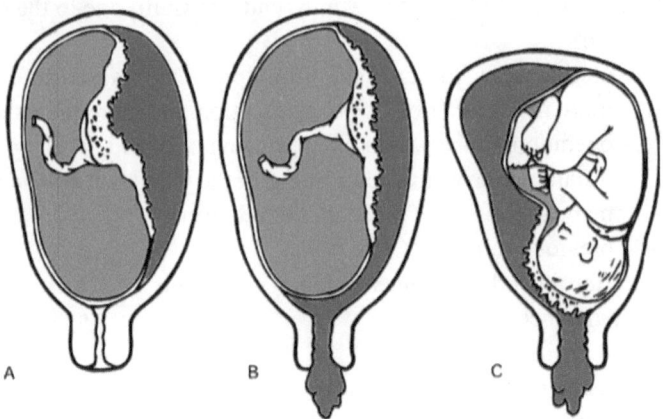

Figure 147. Premature separation of the placenta with bleeding—placenta abruption

RISK FACTORS FOR ABRUPTION

They are as follows:

- previous abruption
- pre-eclampsia
- FGR
- Baby's head is not presenting
- polyhydramnios
- advanced maternal age
- multiparity(when you already have 4 children and more)
- low BMI
- pregnancy following assisted reproductive techniques
- previous infection of the inner lining of the womb.
- when your waters goes early
- abdominal trauma (both accidental and those resulting from domestic violence)
- smoking and drug misuse (cocaine and amphetamines) during pregnancy
- threatened miscarriage
- Sticky blood problems.

Unfortunately, as in placenta praevia, using the above risk factors, APH cannot reliably be predicted, and there is limited evidence to support interventions to prevent it. The risk can be reduced by modifying the risk factors, for example smoking, not using drugs, and so on.

DIAGNOSIS OF PLACENTA ABRUPTION

It is a clinical diagnosis based on the following:

- Continuous abdominal pain.
- Uterus feels tense or 'woody' when feeling the tummy (on abdominal palpation).
- Uterine contractions may be there.
- Foetal compromise—trace of baby's heart may be abnormal.
- Vaginal bleeding.
- Ultrasound is poor at diagnosing placenta abruption; it can, however, easily pick up a big blood clot lying between the placenta and the womb.

SEVERE OR MORBIDLY ADHERENT PLACENTA

This situation exists when the placenta penetrates through the inner lining of the womb called decidua during pregnancy into and then through the muscle layer (myometrium); sometimes, the surrounding organs, for example the bladder in front or bowel in the back, can be invaded by the placenta.

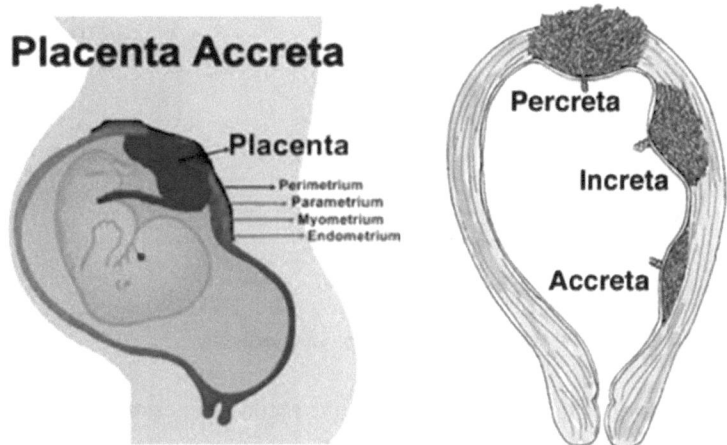

Figure 148a and b. Morbidly adherent placenta

RISK FACTORS FOR MORBIDLY ADHERENT
PLACENTA AND ITS DIAGNOSIS

If you had a previous Caesarean section and in your present pregnancy, you have placenta praevia or an anterior placenta overlying the old Caesarean section scar at 32 weeks of gestation, you are at increased risk of placenta accreta and should be managed as if you have it with appropriate preparations for surgery made. The diagnostic tools to be used are:

- ultrasound during pregnancy
- magnetic resonance imaging, which is a specialised imaging technique

VASA PRAEVIA

Vasa praevia describes foetal blood vessels running through the amniotic membranes over the internal cervical os (entrance into the womb) and below the foetal PP, unprotected by placental tissue or the umbilical cord (Figure xxx). The reported incidence varies between 1 in 2,000 and 1 in 6,000 pregnancies, but the condition may be under-reported.

RISK FACTORS FOR VASA PRAEVIA

- Placenta consisting of 2 lobes (bilobed placenta) or a small portion of it is separated from the main bulk but covered with the same membranes (succenturiate lobe). In this situation, the foetal vessels run through the membranes joining the separate lobes.

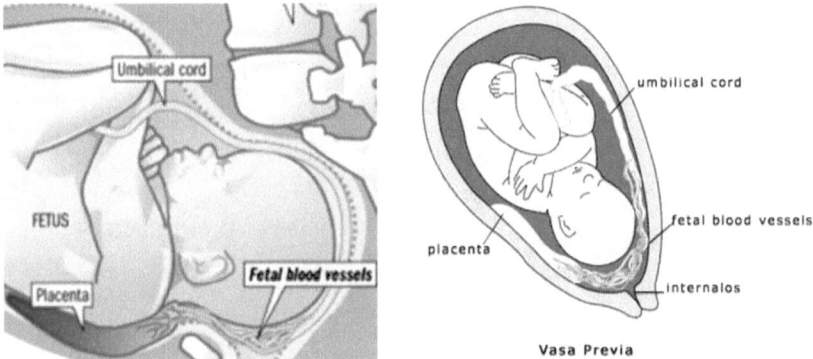

Figure 149a and b. Vasa praevia

- A history of low-lying placenta in the second trimester.
- Multiple pregnancy
- IVF, where the incidence of vasa praevia has been reported to be as high as 1 in 300.

DIAGNOSIS AND PRESENTATION

When the foetal membranes are ruptured, either spontaneously or artificially, the unprotected foetal vessels are at risk of disruption and therefore bleeding from the baby.

- Therefore, vasa praevia often presents at the time of membrane rupture with
  - fresh vaginal bleeding
  - FHR abnormalities on CTG
  - foetal death in around 60 out of 100 cases
- Rarely, bleeding can occur in the absence of membrane rupture.
- Very rarely, FHR abnormalities in the absence of bleeding may be present secondary to compression of the foetal vessels by the foetal PP.

- In the antenatal period, the diagnostic features are
  - vaginal bleeding
  - a colour Doppler transvaginal ultrasound scanning shows the vasa praevia overlying the cervix

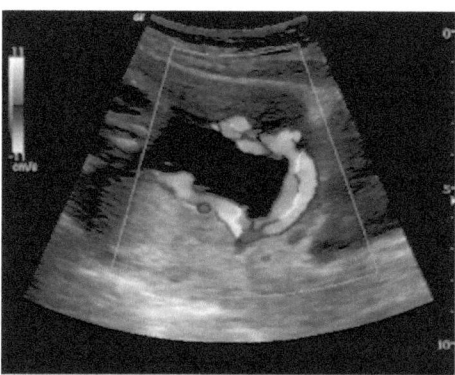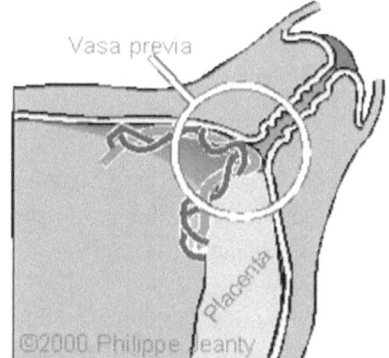

Figure 150a and b. Blood vessels on the outlet of the womb on scan

Survival rates of up to 97 out of 100 cases have been reported, where the diagnosis has been made during the antenatal period.

- In labour, in the absence of vaginal bleeding, vasa praevia can occasionally be diagnosed clinically during vaginal examination by feeling foetal blood vessel in the membranes. This can be confirmed by direct visualisation using an instrument called amnioscope.

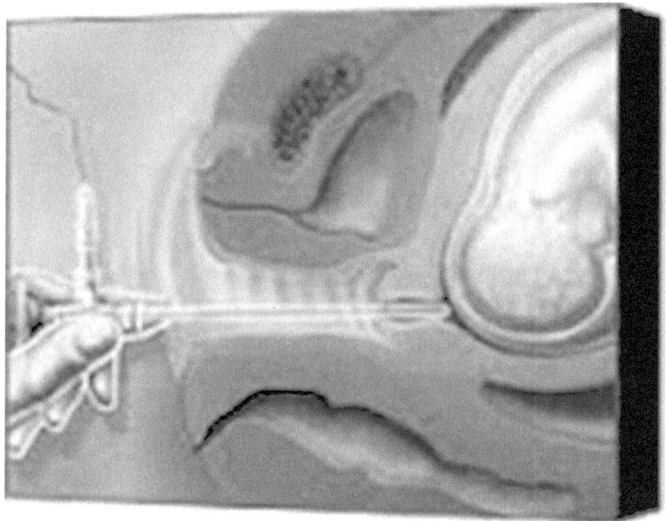

Figure 151. Using amnioscope in labour to look at vasa praevia

255

- Various tests exist which can differentiate between your own blood and that of your baby, but they are often not applicable in clinical situations since the results take a considerable amount of time to be ready, for example Kleihauer-Betke test.

MANAGEMENT OF VASA PRAEVIA

- In the presence of bleeding vasa praevia, delivery will be accomplished by emergency Caesarean section within 30 minutes of the diagnosis.
- If vasa praevia is diagnosed at term, delivery will be carried out by elective Caesarean section in a timely manner.
- If vasa praevia is diagnosed in the second trimester, imaging will be repeated in the third trimester to confirm persistence. As pregnancy advances, vasa praevia can resolve in up to 15% of cases. If persistent, you will be admitted at 28 weeks to a unit with appropriate neonatal facilities that can facilitate quicker intervention in the event of bleeding or labour. You will be given steroid because of the increased risk of PTD, and elective Caesarean section will be performed between 35 and 37 weeks of gestation.
- Foetal well-being will be confirmed at the time of any bleeding during pregnancy and in labour; this is currently best achieved using the CTG and scan.
- Using laser beam to destroy the vasa praevia may have a role in the treatment of vasa praevia.

EFFECTS OF APH ON YOU (THE MOTHER)

It causes the following:
- Anaemia
- Infection
- Shock
- Kidney failure
- Poor clotting of blood and therefore more bleeding
- Bleeding after delivery (PPH)
- Prolonged hospital stay
- Psychological problems
- Complications of blood transfusion
- Death may occur, especially in developing countries

EFFECTS OF APH ON YOUR BABY

- Less blood and therefore less oxygen going to the baby's organs and systems
- SGA baby and FGR
- Preterm labour
- Death during pregnancy and up to 1 month after delivery

GENERAL MANAGEMENT OF APH

- For low-lying placenta without bleeding, please see pages xx.
- It is very important that you report all vaginal bleeding to your antenatal care provider immediately; if you cannot get in touch with them, you should go to the nearest hospital immediately. If you cannot do that, you should call the ambulance immediately.
- If you present to a midwifery-led maternity unit, a GP, or an A&E department, you should be assessed, stabilised if necessary, and transferred to a hospital maternity unit with facilities for your resuscitation and that of your baby if you go into labour.

INITIAL MANAGEMENT IN A MATERNITY UNIT

The main objective of the initial assessment is to determine the severity of the bleeding (minor, major, or massive haemorrhage) and to conduct resuscitation if necessary. It includes the following:

- Resuscitation if the APH is major or massive.
- Monitoring your vital signs, for example BP, pulse, and so on.
- Intravenous assess and blood tests
- A quick history of the bleeding and examination will be performed, including examination of your tummy, speculum examination, and a digital examination if there is no placenta praevia.
- Assessment of the well-being of your baby.

Further management will depend on the severity of the bleeding.

BLEEDING FROM THE CERVIX

If the APH is from a cervical ectropion or suspected cancer of the neck of the womb, you should be referred for colposcopy(examination of the neck of the womb under microscope); subsequent antenatal care need not be altered.

STAINING AND STREAKING OF BLOOD.

If you are no longer bleeding and placenta praevia has been excluded, you can go home after a reassuring initial clinical assessment

MINOR APH (LESS THAN 50 mL BLOOD LOSS)

If APH is heavier than spotting and you are still bleeding, you should remain in hospital at least until the bleeding has stopped. Your blood will be taken for

- assessment of full blood count and your blood group.
- a clotting screen if the platelet count is low.

Major APH (loss of 50-1,000 mL of Blood) with No Clinical Shock

- Admission to the labour ward initially
- Intravenous access
- Intravenous infusion
- Observation of your vital signs
- Your blood will be taken in major and massive APH for
    - full blood count
    - clotting screen
    - cross-matching 4 units of it
    - urea, electrolytes, and LFTs

Massive APH (Blood Loss of Greater than 1,000 mL and/or Signs of Clinical Shock.)

- This is an obstetric emergency and you will see many medical professionals in the room doing one thing or the other to help you.
- The most senior obstetrician available will start the management, and the obstetric, anaesthetic, and haematological consultants will be alerted.
- The management will follow a specific designed protocol that is used in an emergency situation.

Management Applicable to all Severity of APH

- Trace of baby's heart (CTG)
    - CTG is not advised if active obstetric intervention in the interests of the foetus is not planned at less than 26^{+0} weeks of gestation.
    - Ultrasound should be carried out to establish foetal heart pulsation if foetal viability cannot be detected using the CTG external monitor.
- Ultrasound to look for the cause of the bleeding, including checking for the position of the placenta and also check for foetal growth and liquor volume.
- A single course of antenatal corticosteroids should be offered if you are between 24^{+0} and 34^{+6} weeks of gestation. If the most likely cause of the spotting is lower genital tract bleeding, where imminent delivery is unlikely, corticosteroids are unlikely to be of benefit but could still be considered.
- The pregnancy will be reclassified as 'high risk' and antenatal care will be consultant-led following APH from placental abruption or unexplained APH. Serial ultrasound for foetal growth will be performed.
- Anti-D injection should be given if you are non-sensitised RhD-negative women, independent of whether routine antenatal prophylactic anti-D has been administered. In the event of recurrent vaginal bleeding after 20^{+0}

weeks of gestation, anti-D Ig should be given at a minimum of 6 weekly intervals.

- Administration of anti-D after 20^{+0} weeks of gestation should be followed by Kleihauer test to identify foetal blood in your own blood of greater than 4 mL red blood cells; in that situation, additional anti-D Ig will be given as required.

LABOUR AND DELIVERY

- If foetal death is diagnosed on arrival to the hospital, vaginal birth is the recommended mode of delivery for most women (provided the maternal condition is satisfactory), but Caesarean birth will need to be considered for some.
- If the CTG or scan shows that your baby is compromised, a Caesarean section is the appropriate method of delivery with your concurrent resuscitation.
- If you are compromise, you will be resuscitated and baby delivered immediately by Caesarean section.
- If you present with unexplained APH and neither you nor your baby is compromised, management plans are as follows:
  - If you present before 37^{+0} weeks and bleeding has settled, the pregnancy will be allowed to continue.
  - If you present after 37^{+0} weeks and the APH is spotting or the blood is streaked through mucus, delivery will not be conducted. If it is a minor or major APH, IOL will be considered in order to avoid adverse consequences potentially associated with a placental abruption.
- EFM will be necessary in labour.
- Pain relief in labour
  - Regional anaesthetic (epidura or spinal) is recommended for operative delivery unless there is a specific contraindication.
  - If you and/or your baby are compromised and Caesarean section is required, a general anaesthetic will be considered to facilitate your resuscitation and to expedite delivery.
- A baby doctor will be present at birth to take care of your baby

MANAGEMENT OF THE THIRD STAGE OF LABOUR

- PPH should be anticipated.
- Active management of the third stage of labour will be conducted. This is done by giving you hormonal injection to contract the womb immediately after delivery of your baby and delivery of the placenta when it has separated.

Management if you Have APH and you are on a Medication to thin your Blood (Anticoagulant)

- If you are bleeding, you should not take any more dose of anticoagulant medication.
- If you have APH, you should attend hospital urgently where you will be assessed and advice from haematologist should be sought.
- If you are at high risk of APH and continued heparin treatment is considered essential for you, intravenous unfractionated heparin will be used until the risk factors for haemorrhage have resolved.

APH and Extreme Preterm Pregnancy (from 24+0 to 26+0 Weeks of Pregnancy)

- You will be resuscitated and stabilised before any decision is made regarding delivery of the baby.
- A senior paediatrician/neonatologist will counsel you on the possible outcome.
- The pregnancy will be allowed to continue if your condition is stable.
- Consideration will be given to delivering the foetus when the bleeding is considered life-threatening for you or there is evidence of shock that fails to respond to resuscitation.
- Decision to do a Caesarean will be discussed between you and your obstetrician after you have been counselled by a baby doctor if the FHR is abnormal and vaginal delivery is not imminent.

Further Management of Placenta Praevia and Placenta Accreta

Antenatal Management

- During the antenatal period, anaemia will be prevented and treated.
- In the third trimester, there is high risk of PTD and APH.
- If you are managed at home, you should ensure that you have someone available to help you should the need arise and you should have ready access to the hospital.
- If you experience any bleeding, contractions, or pain (including vague suprapubic period-like aches), you should go to the hospital immediately.
- Depending on your personal circumstances, blood may be made available for you during inpatient antenatal care, especially if you have atypical antibodies.
- Prior to delivery, your doctor should go through everything that is likely to happen, including bleeding, blood transfusion, hysterectomy, and your concerns should be addressed.

PRECAUTIONS AGAINST VTE FOR INPATIENTS

- Prolonged inpatient care can be associated with an increased risk of thromboembolism; therefore, mobility should be encouraged together with the use of thromboembolic deterrent stockings and adequate hydration.
- Prevention of blood clots formation using anticoagulants for those at high risk of thromboembolism.
- In the post-natal period, your risk for clots formation will be assessed and thromboprophylaxis given appropriately.

MODE OF DELIVERY

- If your placental edge is less than 2 cm from the internal os in the third trimester, you are likely to need delivery by Caesarean section.
- As the lower uterine segment continues to develop beyond 36 weeks of gestation, a previously diagnosed placenta praevia can migrate upwards. So prior to Caesarean section, a transvaginal scan will be performed, especially if the baby's head is engaged to see if the placenta has moved up.
- Elective Caesarean section is conducted after 39 weeks if you are asymptomatic or before 36-37 weeks if placenta accreta is suspected.

PREPARATIONS BEFORE SURGERY AND ACTUAL SURGERY IN THE PRESENCE OF PLACENTA PRAEVIA AND ACCRETA

- The management will constitute a multidisciplinary team involving the obstetric team, anaesthetist, haematologist, and the paediatric team.
- The team will discuss with you.

This is a specialised field and is not discussed further in this series of the book.

SOURCES

- RCOG Green-top Guideline No. 63. Antepartum haemorrhage, November 2011.
- Royal College of Obstetricians and Gynaecologists. Blood Transfusions in Obstetrics. Green-top Guideline No. 47. London: RCOG; 2008.
- Khan KS, Wojdyla D, Say L, Gülmezoglu AM, Van Look PF. WHO analysis of causes of maternal death: a systematic review. Lancet 2006;367:1066-74.
- Royal College of Obstetricians and Gynaecologists. Placenta Praevia, Placenta Praevia Accreta and Vasa Praevia: Diagnosis and Management. Green-top Guideline No. 27. London: RCOG; 2011.

- Royal College of Obstetricians and Gynaecologists. Prevention and Management of Postpartum Haemorrhage. Green-top Guideline No. 52. London: RCOG; 2009.
- Royal College of Obstetricians and Gynaecologists. Maternal Collapse in Pregnancy and the Puerperium. Green-top Guideline No. 56. London: RCOG; 2011.

Mental Health in Pregnancy

PREDICTION, DETECTION, AND INITIAL MANAGEMENT OF MENTAL ILLNESS IN PREGNANCY

PREDICTION AND DETECTION

At booking appointment to see your obstetrician or your midwife, your risk of developing mental illness in pregnancy will be predicted by asking you the following questions:

- Past or present severe mental illness (outside pregnancy, during the antenatal and post-natal periods).
- Previous treatment by a psychiatrist/specialist mental health team including inpatient care.
- A family history of mental illness during pregnancy and a month after childbirth.

At the same booking appointment, to identify possible depression, you will be asked certain questions, for example

- Whether you have often been bothered by feeling down, depressed, or hopeless during the past month.
- Whether you have often been bothered by having little interest or pleasure in doing things during the past month
- If your answer to any of the above questions is a 'yes', you will be asked if you feel you need help.

REFERRAL AND INITIAL CARE

- If the health care professional has a significant concern, you should normally be referred for further assessment to your General practitioner or a psychiatric team.
- If you have or you are suspected to have a severe mental illness (e.g. schizophrenia), you will be referred to a specialist mental health service, including, if appropriate, a specialist perinatal mental health service.
- If you have a current mental disorder or a history of severe mental illness, you will be asked about your mental health at all subsequent contacts.

- If you have a current or past history of severe mental illness, a written care plan covering pregnancy, delivery, and the post-natal period will be developed in the first trimester for you.
  - Before writing the plan, you, your partner, family, carers, and relevant health care professionals will be consulted.
  - It will include increased contact with specialist mental health services (including, if appropriate, specialist perinatal mental health services).
  - It will be recorded in all versions of your notes (your own records and maternity, primary care, and mental health notes) and communicated to you and all relevant health care professionals.
- If you need an inpatient care for a mental disorder within 12 months of childbirth, you should normally be admitted to a specialist mother and baby unit, unless there are specific reasons for not doing so.

PRINCIPLES OF CARE FOR WOMEN WITH MENTAL DISORDERS PREPREGNANCY, DURING PREGNANCY AND THE POST-NATAL PERIOD

- If you have an existing mental disorder, you should be given sensitive information at each stage of assessment, diagnosis, and treatment about the impact of the disorder and its treatment on your health and that of your foetus or child.
- Health care professionals should work to develop a trusting relationship with you, and where appropriate and acceptable to you, your partner, and family members. Particular attention will be paid to the following:
  - Exploring your ideas, concerns, and expectations and regularly checking your understanding of the issues.
  - Discussing the level of involvement of your partner, family members, and carers and their role in supporting you.
  - Discussing the issues of stigma and shame in relation to the mental illness.
- Your health care professionals should
  - ensure that adequate systems are in place to ensure continuity of care and effective transfer of information, to reduce the need for multiple assessments.
  - discuss contraception.
  - discuss relapse of the condition, risk to the foetus, and risks associated with stopping or changing medication.
- You should discuss your pregnancy plans with your doctor.
- Your health care professionals should assess, and where appropriate address, the needs of your partner, family members, and your carers including
  - the welfare of your infant and other dependent children and adults

263

- – the impact of any mental disorder on relationships with your partner, family members, and carers
- If you are adolescents, your health care professional should
  - – pay attention to confidentiality and your rights for a child.
  - – obtain appropriate consent, bearing in mind your understanding, parental consent and responsibilities, child protection issues, and the use of the Mental Health Act and of the Children Act, if such exist.
- Discussions about treatment options will cover the following:
  - – the need for prompt treatment because of the potential impact of an untreated mental disorder on the foetus or infant
  - – the risk of relapse or deterioration in symptoms and your ability to cope with untreated or subthreshold symptoms
  - – the severity of previous episodes, response to treatment, and your preference
  - – the fact that if you have been taking a drug that can cause abnormality in a baby and then you stop taking it when pregnancy was confirmed, the risk of abnormality may still persist
  - – the risks from stopping medication abruptly
  - – the increased risk of harm associated with drug treatments during pregnancy and the post-natal period, including the risk in overdose
  - – the treatment options that would enable you to breastfeed if you wish to do so
- When prescribing a drug, the prescribers will
  - – choose drugs with lower risk profiles for you and your foetus or infant.
  - – start at the lowest effective dose and slowly increase it.
  - – use one drug in preference to combination treatment.
  - – consider additional precautions for preterm, LBW, or sick infants.
- When stopping a drug, the following will be taken into account:
  - – the risk to the foetus or infant during the withdrawal period
  - – the risk from not treating the disorder

USE OF DRUGS (WHEN TRYING FOR A BABY, DURING PREGNANCY, OR DURING BREASTFEEDING) THAT CAN CAUSE BIRTH DEFECTS

If you were taking drugs such as lithium, valproate, carbamazepine, lamotrigine, and paroxetine at the time of conception and/or in the first trimester, the following will be done:

- The pregnancy will be confirmed as quickly as possible.
- Appropriate screening and counselling about the continuation of the pregnancy, the need for additional monitoring, and the risks to the foetus if you continue to take the medication will be offered.
- A full paediatric assessment of the newborn infant will be undertaken.

- The infant will be monitored in the first few weeks after delivery for adverse drug effects, drug toxicity, or withdrawal (e.g. floppy baby, irritability, constant crying, shivering, tremor, restlessness, increased tone, feeding and sleeping difficulties, and, rarely, seizures).

DEPRESSION

Symptoms of depression are as follows:
- Core (key) symptoms:
    - Persistent sadness or low mood. This may be with or without weepiness.
    - Marked loss of interest or pleasure in activities, even for activities that you normally enjoy.
- Other common symptoms:
    - Disturbed sleep compared with your usual pattern. It may be difficulty in getting off to sleep or waking early and being unable to get back to sleep. Sometimes, it may be sleeping too much.
    - Change in appetite—poor appetite and weight loss; sometimes, the reverse happens with comfort eating and weight gain.
    - Tiredness or loss of energy.
    - Agitation or slowing of movements.
    - Poor concentration or indecisiveness. For example, you may find it difficult to read, work, and so on. Even simple tasks can seem difficult.
    - Feelings of worthlessness, excessive, or inappropriate guilt.
    - Recurrent thoughts of death and dying. For some people, despairing thoughts such as 'life's not worth living' or 'I don't care if I don't wake up' are common. Sometimes, these thoughts progress into plans for suicide.

Symptoms can develop quite suddenly. An episode of depression is usually diagnosed if
- you have at least 5 out of the above 9 symptoms, with at least 1 of these a core symptom.
- the symptoms cause you distress or impair your normal functioning, such as affecting your work performance.
- the symptoms occur most of the time on most days and have lasted at least 2 weeks.
- the symptoms are not due to a medication side effect or due to drug or alcohol misuse or a physical condition such as an underactive thyroid or pituitary gland.

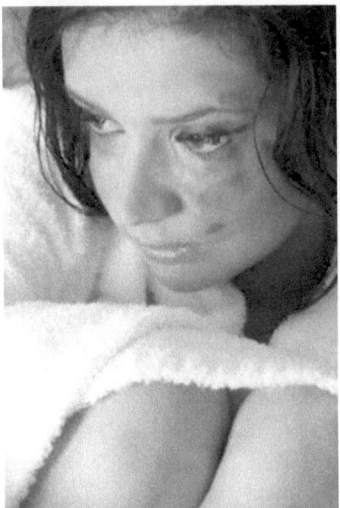

Figure 152. Depression

Some other presentations are as following:
- Worsening of the symptoms in the morning.
- Physical symptoms such as headaches, palpitations, chest pains, and general aches.
- Some people with severe depression develop delusions and/or hallucinations. These are called psychotic symptoms. A delusion is a false belief that a person has. For example, a belief that people are plotting to kill you or that there is a conspiracy about you. Hallucination means hearing, seeing, feeling, smelling, or tasting something that is not real.

SEVERITY OF DEPRESSION
Depression is classified into the following categories of severity:
- Severe depression: You would normally have most or all the 9 symptoms listed above, and they markedly interfere with your normal functioning.
- Moderate depression: You would normally have more than the 5 symptoms that are needed to make the diagnosis of depression. Also, symptoms will usually include both core symptoms, and the severity of symptoms is between mild and severe.
- Mild depression: You would normally have 5 of the symptoms listed above that are required to make the diagnosis of depression; your normal functioning is only mildly impaired.
- Subthreshold depression: You have less than the 5 symptoms needed to make a diagnosis of depression, so it is not classed as depression. However, the symptoms you do have may be troublesome and cause

distress. If this situation persists for more than 2 years, it is sometimes called dysthymia.

CAUSES OF DEPRESSION

The exact cause is unknown. Genetic factor has been implicated. A life event such as a relationship problem, bereavement, redundancy, illness can also trigger an episode of depression.

TREATMENT OPTIONS FOR DEPRESSION

Most people with depression will get better without treatment. However, this may take several months. The average length of an episode of depression is 6-8 months. Meanwhile, living with depression can be difficult and distressing for you and also for your family and friends. Therefore, many people with depression opt for treatment.

Management is based on the prevailing circumstance and scenario.

Scenario 1: You are being treated for depression and you are planning a pregnancy or have an unplanned pregnancy.

A. If you are taking an antidepressant, the medication will be withdrawn gradually and monitoring ('watchful waiting') considered. If intervention is then needed, the following will be considered:
- Self-help approaches
- Brief psychological treatments

SELF-HELP APPROACHES

A guided self-help programme: There are various pamphlets, books, and audio tapes which can help you to understand and combat depression. The best are based on the principles of computer-based cognitive behavioural therapy (C-CBT). The materials are provided by a trained practitioner such as a doctor who monitors your progress. A typical guided self-help programme consists of 6-8 sessions (face-to-face and via telephone) over 9-12 weeks, and you are given tasks to try out between sessions.

Exercise: Some people claim that regular exercise helps to lift their mood and help to combat depression.

BRIEF PSYCHOLOGICAL TREATMENTS

Most psychological treatments for depression last in the range of 12-20 weekly sessions of 1-2 hours per session. Cognitive behavioural therapy (CBT): Briefly, cognitive therapy is based on the idea that certain ways of thinking can trigger, or fuel, certain mental health problems such as depression.

The therapist helps you to understand your thought patterns in particular, to identify any harmful or unhelpful ideas or thoughts which you have that can make you depressed. The aim is then to change your ways of thinking to avoid these ideas. Behavioural therapy aims to change any behaviour which is harmful or not helpful. In short, CBT helps people to achieve changes in the way that they think, feel, and behave.

Interpersonal therapy (IPT): This is sometimes offered instead of CBT. It is based on the idea that your personal relationships may play a large role in affecting your mood and mental state. The therapist helps you to change your thinking and behaviour and improve your interaction with others. For example, IPT may focus on issues such as bereavement or disputes with others that may be contributing to the depression.

B. If you are taking an antidepressant and your latest presentation was a moderate depressive episode, the following options will be discussed with you, taking into account your previous response to treatment, preference, and risk:
- Switching to psychological therapy (CBT or IPT)
- Switching to an antidepressant with lower risk

C. If you are taking an antidepressant and your latest presentation was a severe depressive episode, the following options will be discussed with you, taking into account your previous response to treatment, preference, and risk:
- Combining drug treatment with psychological treatment, but switching to an antidepressant with lower risk
- Switching to psychological treatment (CBT or IPT)

Scenario 2: You are pregnant or breastfeeding and you develop a new episode of depression.

A. If the depression is mild or moderate, the following options should be considered:
- Self-help strategies (guided self-help, C-CBT, or exercise)
- Non-directive counselling delivered at home
- Brief CBT or IPT

B. If the depression is mild but you have a history of severe depression and you decline or your symptoms do not respond to psychological treatments, antidepressant drugs will be considered.

C. If you develop a moderate or severe depressive episode but you have a history of depression, the following options will be considered:
- CBT or IPT
- Antidepressant drugs, if you have expressed a preference for it

- Combination treatment if there is no response or a limited response to psychological or drug treatment alone, provided you understands the risks associated with antidepressant medication

Scenario 3: If you have a treatment-resistant depression, a trial of a different single drug or ECT will be considered before combination drug treatment. A drug called lithium may be used.

ANTIDEPRESSANT DRUGS

They are commonly used to treat moderate or severe depression. However, symptoms such as low mood, poor sleep, poor concentration, and so on, are often eased with an antidepressant. This may then allow you to function more normally and increase your ability to deal with any problems or difficult circumstances.

An antidepressant does not usually work straightaway. It can take 2-4 weeks before the effect builds up fully. A normal course of an antidepressant lasts for at least 6 months after symptoms have eased. Some people stop their medication too early, and the depression may then quickly return. At the end of a course of treatment, it is usual to reduce the dose gradually over about 4 weeks before finally stopping. This is because some people develop withdrawal symptoms if an antidepressant is stopped abruptly.

Some antidepressants work better in some people than in others. Therefore, inform your doctor if symptoms do not start to improve after about 3-4 weeks of taking an antidepressant. In this situation, it is common to advise either an increase in dose (if the maximum dose is not yet reached) or a switch to another type of antidepressant.

GENERALISED ANXIETY DISORDER

Anxiety is normal in stressful situations and can even be helpful, for example, when threatened by an aggressive person. The burst of adrenaline and nerve impulses which we have in response to stressful situations can encourage a 'fight or flight response'. Some people are more prone to normal anxieties, for example been anxious before examinations.

Anxiety is common in pregnancy, especially if you are expecting your first child. There are a number of things that you may feel anxious about; they are enumerated as follows:
- Antenatal test results, because of the possibility that something may be wrong
- Financial problems
- Work

- Accommodation
- Parenthood
- Labour and its problems

You can discuss your problem with your partner, friends, and midwife, and this should make you feel more confident and more in control. You may want to read your pregnancy book. Anxiety is abnormal if it
- is out of proportion to the stressful situation.
- persists when a stressful situation has gone, that is the stress is minor.
- appears for no apparent reason when there is no stressful situation.

CLINICAL PRESENTATION OF GENERALISED ANXIETY DISORDER

It is characterised by the following symptoms:
- Excessive anxiety on most days.
- Feeling fearful and tense when you are anxious.
- Your day-to-day life activities are affected.
- Other symptoms: You may have the following symptoms in addition to the above:
  - Feeling restless, on edge, irritable, muscle tension, or keyed up a lot of the time.
  - Tiring easily.
  - Difficulty in concentrating and your mind going blank quite often.
  - Poor sleep (insomnia). Usually, it is difficulty in getting off to sleep.
- Physical symptoms. Sometimes, you may have one or more of the following symptoms:
  - Fast heart rate
  - Palpitations
  - Feeling sick
  - Shaking (tremor)
  - Sweating
  - Dry mouth
  - Chest pain
  - Headaches
  - Fast breathing

You do not have GAD if your anxiety is about one specific thing. For example, if your anxiety is usually caused by fear of one thing, then you are more likely to have a phobia. GAD develops in about 1 in 50 people at some stage in life. Twice as many women as men are affected. It usually first develops in the 20s and is less common in older people.

Causes of GAD

The cause is not clear. The condition often develops for no apparent reason. Various factors may play a part. For example:

- Genetic make-up may be important.
- Childhood traumas such as abuse or death of a parent may make you more prone to anxiety when you become older.
- A major stress in life may trigger the condition. For example, a family crisis or a major civilian trauma such as a toxic chemical spill. But the symptoms then persist when the trigger has gone.
- People who have other mental health problems such as depression or schizophrenia may also develop GAD.

Diagnosis

If the typical symptoms develop and persist for at least 6 months, then a doctor can usually confirm that you have GAD. However, it is sometimes difficult to tell if you have GAD, panic disorder, depression, or a mixture of these conditions. Sometimes, other conditions may need to be ruled out, for example:

- Drinking a lot of caffeine (in tea, coffee, and cola).
- The side-effect of some prescribed medicines, for example antidepressant drugs.
- An overactive thyroid gland.
- Taking some street drugs.
- Certain heart conditions which cause palpitations.
- Low blood sugar level.
- Tumours which make too much adrenaline and other similar hormones (very rare).

Management

Scenario 1: You have GAD and you are planning a pregnancy or pregnant

If you are on medication, it will be stopped, and CBT will be started. If drug treatment is needed, you will be switched to a safer one.

Scenario 2: You have a new episode of GAD

- CBT: This is probably the most effective treatment. It probably works for over half of the people with GAD to reduce symptoms and improve quality of life.
- Counselling: In particular, counselling that focuses on problem-solving skills may help some people.
- Anxiety management courses: Some people prefer to be in a group course rather than have individual therapy or counselling. The courses may include learning how to relax, problem-solving skills, coping strategies, and group support.

- Self-help: You can get leaflets, books, tapes, videos, and so on, on relaxation and combating stress. They teach simple deep breathing techniques and other measures to relieve stress, help you to relax, and may ease anxiety symptoms.
- Antidepressants: The two drugs licensed to treat GAD are citalopram and paroxetine. It is important to note that when you are started on an antidepressant, the anxiety symptoms may worsen for a few days before they start to improve.
- Benzodiazepines such as diazepam: They are almost not used for GAD. A short course of up to 2-3 weeks may be an option to help you over a particularly bad spell. They are addictive and can cause drowsiness.
- Hydroxyzine: This is an antihistamine which is sometimes used to ease anxiety symptoms. A common side effect, though, is drowsiness.
- A combination of treatments: For example, cognitive behaviour therapy plus an antidepressant medicine may work better in some cases than either treatment alone.

PROGNOSIS

Without treatment, GAD tends to persist for life. It is relatively mild in some cases but for others, it can be very disabling. The severity of symptoms tends to wax and wane; worse during periods of major life stresses.

DREAMS

It is normal to have dreams about your baby. Sometimes, your dreams may reflect your anxieties. This is often because you are thinking much more about your pregnancy and the changes that are happening in your body. Talk to your midwife if you are worried by this.

SOURCES

- Antenatal and postnatal mental health. The UK NICE guideline on clinical management and guidance, 2007.
- Routine Postnatal Care of Women and Their Babies. The UK National Collaborating Centre for Primary Care, July 2006.
- Antenatal Care: Routine Care for the Healthy Pregnant Woman. National Collaborating Centre for Women's and Children's Health. Commissioned by the UK National Institute for Health and Clinical Excellence, March 2008. This is a partial update of the 2003 guideline.
- www.patient.co.uk
- Antenatal and Postnatal Mental Health: Clinical Management and Service Guidance. NICE Clinical Guideline 45, February 2007
- Baby Centre website.

Infection in Pregnancy

URINARY INFECTION IN PREGNANCY

UNDERSTANDING THE URINARY TRACT

There are two kidneys, one on each side of the tummy. They produce urine which drains down the urinary pipe called the ureter into the bladder as shown in Figure 153b. Urine is stored in the bladder and is passed out through the urethra during urination.

Urinary infection is caused by bacteria (germs) that get into your urine, and the presentation depends on the part of the urinary tract that is affected.

FACTORS THAT PREDISPOSE TO URINARY INFECTION

- Germs from the bowel cause no harm in your bowel but can cause infection if they get into other parts of the body. They lie around the back passage after passing stool and sometimes move up the urethra (the tube from the bladder through which urine passes out) and then bladder where they thrive and multiply quickly and cause infection.

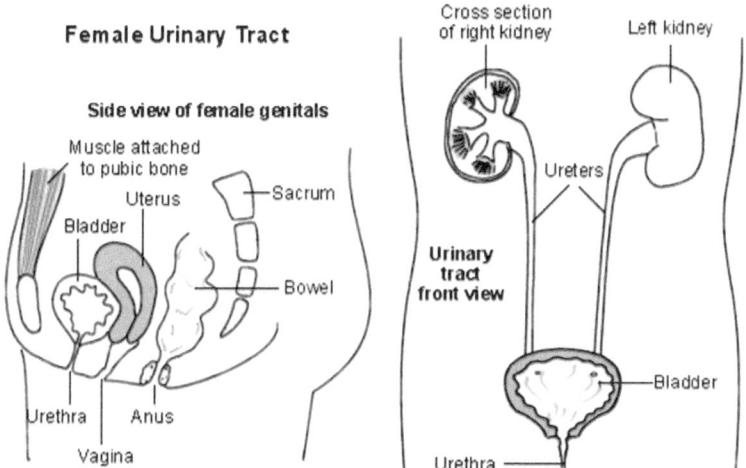

Figure 153a and b. The relative position of the urinary tracts, bowel, vagina/uterus, and urethra/bladder

- Women are more prone to urinary infections than men as their urethra is shorter and opens nearer the back passage.
- Pregnant women are more prone to urinary infections than non-pregnant women. This is due to the hormonal changes of pregnancy that affect the urinary tract and tend to slow down the flow of urine.

PRESENTATION OF WATER INFECTION

- Sometimes no symptom at all.
- **Cystitis (bladder infection):** This is common in both pregnant and non-pregnant women. Symptoms can occur in different combinations including
  - pain when passing urine
  - passing urine more often
  - pain in your lower abdomen
  - blood in urine
  - fever (high temperature)
- **Kidney infection:** This is uncommon and may occur as a complication of cystitis. Symptoms may include
  - pain in your loin (side of the abdomen over your kidney)
  - fever
  - feeling sick, vomiting, and/or diarrhoea
  - blood in your urine
  - symptoms of cystitis

DIAGNOSIS OF URINARY INFECTION DURING PREGNANCY

- Your urine sample will be taken in a container or sample bottle and tested for the germs and the antibiotics that can kill them.

EFFECTS OF URINARY INFECTION ON YOUR PREGNANCY

It may cause problems such as
- early labour
- small baby (SGA or FGR)

TREATMENT

- Urinary infection should be treated by your doctor.
- A 7-day course of an antibiotic is the usual treatment if you have symptoms.
- A 3-day course may be given if you have no symptoms but bacteria are found in your urine, unlike in non-pregnant women when treatment is not given in that situation.
- Symptoms will usually improve within a few days. However, it is very important that you complete the course of antibiotics.
- The antibiotic will not harm your baby.
- Painkillers like paracetamol will usually ease any pain, discomfort, or fever.
- Drinking fluids: If you have cystitis, you will be advised to drink plenty of water which should flush out the bladder. This is particularly so if you have a fever in other to prevent dehydration.
- Repeated urine test is done after the course of treatment to check that your urine is clear of bacteria.

SOURCES

- www.patient.co.uk.
- Guidelines on Urological Infections. European Association of Urology, 2011.
- Urinary tract infection (lower)—women, Prodigy, October 2009.
- Schnarr J, Smaill F. Asymptomatic bacteriuria and symptomatic urinary tract infections in pregnancy. Eur J Clin Invest. 2008;38 Suppl 2:50-7 [abstract].

GROUP B STREPTOCOCCUS INFECTION IN PREGNANCY

GBS is a common germ which lives in the vagina and the large bowel. It is isolated from the vagina and urine of up to 30 out of 100 pregnant women. It causes no harm to the carrier, but if GBS is passed on from you to your baby around the time of delivery, this can occasionally cause serious illness for the newborn; majority of babies will not be harmed. In the UK and Ireland, only 1 out of 2,000 newborn babies is diagnosed with GBS infection.

RISK FACTORS FOR TRANSMITTING GBS TO BABY DURING DELIVERY
You have a high risk of transmitting the infection to your baby during delivery if the following is applicable to you:
- GBS has been found in your urine in your current pregnancy.
- GBS has been found on swabs taken from your vagina and/or rectum
- Previous baby had GBS infection after delivery.
- A high temperature during labour.
- Premature labour (page xxx).
- Labour starts more than 18 hours after your waters have broken.

DIAGNOSIS
GBS carriage can be detected during pregnancy by doing the following tests.
- taking a swab from the vagina and/or rectum for test. It is important to note that a negative swab test, however, does not guarantee that you or your baby is not a carrier of GBS.
- taking a mid-stream urine (MSU) sample for test.
- taking a sample of blood from the vein or a sample of spinal fluid from the backbone of your baby to test for the bug

Taking a swab from the vagina and/or rectum for test. It is important to note that a negative swab test, however, does not guarantee that you or your baby is not a carrier of GBS.

PREVENTING TRANSMISSION OF GBS TO YOUR BABY
- You should be given antibiotic in labour if the risk factors listed above, except the last two, are applicable to you. In the UK, penicillin is

275

normally given, and if you are allergic to it, clindamycin will be given. The antibiotic is normally started from the onset of labour.
- It is possible to be tested for GBS late in pregnancy if you have concerns. Talk to your doctor or midwife.
- It is safe to breastfeed your new baby if you are a carrier.

WHEN ANTIBIOTICS ARE NOT NECESSARY
Antibiotics are not usually needed in the following situations because the risk of your baby becoming infected with GBS is low:
- during pregnancy (not labour), unless you have symptoms or GBS is detected in urine
- if you are to have a Caesarean section and you go into spontaneous labour with intact membrane; caesarean section will be done anyway.

EFFECT OF GBS ON THE BABY
Symptoms occur within 12 hours of birth and include the following:
- Baby may be floppy and unresponsive or irritable
- Poor feeding
- Grunting, high or low temperature, fast or slow heart rates
- Fast or slow breathing rates, low BP, and low blood sugar levels

MANAGEMENT OF YOUR BABY
- If your baby shows any sign of GBS infection, he or she will be treated with antibiotics immediately.
- If you have had a previous baby with GBS, your health care team will either monitor your newborn baby closely for at least 12 hours after birth or treat him or her with penicillin until blood tests confirm whether or not GBS is present.
- If you have any of the other risk factors listed above, your baby will be monitored for 12 hours before discharge from the hospital.

If you need antibiotics during labour, there may be some concern about your baby been infected if for some reason:
- You were not able to receive them.
- You receive them more than 4 hours after your waters have gone.
- You delivered very soon after receiving them.

The best approach in these circumstances is not clear. The options of monitoring the health of your baby or of treating him or her with penicillin will be discussed between you and the medical staff, taking into account the potential risks and benefits of each approach.

SOURCES
- Prevention of early onset neonatal Group B streptococcal disease. Royal College of Obstetricians and Gynaecologists (RCOG), November 2006.
- Preventing GBS infection in newborn babies. Information for you. Royal College of Obstetricians and Gynaecologists (RCOG), January 2007.

HEPATITIS B

Hepatitis B caused by the hepatitis B virus (HBV) is the most common serious liver infection in the world. It can lead to liver failure, scarring, or cancer of the liver later in life. Most adults who contract the disease make a full recovery, but a small number become carriers of the virus and may develop the serious liver diseases.

MODE OF TRANSMISSION (HOW THE INFECTION IS SPREAD)

You can become infected with hepatitis B if you are not immune (resistant) to the virus and you come into contact with the blood or body fluids of an infected person. Many people with hepatitis B do not know that they are infected. You are at risk of catching the disease in the following situations:

- Exposure to blood
  - injecting drugs and sharing needles and other equipment, such as spoons or having a sexual relationship with someone who injects drugs
  - if you have an open wound, cut or scratch, and come into contact with the blood of someone with hepatitis B
  - medical or dental treatment in a country where equipment is not sterilised properly
  - working closely with blood e.g., healthcare workers and laboratory technicians are at increased risk of injury when the skin is accidentally punctured by a used needle
  - having a blood transfusion in a country where blood is not tested for hepatitis B
  - having tattoo or body piercing in an unsafe, unlicensed place
  - sharing toothbrushes, razors and towels that are contaminated with infected blood
- Exposure to infected body fluid
  - having sex (anal and oral sex) with an infected person or several different partners without using a condom
  - Prostitutes (both women and men).
- Geographical risk
  - You have an increased risk if you (or your sexual partner) grew up, lived or worked in a part of the world where hepatitis B is relatively common, namely sub-Saharan Africa, South Asia (India, Pakistan, Sri Lanka and Bangladesh) and China.

- Infections in Pregnancy
    - A mother who is infected passes the virus to her baby during delivery.
    - Hepatitis B virus is large and does not cross the placenta; hence, it cannot infect the foetus unless there have been breaks in the maternal-foetal barrier, which can occur during amniocentesis and bleeding associated with childbirth.

EFFECTS ON INFECTED MOTHERS

It takes between 40 and 160 days for any symptoms to develop after exposure to the virus. Most cases present with the following symptoms for a few days:

- feeling sick
- being sick
- lack of appetite
- flu-like symptoms, such as tiredness, general aches and pains, headaches
- yellowing of the skin and eyes (jaundice)

In 1 out of 20 cases the virus stays in the body for 6 months or longer, usually without causing any noticeable symptoms. It is this chronic disease that can cause scarring of the liver and liver cancer.

EFFECTS ON NEWBORN AND CHILDREN

About 9 in 10 children infected at birth and around 1 in 5 children infected in early childhood will develop a long-term infection.

TREATMENT

There is currently no specific treatment for acute hepatitis B, other than using painkillers to relieve symptoms. However, chronic hepatitis B can be treated using a combination of antiviral medications designed to slow the spread of the virus and prevent damage to the liver.

TESTING FOR HEPATITIS B IN PREGNANCY

Testing for hepatitis is recommended when you are planning for pregnancy.

Furthermore, all pregnant women are offered a blood test for hepatitis B as part of a routing screening in the first trimester. If you screen positive for the infection, the following will be done:

- You will be referred to a specialist who will be monitoring your liver and the disease throughout the pregnancy.
- The risk of transmitting the infection to your baby will be assessed from the blood that you have already given.
- Measures will be put in place to protect your newborn baby from the infection.

PREVENTION OF HEPATITIS B INFECTION IN THE NEWBORN

Newborn at risk of being infected during delivery are given a course of hepatitis B vaccine and immunoglobulin soon after birth. Immunoglobulin is given within 12 hours of birth, while the first dose of the vaccine is to be given within 24 hours of birth. Two more doses of the vaccine are given at 1 and 2 months, with a booster dose at 12 months. Your baby will be tested for hepatitis B infection at the twelfth month.

Out of 100 newborn at risk who receive the treatment, 5-10 will still go on to develop the disease, while the rest will not. Babies who have become infected will be referred for specialist assessment and follow-up. Irrespective of the benefits of breastfeeding, it is not safe to breastfeed.

OTHER ASPECTS OF PROTECTION AGAINST HEPATITIS B INFECTION

In a situation where another family member is infected with hepatitis B, all who are in contact with the infected family member, including babies, will be vaccinated against hepatitis B.

HEPATITIS C

This is another virus that affects the liver. The virus is transmitted the same way as hepatitis B. If you have hepatitis C infection, you may have no symptoms and unaware that you have been infected. You may pass the infection to your baby, although the risk is much lower than with hepatitis B or HIV. Unfortunately, the infection cannot be prevented at birth. Your baby can be tested for hepatitis C after delivery, and if he or she is infected, she can be referred for a specialist assessment.

SOURCES

- www.patient.co.uk
- The Pregnancy Book. Your complete guide to: a healthy pregnancy, labour and childbirth. The first weeks with your new baby, UK, 2009.
- NHS Choices, Your health, your choices, 2010.
- Hepatitis B Foundation at www.hepb.org.
- Centers for Disease Control at www.cdc.gov/hepatitis

CHICKENPOX IN PREGNANCY

INTRODUCTION

Chickenpox, also called varicella, is a very infectious and common childhood illness caused by a virus called herpes zoster. It presents with a rash on part or the whole body. Once you have had chickenpox, you cannot develop the disease in the future even if you are in contact with the virus. However, after you have had chickenpox, the virus stays in your body and can become active later, and this time it causes shingles. Shingles is a patch of itchy blisters on the skin that dry out and crust over in a few days. It can be very painful.

PREVALENCE OF THE DISEASE

Many people are immune to chickenpox; for instance, in the UK, 9 out of 10 pregnant women are immune. For this reason, primary infection is uncommon in pregnancy and is estimated to occur in 3 out of 1,000 pregnancies. The disease is less common in a tropical or subtropical region, for example Africa. Therefore if you move form a tropical to a temperate region, for example the UK, you havea greater risk of catching chickenpox than those who are born and grown up in a temperate region. So testing for the disease and immunisation if not already immunised, is vital when travelling from a tropical to a temperate region.

MODE OF TRANSMISSION OF THE DISEASE

About 90 out of 100 people who have not previously had chickenpox will become infected when they come into contact with the disease. The virus is spread in the same ways as the flu virus.

- Tiny droplets from the nose and mouth of infected person when he or she sneezes or coughs contain the virus. Mode of transmission is therefore by breathing in these droplets from the air. So one can catch the disease if you are
    - in close contact with infected person
    - face to face with the person for at least 5 minutes
    - in the same room with the person for at least 15 minutes
- Handling a surface or object that these droplets have landed on, then transferring the virus to yourself by inserting your hand into the nose or mouth.
- One can acquire chickenpox from someone with shingles (an infection caused by the same virus), but you cannot acquire shingles from someone with chickenpox.

It takes 10-21 days for the symptoms of chickenpox to manifest after you have come into contact with the virus. Someone with chickenpox is most infectious from 1 to 2 days before the rash appears until all the blisters have crust over, which is 5-6 days from the start of the rash but may take up to 2 weeks.

People at risk of serious problems if they catch chickenpox are as follows:
- Pregnant women
- Newborn babies
- People with a weakened immune system
- Smokers

- People who have certain lung diseases
- People who have been on steroids in the last 3 months

You should, therefore, seek medical advice as soon as you are exposed to chickenpox virus or develop symptoms.

EFFECT OF CHICKENPOX ON MOTHERS

It presents with mild flu-like symptoms and signs including the following:
- feeling sick and unwell
- headache
- loss of appetite
- fever and
- aching, painful muscles

These symptoms, especially fever, tend to be worse in adults than in children. They are followed by the formation of itchy blisters, which can appear anywhere on the body. Most healthy children (and adults) recover from chickenpox with no lasting ill effects simply by resting, but some have a severe infection than usual.

Complications can occur in pregnancy and include
- chest infection (pneumonia). The further you are into your pregnancy, the more serious the risk of pneumonia tends to be.
- inflammation of the liver (hepatitis).

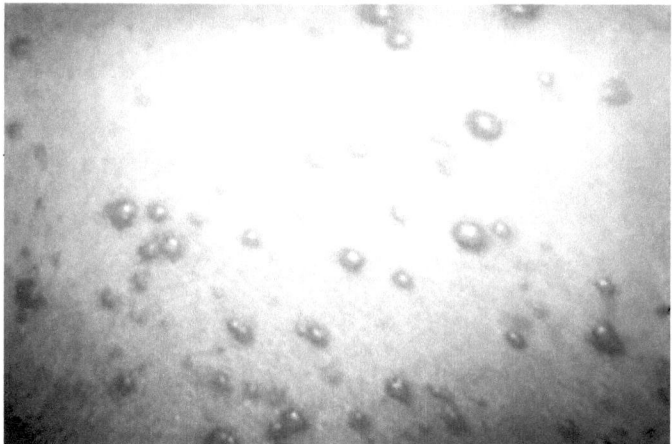

Figure 154. Chickenpox rash

- inflammation of the brain (encephalitis).
- death due to complications, but very rare.

MANAGEMENT OF MATERNAL INFECTION

- Contact your doctor immediately if you develop the rash of chickenpox.
- Avoid contact with susceptible individuals, that is other pregnant women and newborns, until the rash crusts over.
- The symptoms will be treated and personal hygiene is advised in other to prevent secondary bacterial infection of the rash.
- You will be given a drug called aciclovir (acyclovir) if you present within 24 hours of the onset of the rash and you are more than 20 weeks pregnant. If you need to take acyclovir before 20 weeks of pregnancy, your doctor will discuss with you its implications. Acyclovir reduces the severity of the infection but does not prevent transmission of the infection to your baby.

Your doctor should refer you to a hospital if any of the following is applicable to you:

- chest and breathing problem.
- headache, drowsiness
- vomiting, or feeling sick
- vaginal bleeding.
- rash that is bleeding. the skin surrounding the blisters becomes red and painful.
- you are immune-suppressed.
- you smoke cigarettes, have chronic lung disease, are taking a drug called corticosteroid or you are in the later half of your pregnancy.

In these situations, appropriate treatment will be decided in consultation with a multidisciplinary team.

EFFECTS OF CHICKENPOX ON YOUR BABY AND MANAGEMENT

The chance of you infecting your baby depends on the stage of pregnancy when you develop the infection.

UP TO 28 WEEKS OF PREGNANCY

A condition called 'foetal varicella syndrome' (FVS) can develop. It does not happen at the time when the baby is first infected in the womb; it occurs as a result of the virus reactivating itself in the foetus. It is this reactivated virus that causes the damage in the foetus. It occurs in 1-2 out of 100 foetuses of infected mothers. It has been reported in women as early as 3 weeks of pregnancy but rare from 20 to 28 weeks. FVS, unfortunately, is characterised by the following complications:

- damage to the head and brain, eyes, heart, limbs, skin, bowel, genitals, and urinary tracts
- restricted foetal growth
- developmental delay after birth

You will be referred to a specialised unit called 'foetal medicine unit' at 16-20 weeks or 5 weeks after infection for ultrasound scans and counselling. In the presence of ultrasound abnormalities in a pattern consistent with FVS and a confirmed diagnosis of chickenpox in the mother prior to 28 weeks of pregnancy, a severely affected baby is likely and TOP may be offered. In the absence of ultrasound abnormalities on serial ultrasound scans performed in the specialised unit, reassurance may be all that is needed.

BETWEEN 28 AND 36 WEEKS OF PREGNANCY
The virus stays in the baby's body but will not cause any symptoms. It may become active again, causing shingles in the first few years of the child's life.

AFTER 36 WEEKS AND UNTIL BIRTH
After 36 weeks, or when delivery occurs within 4 weeks of you developing the disease, your baby may become infected and could be born with chickenpox or shingles.

CHILDBIRTH WITHIN 7 DAYS OF DEVELOPMENT OF CHICKENPOX RASH OR DEVELOPMENT OF THE RASH WITHIN 7 DAYS OF CHILDBIRTH
If the above is applicable to you, your baby may develop a severe infection and therefore should be given a drug called varicella-zoster immunoglobulin (VZIG) and be monitored for signs of infection until 28 days after the onset of your infection.

If your newborn baby has come into contact with chickenpox in the first 7 days of life and you are immune, then the baby will be protected by your immunity, and there is nothing to worry about. If you are not immune or the newborn was delivered prematurely, then the baby should be given VZIG. If your baby is already infected, he or she will be treated with the drug aciclovir following discussion with a specialist in children and viral diseases.

CHILDBIRTH AND AFTER IT
- After the onset of your chickenpox rash, elective delivery will normally be avoided until 5-7 days to allow your immunity to pass to the baby.
- If you are very ill with chickenpox infection, particularly with any of the complications, your obstetrician will discuss whether you should have the baby early.
- After birth, baby will have an eye examination and blood tests to check whether it has been infected. When the baby is 7 months of age, a follow-up blood test can be performed to check if the baby has antibodies (immunity) to chickenpox.
- If you have or have had chickenpox during pregnancy, breastfeeding is safe.

PREVENTION OF CHICKENPOX

PREPREGNANCY CARE—PLEASE SEE CHAPTER 1.

BOOKING CLINIC

At your booking clinic, a blood test can be performed to check if you are immune to chickenpox or not; if you are not, you will be advised to avoid contact with chickenpox and shingles during pregnancy and to immediately inform health care workers of a potential exposure. After delivery, you will be given the vaccine VZIG.

CONTACT OF A PREGNANT WOMAN WITH CHICKENPOX OR SHINGLES

If the contact is applicable to you, a careful history will be taken with particular attention to the age of the pregnancy, the degree of your closeness with the infected person, and the duration of contact. A blood test will be performed to confirm your immunity. If you are not immune to chickenpox and you have a significant exposure, you will be given an injection of VZIG.

VZIG is a human blood product which strengthens the immune system for a short time but does not necessarily prevent chickenpox development. It can make the infection milder and not last long. The injection can be given for up to 10 days after the contact and before any symptom of the disease appears. If after being given VZIG you come into contact with chickenpox again, a second dose of VZIG should be given if it is 3 weeks or longer since your last injection.

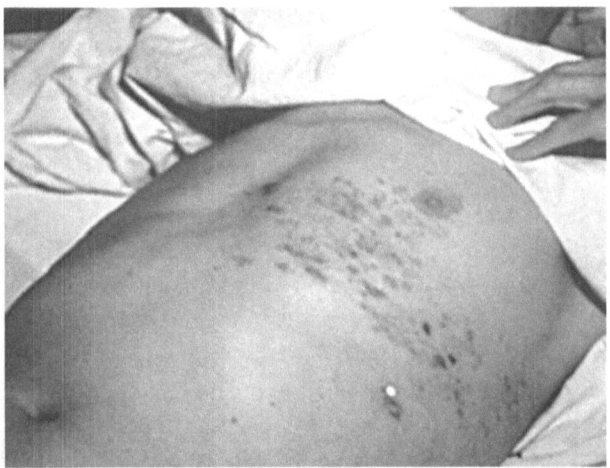

Figure 155. Shingles

After significant contact and VZIG is given, you should be managed as potentially infectious from 8 to 28 days after the contact (8-21 days if VZIG is not given). Regardless of whether or not you are given VZIG, after exposure, you should notify your doctor or midwife early if a rash develops.

SHINGLES DURING PREGNANCY

If you get shingles while you are pregnant, it is usually mild and there is no risk for you or your baby.

SOURCES

- To M, Kidd M, Maxwell D. Prenatal diagnosis and management of fetal infections. The Obstetrician & Gynaecologist. 2009;11:108-16.
- Chickenpox. NHS Choices, Your health, your choices, 2010.
- Chickenpox in Pregnancy. Royal College of Obstetricians and Gynaecologists (RCOG). March 2007.
- Chickenpox in Pregnancy: What You need to Know. RCOG. November 2008.

GENITAL HERPES IN PREGNANCY

INTRODUCTION

Genital herpes is a common infection caused by the herpes simplex virus (HSV) type 1 or type 2. They are found

- in the genital and anal area (genital herpes)
- around the mouth and nose (cold sores)
- in fingers and hand (herpetic whitlows)

MODE OF TRANSMISSION

HSV is highly contagious and can be passed easily from one person to another. The following are the ways through which HSV gets transmitted:

- through skin-to-skin contact (through small cracks in the skin)
- by having vaginal, oral, or anal sex or sharing sex toys
- by a mother to her baby at the time of birth

Once you have the virus, it stays in your body for life. However, certain triggers can activate the virus, causing an outbreak of recurrent genital herpes.

EFFECT ON YOU

The time that elapses from contact with the virus to appearance of symptoms can be 4-7 days, weeks, months, or years. Sometimes, there may be no symptom at all.

PRIMARY INFECTION

This is the first infection. It presents with more severe symptoms than recurrent infections and includes the following:

- painful blisters that burst to leave open sores around the genitals, rectum (back passage), thighs, and buttocks
- vaginal discharge
- pain when passing urine
- fever
- feeling generally unwell, with aches and pains

These symptoms may last for up to 20 days. However, the sores will eventually scab and heal without leaving any scarring.

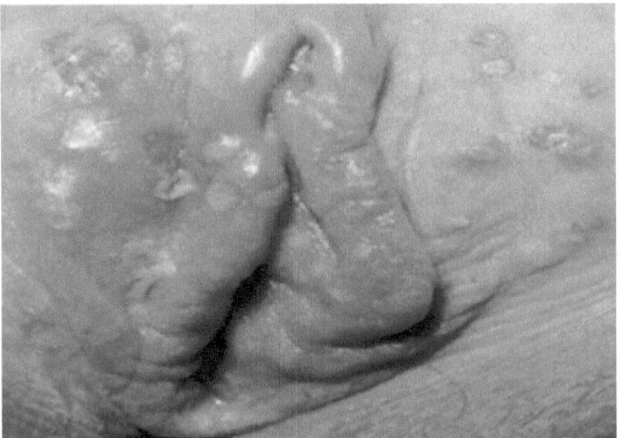

Figure 156. Genital herpes infection

RECURRENT INFECTIONS

Once a primary infection of genital herpes has subsided, symptoms disappear, but the virus remains inactive in the body. It may be reactivated from time to time due to certain triggers, to cause recurrent infections. The triggers are as follows:

- friction in your genital area during sexual intercourse
- being unwell
- stress
- excess amounts of alcohol
- exposure to ultraviolet light, for example, using sunbeds
- surgery on your genital area
- having a weakened immune system (the body's natural defence system), for example as a result of treatment for cancer or HIV infection

THE SIGNS AND SYMPTOMS OF RECURRENT INFECTION

- A tingling, burning, or itching sensation around your genitals, and sometimes down your leg, before the blisters appear.
- Blisters occur as in primary infection but less severe.

Recurrent infections are usually shorter, lasting up to 10 days and less severe than primary infections. This is because your body has produced protective antibodies as a result of the previous infection. In some cases, the blisters and sores may also occur in the same area each time you have a recurrent infection. Over time, the infections become less frequent.

EFFECTS ON YOUR UNBORN BABY AND NEWBORN

If you get genital herpes before you become pregnant, your immune system will provide protection to your baby when you become pregnant. Recurrent episodes of genital herpes during pregnancy do not affect the baby. If you get genital herpes for the first time after you become pregnant, this can be serious. The seriousness will depend on the stage of pregnancy at which the infection occurs.

- First 3 months of pregnancy—small chance of miscarriage.
- Within 6 weeks of birth—there will not be enough time for your immune system to provide adequate protection for your baby. If you then give birth vaginally, there will be about a 4 in 10 chances of passing the virus to your baby.

NEONATAL HERPES

If a baby catches the HSV at birth, this is known as neonatal herpes. It is very rare in developed countries; in the UK, it occurs in 1-2 out of every 100,000 newborn babies. It can affect the following organs:

- skin and eyes
- brain
- other body organs

It can be serious, and baby can die within the first 7 days after birth. Treatment may help to prevent or reduce damage to the baby.

DIAGNOSIS

If you have the symptoms, you should visit your local sexual health clinic. In developing countries where there is no such clinic, you can see your doctor. A history of your sexual partners and STIs will be taken, and you will be screened for them. In most cases, the diagnosis is based on the obvious symptoms alone. The doctor may take a swab from a blister and send it for test to detect the virus. A blood test to differentiate between primary and recurrent infections may be taken if you present with a first episode of genital herpes in the third trimester.

MANAGEMENT

PRIMARY HERPES
- Antiviral drug called acyclovir may be offered.
- You will be admitted into hospital if the rash is severe and you cannot pass urine.
- Caesarean section will be performed if you present with the infection at the time of delivery or within 6 weeks of the EDD. If you present within 6 weeks of delivery and opt for a vaginal birth, your waters will not be broken and invasive procedures will not be performed in labour. Intravenous aciclovir may be given to you during labour and subsequently to your baby after delivery.

RECURRENT HERPES
- Your doctor may suggest some measures to help ease your symptoms.
- Antiviral drugs are rarely used.
- The chance of your newborn developing herpes is very small if you have genital herpes blisters and sores at the onset of labour. Caesarean section is not routinely recommended.
- Suppressive aciclovir treatment will be given daily from 36 weeks of pregnancy until delivery if you would opt for Caesarean delivery and if infection occurs at the onset of labour; the treatment should reduce the likelihood of baby catching the infection, and vaginal birth can still be offered.
- Invasive procedures will be avoided in labour and delivery will be expedited by the appropriate means if your waters break at term.

MEASURES NEEDED TO REDUCE THE RISK TO YOUR BABY
- You should tell your midwife at your first antenatal appointment if you and/or your partner have ever had the HSV (cold sores, whitlows, or genital herpes).
- You Should avoid skin-to-skin contact with the affected area if you or your partner is having an episode of genital herpes. This might include avoiding
  - vaginal intercourse
  - anal intercourse
  - oral intercourse
- You may consider using condoms throughout your pregnancy, particularly in the last 3 months, even if neither you nor your partner has blisters or sores.

- You Should avoid skin-to-skin contact between your baby and anyone with an active herpes simplex infection, such as a cold sore on the mouth or nose or herpetic whitlow on the hand.
- You should ensure that you wash your hands after touching any sores.
- You should avoid sharing towels or flannels to ensure that you do not spread HSV to others.

Sources

- Genital herpes. NHS Choices, Your health, your choices, 2010.
- Genital herpes in pregnancy. RCOG. February 2005.
- Genital herpes in pregnancy. Information for you. RCOG. February 2009.

TORCH Infections

The following infections belong to a group called TORCH infections:
- Toxoplasmosis
- Rubella
- CMV
- Parvovirus B19

They have common characteristics which are as follows:
- They cause minimal or no symptoms in the mother but may be severe in people with deranged immune system, for example HIV/AIDS.
- They have devastating effect on the baby.
- Foetal effects can be picked up on ultrasound assessment.
- Invasive testing may be needed to confirm foetal infections.
- Their investigation can be conducted with similar tests—TORCH screen.
- They are common infections.
- Testing for the infections in pregnancy is usually carried out as a result of the following reasons:
  - Incidental finding of ultrasound markers of foetal infection during a routine ultrasound scan.
  - As part of investigation of early onset FGR baby.
  - If you are exposed to the infection.
  - Rarely, when a pregnant woman is suspected of having symptoms.

	Toxoplasmosis	Rubella	Cytomegalovirus	Parvovirus
Causes	*Toxoplasma gondii*. Lives in cats. No lifelong immunity to the infection, that is no protection against the infection after the first episode.	Rubella virus. Immunity is lifelong, that is there is lifelong protection against the infection after the first episode.	CMV. No lifelong immunity to the infection.	Parvovirus B19. Immunity is lifelong.
Mode of transmission	1. Ingestion of *Toxoplasma gondii* eggs by exposure to soil or water infected with cat's faeces. 2. Ingestion of infected raw or undercooked meat. 3. Mother-to-foetus transmission through the placenta occurs at your first infection. 4. Organ transplant if the donor is infected.	Spread through droplets from the nose or throat of infected persons into the air or surface when they cough, sneeze, or talk by 1. inhaling the droplets through face-to-face contact with infected person or from just being together in the same room. 2. transfer of infection from infected surface to the nose or mouth.	Spread through saliva, semen, blood, urine, vaginal fluids, breast milk by 1. Close contact with the source of infection, for example when infected person coughs or sneezes. 2. Transfer of infection from a contaminated surface to the nose or mouth. 3. Sexual act 4. Activation of a dormant infection.	1. As in rubella virus infection. 2. Via contaminated blood products, such as clotting factor.
Period from infection to symptoms	5-23 days	14-21 days, and women are infectious from 7 days before until 7 days after the onset of the rash.	3-12 weeks	5-7 days. Women are infectious for 3-10 days post-exposure or until the rash appears.

Prevention	1. Wash hands after handling soil, raw meat, pets and animals, esp. cat 2. Wash salads, fruits, and vegetables. 3. Cook raw meats and ready-prepared chilled meals thoroughly. 4. Wear gloves when handling soil and gardening. 5. Avoid sheep, especially during the lambing season, and cat faeces in cat litter or in soil.	1. Stay off work for 6 days after the start of the rash. 2. Keep your child off school if your child has rubella, 3. Minimise the time spent in places where there are many children. 4. Wash hands regularly. 5. If you are not immune, you will be offered MMR in the first week after birth. Children are also offered the same vaccine at 13 months and a second before they start school.	1. Wash your hands with soap and hot water, before preparing food, eating, and after close contact with children. 2. Avoid kissing a young child on the face. 3. Do not share eating utensils with young children. 4. Minimise the time spent in places where there are many children.	1. Stay off work after exposure till symptoms appear. 2. Keep your child off school and if your child has parvovirus, and avoid contact for this period as well. 3. Minimise the time spent in places where there are many children. 4. Wash hands regularly.
Susceptibility to the infection	4-90 out of 100 women. Highest in tropical regions and lowest in cold regions of the world.	1-2 out of 100 women of reproductive age.	30-50 out of 100 women in Europe and the USA.	40 out of 100 women.

Foetal effect	Ultrasound features include defects of the skull and brain. Other features are cataract, blindness, excess fluids in the abdomen (ascites), learning difficulty, convulsions, enlarged liver, jaundice, anaemia, rash and inflammation of the lungs. Any organ can be affected.	Heart defects, small eye sockets, small head and brain, polycystic kidney, FGR, enlarged liver and spleen. Other features are deafness, learning disability, rash, jaundice, anaemia, and easy bruising (thrombocytopenic purpura).	Head and brain defects, FGR, bowel more dense on ultrasound, calcifications in the liver. Other features: eye defects, enlarged spleen and liver, jaundice, easy bruising,	Miscarriage, foetal anaemia leading to heart failure, hydrops 2-12 weeks after maternal infection, and foetal death.

Table 10. General review of TORCH infections

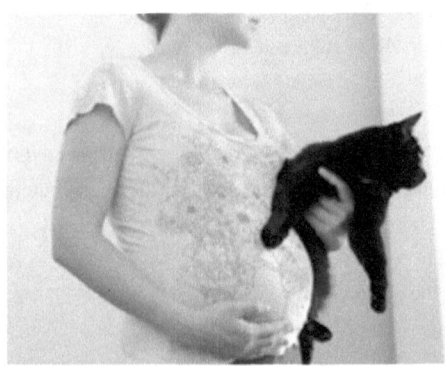

Figure 157. Cat as a source of toxoplasmosis

FURTHER MANAGEMENT

Further management of TORCH infections is not discussed in this book. It belongs to a specialised aspect of obstetrics called foetal medicine.

SOURCES

- To M, Kidd M, Maxwell D. Prenatal diagnosis and management of fetal infections. The Obstetrician & Gynaecologist. 2009;11:108-16.
- www.patient.co.uk
- Patient leaflets from the BMJ Group. Toxoplasma in pregnancy. BMJ Publishing, March 23, 2009, p. 4.

- Rubella. Clinical Knowledge Summaries, December 2009.
- Guideline on Rubella, Health Protection Agency, 2009.
- Cytomegalovirus. NHS Choices, Your health, your choices, 2011.
- Slapped cheek syndrome. NHS Choices, Your health, your choices, 2009.

SYPHILIS

Syphilis is a STI caused by a bug called *Trepanema pallidum*. Its occurrence is higher in developing countries than in developed ones, where it is rare.

MODE OF TRANSMISSION

The bug is spread through blood and from the sore in primary syphilis in the following ways:
- Close contact with an infected sore, normally during vaginal, anal, or oral sex or by sharing sex toys.
- Through blood in drug users who share needles with an infected person.
- Through blood transfusions; this is rare in developed countries as blood for transfusion is routinely tested for syphilis.
- Passing the infection to your baby if you are infected.
    - During pregnancy, through the placenta
    - During childbirth when baby passes through the birth canal, through contact with a sore

The bug cannot survive for long outside the human body, and so syphilis cannot be spread through using the same toilet, clothing, cutlery, orbathroom with an infected person. Breastfeeding does not result in the transmission of syphilis unless an infectious lesion is present on the breast.

SYMPTOMS OF SYPHILIS

The symptoms are the same for men and women and can be difficult to recognise. They are often mild, which means you can pass on the infection without knowing you have got it. The infection develops in four stages namely:
- Primary syphilis
- Secondary syphilis
- Latent syphilis
- Tertiary syphilis

PRIMARY SYPHILIS

- Initial symptoms appear 10 days to 3 months after exposure to the infection in the form of a small painless sore or ulcer (called chancre) on the part of the body where the infection was transmitted, typically the penis, vagina, back passage, tongue or lips. Most people have only one sore, but some may have more.

- Lymph glands (small organs found throughout the body, such as in the neck, groin, or armpit) may be swollen.
- The sore disappears within 2-6 weeks, and if the condition is not treated, syphilis will move into its second stage.

SECONDARY SYPHILIS

- Symptoms begin a few weeks after the disappearance of the sore and include the following:
- non-itchy skin rash appearing anywhere on the body, but commonly on the palms of the hands or soles of the feet

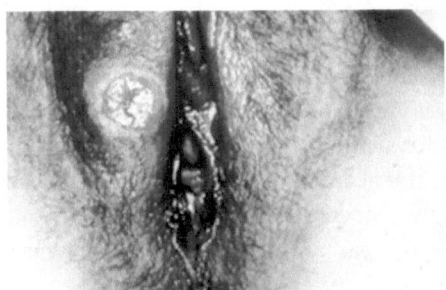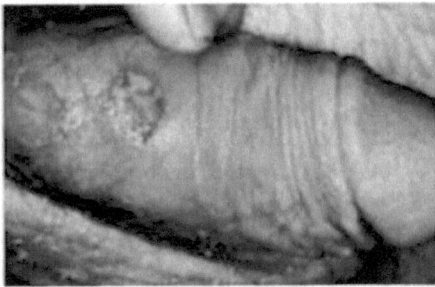

Figure 158a and b. Primary syphilis on the genital organs

- tiredness
- headaches
- swollen lymph glands

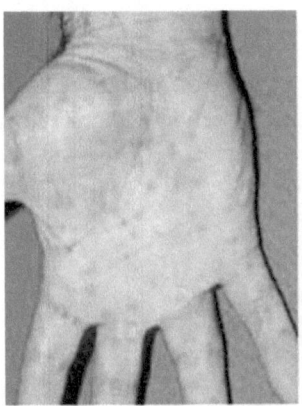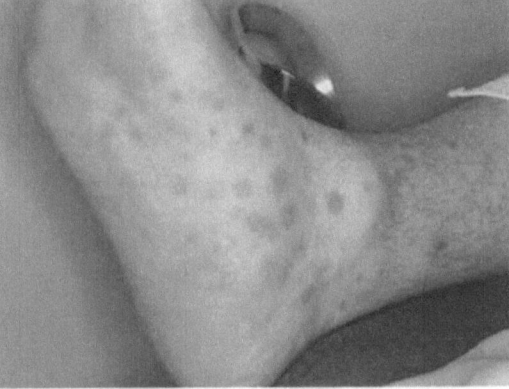

Figure 159 and 160. The rash of secondary syphilis

Less common symptoms include fever, weight loss, patchy hair loss, and joint pains. These symptoms may disappear within a few weeks or come and go over a period of months.

LATENT PHASE

Syphilis will then move into its latent (hidden) phase, where you will experience no symptoms, even though you remain infected, and it can be passed on during the first year of this phase through sexual or close physical contact. After a couple of years, one that remains in the latent phase cannot pass the infection to others, even though they remain infected.

The latent stage can continue for many years (even decades). It is divided into early (within 1 year of the infection) and late (after 1 year of the infection) latent disease. Without treatment, there is a risk that the latent phase will move on to the most dangerous phase—tertiary syphilis.

TERTIARY SYPHILIS

The symptoms depend on the part of the body that the infection has spread to. For example, it may affect the brain, nerves, eyes, heart, bones, skin, or blood vessels; potentially, any organ or system can be affected. Possible symptoms are stroke, loss of memory, loss of coordination, numbness, paralysis, blindness, and so on. Death can also occur.

DIAGNOSIS OF MATERNAL INFECTION.

If you suspect you have syphilis, visit a sexual health clinic or your GP as soon as possible. The following will be done:
- Examination of the genitals and the back passage for the sores of primary syphilis.
- Blood test: Testing for syphilis is one of the screening tests that is normally carried out in the first trimester. If the test is positive, treatment will be given. If you are infected with syphilis, your body will produce antibodies (substances released as part of your immune response) against the bug. Therefore, one way to determine whether you have syphilis or not is to have a sample of your blood tested for the presence of these antibodies—this is a screening test.

  A negative result does not necessarily mean that you do not have syphilis; the antibodies may not be detectable about 3 months after the infection. You may be advised to repeat the test in 3 months' time. A positive result (antibodies present) indicates that you either have the infection or you used to have it (since the antibodies can remain in your body for years, even after a previous infection was successfully treated).

So if the test is positive, the next step is to confirm the results with a confirmatory specific syphilis test.

- Swab test: If sores are present, a swab (like a cotton bud) will be used to take a small sample of fluid from it. This is then sent to a laboratory for examination.
- Test for other STIs such as HIV, chlamydia, and gonorrhoea as it is possible to have more than one STI at a time. People with syphilis are 3-5 times more likely to catch HIV. This is because the genital sores caused by syphilis can bleed easily, making it easier for the HIV virus to enter the blood during sexual activity.

IMPACT OF SYPHILIS ON YOUR FOETUS AND NEWBORN

CHANCE OF YOUR CHILD GETTING THE INFECTION

- If you are pregnant, the bug that causes syphilis crosses the placenta and foetal infection may occur at any stage in pregnancy from 9-10 weeks. Your baby is at a significant risk if you are infected in the first and the third trimesters.
- If you develop primary or secondary syphilis during pregnancy, your baby can be infected (90 out of 100 women who have been infected). About 50 out of 100 infected babies will present with symptoms of syphilis at birth. The rest will develop infection during the first week of life or early latent or late syphilis.
- If you already have primary or secondary infection and you become pregnant, all babies will be infected and approximately 50% will be dead in the womb, prematurely born or dead shortly after delivery. It is therefore always necessary to be screened for syphilis in the prepregnancy clinic if you live in an area with a high prevalence of the disease.

EFFECT OF UNTREATED SYPHILIS ON YOUR FOETUS AND BABY

The presentations are as follows:
- Anaemia in the foetus and newborn
- Too much waters around your baby (polyhydramnios)
- Large placenta
- Large liver
- Hydrops (accumulation of fluid in the abdomen, around the heart, in the lungs and generalised swelling of your foetus)
- Restricted foetal growth due to the involvement of the placenta.
- Dilatation of foetal bowel
- Death

- Involvement of the lungs, heart, kidneys, bones, eyes, blood, face, lymph glands, and many other organs in the newborn
- The World Health Organisation (WHO) estimates that each year, maternal syphilis is responsible for
  - 460,000 abortions
  - 270,000 cases of infection of the baby in the womb (congenital syphilis)
  - the birth of 270,000 LBW or premature babies

DIAGNOSIS OF FOETAL INFECTION IN YOUR BABY

You should be referred to a foetal medicine specialist who will carry out several investigations including the following:
- Taking fluid from the sac surrounding your baby (amniocentesis) for test
- Taking blood from the umbilical cord (cordocentesis) for test
- Ultrasound to pick up the signs enumerated above, especially an enlarged liver, which is the most sensitive ultrasonographic finding suggesting foetal infection.

TREATMENT

- Primary and secondary syphilis can be successfully treated with a single dose of penicillin (which is given as an injection into the buttock). You will be prescribed another antibiotic if you are allergic to penicillin.
- Later stages of the disease need to be treated with three penicillin injections, which are given at weekly intervals.
- Follow-up test: Once the course of antibiotics is completed, you will be asked to return to the sexual health clinic or to your doctor so that a follow-up blood test can be carried out to check that the infection has gone. You can still catch syphilis again, even after you have been successfully treated for it.
- Treatment of tertiary syphilis requires longer courses of antibiotics and may need intravenous treatment (administered directly into the vein). While treatment can stop the infection, it cannot repair any damage that has already been caused by the tertiary syphilis.
- You should refrain from any kind of sexual activity or close physical contact with another person until your treatment is complete and your sexual partner has been tested and treated.
- You can ask your sexual partner to go for a test, but you are not under any obligation to inform him that you have the infection. If you would prefer, the clinic can contact your recent partner(s) for you without informing him about yourself.

PREVENTION OF SYPHILIS

- The only guaranteed way to prevent a syphilis infection is to avoid sexual contact or to only have sexual contact with a faithful partner who has been tested and is clear from the infection.
- Simultaneous use of condoms and dental dam (square of plastic) during intercourse may be helpful.
- Sex toys should not be shared. If you do, wash them or cover them with a condom before each use.
- Other people's needles should not be used if you are an injecting drug user.

REFERENCES

- Syphilis. NHS Choices, Your health, your choices, 2010.
- Tramont EC. *Treponema pallidum* (syphilis). In: Mandell GL, Bennett JE, Dolin R, eds. Principles and Practice of Infectious Diseases. 7th ed. Philadelphia, PA: Elsevier Churchill Livingstone; 2009: chap 238.
- Puder KS, Treadwell MC, Gonik B. Ultrasound characteristics of in utero infection. Infect Dis Obstet Gynecol. 1997;5:262-70.
- The Pregnancy Book. Your complete guide to: a healthy pregnancy, labour and childbirth. The first weeks with your new baby, UK, 2009.

HIV IN PREGNANCY

The HIV is a special type of virus called retrovirus. It prevents the body's immune system from providing a natural defence against infections. The virus infects special cells that are found in the blood known as CD4 cells, multiplies in them, and destroys them.

Although the body will attempt to produce more CD4 cells, their numbers will eventually decline, and the immune system will stop working; this is the end stage of the disease called AIDS. The disease occurs more in developing than in developed countries and it is more prevalent in the sub-Saharan Africa than in any other part of the world.

MODE OF TRANSMISSION AND RISK GROUP

HIV can be passed from one person to another through body fluids, namely

- blood
- semen
- vaginal fluids
- breast milk

Therefore, HIV can spread through

- unprotected sexual contacts, such as vaginal, oral, and anal sex
- drug injection, sharing of needles
- a mother to her unborn child during pregnancy, childbirth, and breastfeeding
- blood transfusions

PEOPLE WHO ARE AT RISK OF CATCHING HIV INCLUDE
- men who have had unprotected sex with men
- women who have had unprotected sex with men who have sex with men
- people who inject illegal drugs
- people who have had unprotected sex with somebody who injects illegal drugs
- people who have caught another STI
- people who have received a blood transfusion while in Africa, Eastern Europe, the countries of the former Soviet Union, Asia, or Central and South America.

PRIMARY HIV INFECTION OR SEROCONVERSION
This is when one gets the infection the first time. Symptoms usually occur 2-6 weeks after infection with the virus and include the following:
- fever
- tiredness
- a blotchy rash
- sore throat
- swollen glands (nodes)
- muscle and joint pain

These early symptoms are often very mild, so it is easy to mistake them for another condition such as a cold or glandular fever, so if you are concerned about the risk of HIV infection, you should request a blood test. After the initial symptoms have gone, HIV will often not cause any further symptoms for many years. During this time, the virus will reproduce and damage your immune system.

LATE-STAGE HIV INFECTION
Late-stage HIV infection is also known as AIDS. This happens when your CD4 count drops below 200. It typically takes about 10 years for the virus to damage the immune system in this way. However, if you stick to your HIV treatment, the likelihood of reaching an end stage is low.

AIDS presents with lymphoma which is a blood cancer and opportunistic infections(that is infections that take advantage of an HIV-weakened immune system). The four main types of the infections are

- bacterial infections, such as pneumonia or tuberculosis
- fungal infections, such as thrush and pneumocystis carinii pneumonia (PCP)
- parasitical infections, such as toxoplasmosis and
- viral infections, such as hepatitis

INTERVENTIONS TO PREVENT TRANSMISSION OF HIV.

PREVENTION AFTER EXPOSURE TO THE VIRUS

The exposure can be in the form of having sex with someone who has HIV and the condom broke, or you were accidentally stabbed with an HIV-infected needle. The measure involves taking anti-HIV medicines within 72 hours of exposure to the virus and continuing on it for 4 weeks. Since it is not guaranteed that this measure will be successful, it is recommended that you go to your local sexual health clinic immediately if exposed to the virus.

PREVENTION OF TRANSMISSION OF HIV IN A COUPLE—SAFER SEX.

- This is achieved by using condoms (for penetrative and oral sex on penis) and dental dams (for oral sex on vagina or anus). It is important to continue to practise safe sex even if you and your sexual partner both have HIV. This is because it is possible to expose yourself to a new strain of the virus that your antiretroviral drugs will not be able to control.
- Using lubricants—They can enhance the safety of intercourse by reducing the risk of vaginal or anal tears being caused by dryness or friction. It can also reduce the likelihood of a condom tearing. A water-based lubricant (such as K-Y Jelly) is better than an oil-based lubricant (such as Vaseline or baby oil), which weakens the latex in condoms and can cause them to break or tear.

Prevention in intravenous drug users—Do not share needles. In developed countries, many local authorities and pharmacies offer needle exchange programmes, where used needles can be exchanged for clean ones. If you are a heroin user, consider enrolling in a methadone programme, whereby you take methadone instead of heroin. Methadone can be taken as a liquid, so it reduces your risk of getting HIV.

THE IMPACT OF HIV INFECTION ON YOU AND YOUR BABY DURING PREGNANCY

The main problems in pregnancy are

- Worsening of the infection
- Mother-to-baby transmission of HIV

MOTHER-TO-BABY TRANSMISSION OF HIV

You can pass HIV on to your baby through

- the placenta while you are pregnant
- childbirth
- breastfeeding

A number of factors can increase the risk of passing on HIV to your baby. They include the following:

- being ill because of HIV
- having a high viral load (number of virus in your blood) and a low CD4 cell count
- waters breaking 4 hours or more before delivery
- having an untreated STI at the time of delivery
- using recreational drugs, particularly injected drugs, during pregnancy
- having a vaginal delivery (rather than a Caesarean delivery) if HIV viral load is detectable
- having a difficult delivery, requiring, for example, the use of forceps
- breastfeeding

ANTENATAL HIV SCREENING

- If you are pregnant, you will be offered screening for HIV infection, syphilis, hepatitis B, and rubella in every pregnancy at your booking antenatal visit. If you decline an HIV test, your reasons will be explored and screening offered again at around 28 weeks. Screening can also be conducted at your GP clinic, at your local sexual health clinic, or at a hospital.
- If you test HIV negative at booking but your doctor feels you are at continued high risk of acquiring HIV, a repeat HIV test will be considered later in pregnancy.
- If you book for antenatal care late, the test should be requested urgently and the result issued within 24 hours.
- If you present for the first time in pregnancy in labour, you will be offered a rapid HIV test, which delivers results within 20 minutes of the sample being taken.
- If you test HIV positive, you will be seen by a special counsellor and then a team of doctors who will take care of you during your pregnancy.

THE BENEFITS OF ANTENATAL SCREENING

- Twenty percent of HIV-infected babies develop AIDS or die within the first year of life. Interventions will be put in place to prevent you from transmitting the infection to your baby. They are as follows:
  - Avoidance of breastfeeding.
  - Antiretroviral treatment (ART) during pregnancy.

- Delivery by Caesarean section at 39 weeks and vaginal delivery when safe to do so.
- Appropriate care of your baby after delivery.
  - ➤ Your baby's umbilical cord will be clamped as soon as possible after the birth.
  - ➤ Baby will be bathed immediately after the birth.
  - ➤ Your baby will be treated with anti-retroviral drug within 4 hours of birth and that will be continued for 4 weeks after delivery.

The above measures have reduced mother-to-child transmission rates from 25-30 in a 100 to 1 in a 100.

- Appropriate measures will be put in place if it is believed that your baby is infected. They are as following:
  - As above.
  - Baby will be given a drug called co-trimoxazole as a prophylaxis against PCP.
  - Your baby should be tested at day 1, 6 weeks, and 12 weeks of age. If all these tests are negative and the baby is not being breastfed, it means your baby is not HIV-infected. A confirmatory HIV antibody test is performed at around 18 months of age since loss of antibodies that your baby acquired from you often occurs by 18 months of age but may take longer.
- Interventions to reduce disease progression in you will be put in place.
- Possible complications in pregnancy will be treated appropriately in order to decrease the risk to you and your baby.
- Your prepregnancy advice before your next pregnancy will be modified in order to maximise your chance of getting pregnant and also reduce the risk of passing on the disease to your partner.

MODIFICATION OF YOUR ANTENATAL CARE

- A multidisciplinary team including a HIV physician, obstetrician, specialist midwife, health advisor, and paediatrician should take care of you.
- Early assessment of your social circumstances will be conducted and help should be offered if needed, for instance relationship break-up, domestic violence, drug abuse.
- HIV test should be done for your other children of unknown HIV status if you test positive.
- Blood tests for viral infections (hepatitis C, varicella-zoster, and measles) and toxoplasma will be offered apart from the infection screening that is normally carried out at booking clinic. You should be offered additional treatment on the basis of the blood results if you need it. The tests will usually be repeated around the twenty-eighth week of your pregnancy.

Any genital infection that is detected will be treated even if there is no symptom.

- Jabs will be given to protect you against infections namely hepatitis B, pneumonia, and also influenza (to be given during the cold season.) Jabs against other infections namely chickenpox and MMR are contraindicated in pregnancy; if you are not already immunised, the vaccines will be given after delivery.
- Intervention to reduce mother-to-child transmission of the disease as above will be conducted.
- Interventions to prevent progression of the infection will be embarked upon.
- Screening for gestational diabetes, which is one of the complications of HAART, should be carried out if you are already taking HAART at the time of booking.
- Dating and anomaly scans and screening for chromosomal abnormalities will be performed as in non-infected women.
- Invasive tests (CVS and amniocentesis) may increase the risk of transmitting the disease to your baby. Therefore, if you need invasive procedure, you may be offered treatment with HAART if you are not already taking it. This reduces the risk of the HIV virus infecting your baby.
- A plan for mode of delivery will be made at 36 weeks.

INTERVENTIONS TO REDUCE DISEASE PROGRESSION

- HAART: The intervention involves giving you a combination of drugs against HIV called HAART. You will start taking it when you are 12 weeks into your pregnancy (earlier administration of the drugs may have ill effects on early foetal development) if your specialist believes that you need it based on your blood results. Otherwise, you will start taking it between 20 and 28 weeks and discontinue at delivery.
- Opportunistic infections: Furthermore, if your specialist feels that you are at risk of opportunistic infections, e.g. PCP, you will be given medication against it.
- Monitoring disease progression: This is necessary to determine your risk of developing an HIV-related infection and to determine when to change your drugs and also the mode of delivery. The tests used are as follows:
  - CD4 cell count
  - viral load levels (the quantity of the virus in your blood)

SPECIFIC SITUATIONS AND MANAGEMENT

Many of these situations are not fully treated in this book. So if any of them is applicable to you, you should call your obstetrician immediately. They are enumerated below.

- Increased risk of opportunistic infections in advanced disease. This is particularly so for the atypical chest infection. Symptoms include fever, dry cough, shortness of breath, and deprivation of oxygen.
- Side effects of HAART: The side effects include bowel disturbances, skin rashes, gestational diabetes, and liver problems. So symptoms suggestive of other pregnancy problems like PE, cholestasis, or liver dysfunction may indicate drug side effects. In that situation, your obstetrician will liaise with HIV physicians in the management of the disease.
- Preterm labour.
- PPROM after 34 weeks of pregnancy.
- PPROM before 34 weeks of pregnancy.
- PPROM at term.
- Post-term pregnancy
- Vaginal birth after previous Caesarean section.
- HIV diagnosed late in pregnancy.
- HIV diagnosed during labour.

MODE OF DELIVERY

A decision about mode of delivery will be made by 36 weeks of gestation. This decision will be reviewed when you are in labour. Your obstetrician in collaboration with other members of HIV team specialists will assess your situation and propose to you appropriate mode of delivery based on your blood tests—CD4 count and viral load. Delivery is by either Caesarean section at 39 and more weeks or vaginal delivery at term with precautions taken to reduce mother-to-child transmission of the disease.

YOUR CARE AFTER THE DELIVERY

- You should continue with HAART if you were taking it before delivery.
- You should neither breastfeed nor express your milk for your baby. You should be given supportive advice about formula feeding.
- You will be recommended for the suppression of milk production. In the UK, a drug called cabergoline 1 mg orally is given within 24 hours of birth.
- You should receive guidance about contraception after delivery.
- You should be given a jab against MMR if your CD4 count is above 200 and against chickenpox if your CD4 cell count is above 400; this should happen only if you are not immune to these infections.

CARE OF YOUR BABY AFTER THE DELIVERY

Please see under benefits of antenatal screening.

PREPREGNANCY CARE

The care is the same as in non-HIV positive woman but with some modifications. Your health and HAART regimen should be optimised before conception. It is recommended that you delay pregnancy until your viral load is low, preventive measures against atypical lung infection is not needed, and any opportunistic infections have been treated. Furthermore, annual cervical smear test is indicated because of the positive association of HIV and precancerous changes in the cervix.

If you are HIV positive but your partner is HIV negative and you choose to have sexual intercourse, condoms should be used. Consistent use of condoms in this situation is associated with an 80% reduction in transmission of the disease to your partner. If you choose to have children, your doctor should explain to you the process of self-insemination during the fertile time of the cycle using quills, syringes, and sterile containers, or you can go for a test-tube baby.

If you are HIV negative but your partner is HIV positive, then assisted conception with sperm washing is significantly safer than timed unprotected intercourse. If you do engage in sexual act, the risk of transmission for each act of sexual intercourse is estimated to be between 3 in 10,000 and 1 in 100,000. This risk is significantly reduced, although not eliminated, if the male partner has a viral load of less than 50 copies/mL and is taking HAART. The risk can be further reduced by limiting exposure to the fertile period of your menstrual cycle and ensuring that all genital infections have been treated.

ETHICAL ISSUE AND CONFIDENTIALITY IN PREGNANCY

Your health care team need to know that you are HIV positive so that your care can be planned appropriately. The team will encourage you to inform your sexual partner about your HIV status in order to reduce the risk of passing on the HIV virus to him. They should not tell anyone about your status, without your permission. The only exception to this is when your health care team thinks that by not telling a sexual partner that you are HIV positive, you are putting that person's life at serious risk. In these circumstances, your health care professionals may tell a sexual partner about your status.

This is what happens in developed countries, including the UK, where the body that regulates doctor's registration 'The General Medical Council' supports such action. Your health care team must discuss this with you first. They must weigh up any risks involved for you (such as violence and/or abuse) before they decide on what to do. In rare cases where you refuse interventions to reduce the risk of mother-to-child transmission, a pre-birth planning meeting will be held with social services to discuss safeguarding issues. Legal permission may be sought at birth to treat the infant for 4 weeks with ART and to prevent breastfeeding.

Sources

- HIV in Pregnancy. Royal College of Obstetricians and Gynaecologists (RCOG) Guideline, 2010.
- NAM (National Aids Manual), a UK-based organisation at: www.aidsmap.com
- Routine antenatal care for healthy pregnant women, NICE website at: www.nice.org.uk
- HIV in pregnancy: information for you. Published February 2005 by the RCOG Genital Herpes.
- HIV. NHS Choices, Your health, your choices, 2010.

Malaria in Pregnancy

Malaria is caused by parasites called plasmodia (P). They are as follows: *P. falciparum, P. vivax, P. malariae, P. ovale,* and rarely *P. knowlesi.*

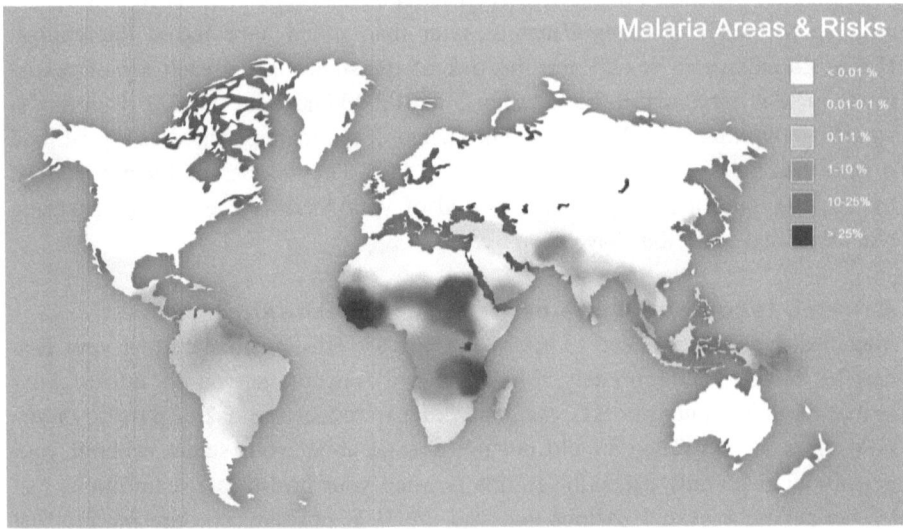

Figure 161. Malarial endemic regions

They live in water or at least where it is damp, human body and mosquitoes. Malaria remains one of the leading causes of illness and death in Africa and some Asian countries. In Nigeria, for instance, it is responsible for

- 60 out of every 100 clinic attendance to hospitals
- 11 out of every 100 maternal deaths

The non-*falciparum* species are rarely fatal. The most vulnerable groups are as follows:
- children below 5 years of age
- pregnant women
- immigrants returning home from Western countries

TRANSMISSION OF MALARIA AND LIFE CYCLE OF PLASMODIUM

The female mosquito called anopheles bites an infected person and sucks human blood containing one form of the parasite. The parasite develops in the mosquito which then bites another human and transfers the parasite into her or his blood. In human, the parasite moves into the liver and develops into a form which is released into the blood; the parasite is then taken up by the red blood cells. The parasite bursts the red blood cell and is released into the bloodstream again; this coincides with increase in temperature that occurs in malaria.

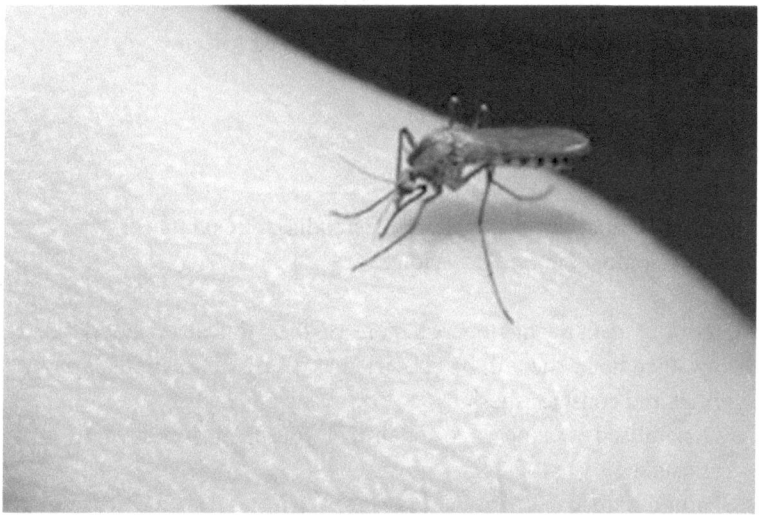

Figure 162. Blood meal by malarial parasite

In falciparum malaria, part of the infected and also non-infected red blood cells become stuck inside small blood vessels of the brain, kidneys, and other affected organs including the placenta. This process is called sequestration. The interval from mosquito bite to manifestation of the disease is usually about 10-15 days. *Plasmodium ovale* and *Plasmodium vivax* can produce a dormant form in the liver that can cause relapses of the disease months and even years after the original disease (relapsing malaria).

FALCIPARUM MALARIA

EFFECTS OF MALARIA ON YOU
Malaria can be uncomplicated or complicated (severe).

UNCOMPLICATED MALARIA
This occurs when there are general symptoms of malaria but no evidence of organ dysfunction. The presentation is as follows:

- Fever/chills/sweats
- Headache
- Elevated temperature
- Muscle pain
- General malaise
- Difficulty breathing

- Cough
- Feeling sick
- Vomiting
- Diarrhoea
- Looking pale
- Enlarged spleen

SEVERE OR COMPLICATED MALARIA
It is caused by the following:
- *P. falciparum*
- mixed *P. falciparum* and other plasmodia, for example *P. vivax*
- *P. vivax* alone, in rare occasions

If a patient with malaria has one or more of the clinical or laboratory features given below, then he or she will be classified as a case of severe malaria.
- Impaired consciousness
- Generalised weakness, so much that you cannot walk or sit up without assistance
- Failure to feed
- Multiple convulsions, more than two episodes in 24 hours
- Brisk reflexes
- Deep breathing, difficulty breathing
- Shock
- Jaundice (yellow eyes)
- Spontaneous bleeding
- Swelling of the lungs seen on X-rays
- Severe anaemia
- Acute kidney failure
- Secondary bacterial infection

- Specific laboratory findings which should be assessed by a specialist in malaria
- Death

DIFFERENCES IN THE PRESENTATION OF MALARIA IN ENDEMIC AND IN NON-ENDEMIC AREAS

Endemic area is a place of high transmission rate of malaria, for example some Asian countries and Africa. In these areas, people including pregnant women have acquired immunity to malaria. Malaria, therefore, does not present with symptom, and if it does, they are mild. It, however, causes anaemia and also placental sequestration of the parasite which leads to LBW babies. In low-transmission or non-endemic areas, there is an increased risk of severe malaria and death because of the absence of immunity or low immunity to the disease.

EFFECTS OF MALARIA ON YOUR PREGNANCY

In pregnancy, the adverse effects of malarial infection are as follows:
- Effects due to high temperature:
  - Foetal death
  - Foetal distress shown by abnormal trace of baby's heart
  - Stillbirth
  - Miscarriage
  - Premature birth
- Effects due to the presence of the parasite in different parts of the body and interaction with HIV infection:
  - FGR (malaria is responsible for 50 out of 100 cases of FGR in endemic regions) and LBW
  - Anaemia in you and your baby
  - Interaction with HIV—malaria occurs more in patients with HIV
- Transmission of the disease during pregnancy or during childbirth to your baby, giving rise to congenital malaria

EFFECTS OF PREGNANCY ON MALARIAL INFECTION

- Pregnancy increases four-fold a woman's risk of catching malarial illness and doubles her risk of death.
- The symptoms of severe malaria are more grievous in the pregnant women than in the non-pregnant women.

DIAGNOSIS OF MALARIA IN PREGNANCY

The diagnosis is based on the clinical presentation as listed above and results of investigations. The investigations are as follows:
- Blood tests to check for the following:
  - the parasite, this confirms the diagnosis

- anaemia
- glucose levels
- liver function
- Urine test (urine dipstick) and stool tests
- Chest X-ray if breathing problem is present (precautions apply in pregnancy)
- Obstetric ultrasound to assess your baby

TREATMENT

Different drug combinations are used, but the ones recommended by the WHO are outlined below.

FIRST TRIMESTER

- Quinine plus clindamycin is given for 7 days; this regime is used in the UK.
- Artemisinin-based combination therapy (ACT) is primarily an alternative to the above regime; it is the drug combination used in Africa.
- Atovaquone-proguanil combination is also used.

Your doctor should prescribe the drugs for you.

SECOND AND THIRD TRIMESTERS

- ACT
- Quinine plus clindamycin for 7 days

Maximum benefit can be derived if the drugs are taken within 24-48 hours of the onset of malarial symptoms. The drugs have their specific complications, and therefore the treatment should be monitored by your doctor. In endemic regions of Africa and part of Asia, most cases are managed as outpatients, and treatment regime is given not for 7 but 3 days. In developed countries, for example the UK, all pregnant women with *P. falciparum* are admitted into hospital, as the clinical condition can deteriorate rapidly.

OTHER IMPORTANT CO-TREATMENT OF MALARIA IN PREGNANCY

Different symptoms are treated. These are as follows:
- Fever—paracetamol.
- Vomiting—anti-vomiting drugs.
- Seizures (convulsion), which occurs more in children—specific treatment will be given.
- Anaemia—ferrous sulphate, folic acid, and blood transfusion.
- Low blood sugar level—a drip of dextrose infusion is given.

TREATMENT FAILURE

Recurrence of *P. falciparum* malaria can be as a result of

- failure of treatment if symptoms are back within 2 weeks of the initial treatment.
- a reinfection if treatment failure happens after 2 weeks of the initial treatment. Most cases occur around day 28-42 from the onset of symptoms, but late cases have been reported for different drug combinations.

Treatment failures may result from

- drug resistance
- poor adherence
- substandard medicine
- inadequate drug exposure (from under-dosing, vomiting, or unusual body handling of the drug in that individual)

MANAGEMENT OF TREATMENT FAILURE

If your treatment fails, you will be treated with a second-line antimalarial drugs, which are as follows:

- a 7-day regime of an alternative ACT regime which is known to be effective in the endemic region.
- quinine plus clindamycin (given for a total of 7 days) if ACT was used in the initial treatment.

If you have a reinfection you will be treated with the first-line ACT regime.

HOW PREGNANCY MODIFIES THE
EFFECT OF ANTIMALARIAL TREATMENTS

- The treatment in pregnant women is less effective than in non-pregnant patients, probably because of the lower concentrations of antimalarial drugs in pregnancy.
- The ability of *P. falciparum* to sequester (hide) in the placenta enhances recurrence of the disease in pregnancy.

THE PECULIARITIES OF TREATMENT OF SEVERE FALCIPARUM MALARIA

- Many tests will be done in order to rule out other medical conditions that present similarly like severe malaria and to confirm the severity of the infection. Management is undertaken by the intensive care unit, obstetricians, and other associated specialists.
- Initial treatment involves resuscitation. So the specialist will ensure that your airway is open, you are breathing, and your blood circulation

is maintained and will take the necessary precautions if you are unconscious.

- Pre-transfer treatment is applicable in developing countries. The risk of death from severe malaria is greatest in the first 24 hours, yet in most malarial endemic countries, the transit time between referral and arrival at health facilities that is able to administer intravenous treatment is usually prolonged. This delays the commencement of appropriate antimalarial treatment. It is, therefore, recommended that patients should be treated with the first dose of one of the recommended treatments before transfer unless the transfer time is less than 6 hours. Example is the administration of one of the components of ACT called 'artesunate' or 'artemether' into the back passage. If, however, referral is impossible, this treatment will be continued until you can tolerate oral medication; at this point, a full course of the recommended ACT for uncomplicated malaria in the locality can be administered.
- Intravenous artesunate is used in preference to quinine for the treatment of severe *P. falciparum* malaria in a hospital facility; it is used for a minimum of 24 hours, and then oral medication follows when tolerated.
- Subsequent management depends on the presentation and is for prevention of disabilities and failure of treatment.

Specific Obstetric Management of Malarial Infection in Pregnancy

Prompt treatment of malaria reduces the systemic effects of the parasite in your blood, placental sequestration, and consequently the adverse effects on the foetus.

Antenatal Care After Recovery from an Episode of Malaria in Pregnancy

- Regular antenatal appointments, including assessment of your haemoglobin, platelets, and glucose, should be followed.
- The chances of recurrence are low when you have completed an effective course of antimalarial drugs. Should symptoms return, prompt confirmation with blood test and treatment is essential.
- The risk of preeclampsia may increase significantly if the parasite has infected the placenta (placental malaria). Therefore, regular checks for PE will be conducted by doing urine dipstick for protein and measuring your BP.
- Foetal distress is common and is due to malarial fever, FGR, and low glucose levels, especially if quinine has been used in the treatment. Therefore screening for these problem and regular trace of baby's heart are indicated.

IOL and Mode of Delivery

- Vaginal birth is allowed.
- Uncomplicated malaria in pregnancy is not a reason for IOL.
- Preterm and threatened preterm labours are managed as in non-infected patients.
- Instrumental birth in the second stage of labour in the presence of maternal or foetal distress is indicated if there are no contraindications.
- The role of early Caesarean section for the viable foetus is unproven in severe malaria.
- Acute malaria can cause low platelets in pregnancy, so significant bleeding after delivery will be expected.
- Prevention of blood clots formation in the lungs or legs with drugs that thin the blood will be weighed up against the risk of bleeding; if the platelet count is falling or less than 100, preventive measures will be withheld.

Congenital Malaria

- Your baby can be infected and he or she can develop congenital malaria if you get the infection close to delivery. The parasites cross the placenta to your baby, either during pregnancy or at the time of birth.
- It occurs in 8-33 out of 100 infected mothers but more in non-endemic than in endemic regions. This is because your high immunity to the disease in endemic region is transferred to your baby.
- It occurs in all the four types of plasmodia, but more in *P. falciparum* and *P. malariae*.
- It may present in the first week to months of life with symptoms such as
    - fever
    - feeling lethargic
    - anaemia
    - enlarged liver and spleen
    - features suggestive of neonatal sepsis such as irritability, poor feeding, vomiting, loose stools, jaundice, drowsiness, and restlessness
- You and your baby will be tested to confirm the diagnosis if you have had malaria in pregnancy. Blood will be taken from the placenta, umbilical cord, and your baby for test. Furthermore, your baby will be screened weekly for 28 days for the parasite. The placenta will also be sent for a test called histology to analyse its tissue for the parasite.

PLASMODIUM VIVAX, PLASMODIUM OVALE, PLASMODIUM MALARIAE MALARIA AND MIXED MALARIAL INFECTION

The effects of these infections on pregnancy are the same as in falciparum infection, but less severe. *Plasmodium vivax*, the second most important species causing human malaria, accounts for about 40% of malarial cases worldwide; it is the dominant malarial species outside Africa. It is prevalent in endemic areas of Asia, Central and South America, Middle East, and Oceania but rare in Africa. Transmission rates are low, and the affected populations, therefore, achieve little immunity to the disease. Consequently, people of all ages are at risk. *Plasmodium Malariae* and *Plasmodium ovale* are less prevalent, but they are distributed worldwide, especially in the tropical areas of Africa.

Plasmodium vivax and *Plasmodium ovale* form parasite stages in the liver, which can result in multiple relapses of infection weeks to months after the primary infection. The objective of their treating, therefore, is to get rid of both the blood and the liver stages of the infection and thereby prevent treatment failure. The only drugs with significant activity against the liver stages are a group of drugs called 8-aminoquinolines (buloquine, primaquine, and tafenoquine).

TREATMENT

- The treatment for all types of plasmodia parasites is the same but for *P. ovale* and *P. vivax* infections, primaquine which kills the liver form and prevents relapse is to be added to the regime. Unfortunately, primaquine has significant side effects and therefore contraindicated in pregnancy but not in breastfeeding. Chloroquine can also be used for treatment.
- *Plasmodium malariae infection* is treated with the standard regimen of chloroquine.
- ACT is the treatment of choice for mixed infection.

MALARIAL INFECTION IN DIFFERENT SITUATIONS

TREATMENT OF MALARIA WHEN YOU ARE BREASTFEEDING

- The amount of antimalarial drugs that enter breast milk and is consumed by the breastfeeding infant is relatively small.
- You can receive the recommended antimalarial treatment (including ACTs), except tetracycline and dapsone. Tetracycline has bad effect on infant's bones and teeth while dapsone can suppress the growth of the bone marrow.
- Primaquine can be taken if you and your baby do not have a condition called glucose-6-phosphate dihydrogenase deficiency (G6PD-deficient). It causes breakdown of red blood cells, giving rise to anaemia if you are

G6PD-deficient. Therefore, before you take it, both you and your baby should be tested for the condition.

MALARIA IN TRAVELLERS

The following category of people are likely to develop severe malaria:
- those who do not have immunity against malaria and live in a city with little or no transmission within endemic country
- visitors from non-endemic countries who travel to endemic area

If you belong to any of these two categories of people and develop malaria, you should be treated promptly.

Another scenario is a situation whereby travellers who, having travelled to an endemic area, return home in non-endemic region and develop malaria. In this situation, the malaria is likely to be severe. This is applicable to people from Europe, the USA, or other non-endemic regions and also Africans and Asians who have lived in non-endemic area for a long time. The peculiarities in this situation are as following:
- Doctors in non-malarious areas may be unfamiliar with malaria so the diagnosis may be delayed.
- The same medicine that you used fro prophylaxis should not be used for treatment.
- The treatment should be as per severe malaria and is the same as practiced in endemic area with little modifications. The treatment will be in intensive care unit.

HIV INFECTION AND MALARIA

- Worsening HIV infection may lead to more severe manifestations of malaria. This is worse in non-endemic regions; therefore, prompt and effective antimalarial treatment regimens should be initiated when the diagnosis has been made.
- The response to treatment of malaria is low and the adverse effect of placental malaria on birth weight is high in HIV patients. So ultrasound monitoring is essential.
- There is limited information at present on the interactions between antimalarial and anti-HIV drugs. Therefore, your medication for HIV and malaria will not be modified. The only exceptions are as follows:
  - Prevention of malaria in pregnancy by taking the WHO recommended 'intermittent preventive treatment—sulphadoxine-pyrimethamine (SP)' will not be given to HIV patients receiving preventive treatment against a type of pneumonia called PCP. This is because the drug used for PCP treatment (co-trimoxazole) and SP belong to the same family of drugs.

315

– ACT containing amodiaquine will not be used because it decreases white blood cells count.

PREVENTION OF MALARIA DURING PREGNANCY

PREVENTION IN WOMEN LIVING IN ENDEMIC REGION

If you live in endemic region, for example West Africa, you should be managed with the following malarial prevention strategy aimed at making pregnancy safe:

- WHO recommended intermittent preventive treatment
  – SP is given as two doses: the first at 18-20 weeks and the second a month later. A third dose is given in HIV-positive patients.
  – Major part of foetal growth occurs between 24 and 36 weeks of gestation. So if you receive the two doses of SP at the specified time, the parasites should be cleared from the placenta and therefore less FGR will occur.
  – SP acts against folic acid and therefore will not be given to you in combination with it. So if you take folic acid regularly, it will be withheld for 7 days after taking the SP.
- Insecticide-treated nets (ITNs) are used throughout pregnancy and puerperium (6 weeks after delivery).
- Prompt and effective management of malaria.
  – Treatment of a case
  – Screening and treating the positive cases
- Prophylaxis (iron and folate) and treatment of anaemia.
- Nutritional counselling.
- Anti-worm drugs (e.g. mebendazole 500 mg) in second or third trimesters.

PREVENTION IN WOMEN LIVING IN NON-ENDEMIC REGION

This advice is applicable to those living outside an endemic area and travelling to endemic zone. They include the following:
- Europeans
- North Americans
- Other non-endemic people, for example the Japanese
- People who had lived in the endemic areas in the past but presently living in the non-endemic area, for example immigrants from Africa, India, and so on

The advice covers malarial prevention and travel recommendations to
- women planning a pregnancy and
- those already pregnant or breastfeeding

If you belong to one of these two groups, you should not travel to a malarial endemic region because you have low immunity to the disease; you are highly susceptible to it. If travelling is unavoidable, then you have to adhere to the following regime:

- Prevention of malarial infection should be followed strictly using the following guide:
    - Awareness of the high risk of being infected with malaria.
    - Bite prevention - You should use skin repellents, knock-down mosquito sprays ITNs and clothing when you are in an endemic region.
    - Your should take a prophylactic drug before travelling to endemic region.
    - D*iagnosis* and prompt treatment of a case of malaria in the endemic region.
- You should be aware that a fever or flu-like illness while at your destination or 1 year or more after returning home may be due to malaria and requires urgent medical attention.

PROPHYLACTIC DRUGS.

A drug called Malarone (contains Atovaquone and Proguanil) is used.

- It kills the liver stage of the disease called schizont, which takes approximately 7 days after been infected to develop. So this drug needs to be taken on the day of travelling to an endemic region and continued for 7 days after leaving the area.
- It is safe in all trimesters of pregnancy.

Mefloquine is also used.

- It kills the red-blood-cell stages of the malarial parasite and so will be taken while in the endemic region and continued for 4 weeks after leaving the area.
- It is safe in all trimesters of pregnancy.
- It will not be given in the following situations:
    - if you have current or previous history of depression or psychiatric disorders
    - if you have epilepsy
    - if you have allergic reaction to quinine or mefloquine
    - if you are breastfeeding

EMERGENCY STANDBY TREATMENT IN PREGNANCY

- If you are pregnant and travelling to a malarial endemic area, your doctor should give you a written instructions regarding emergency standby malarial treatment in the event of suspected malaria without access to medical care within 24 hours.

- If malaria is suspected (flu-like illness) and temperature is 38°C or above, standby treatment should be started, after which a full investigation can follow.
- If you are infected, the recommended regime in most developed world e.g. the UK for pregnant women is a combination of quinine and clindamycin given for 7 days. Suppressive prophylaxis with mefloquine is normally commenced 1 week after the last treatment dose. Instead of the above regime, artemether/lumefantrine (Coartem) can be used.

SOURCES

- Guidelines for Malaria Prevention in Travellers from the United Kingdom. London: Health Protection Agency; January 2007.
- The prevention of malaria in pregnancy. RCOG guideline, April 2010.
- Diagnosis and treatment of malaria in pregnancy. RCOG guideline, April 2010.
- Guideline for the Treatment of Malaria, WHO, 2010, 2006.
- National Guidelines and Strategies for Malarial Prevention and Control during Pregnancy. Federal Ministry of Health, Nigeria, May 2004.

Medical Problems in Pregnancy
OBESITY IN PREGNANCY

Obesity can be defined as weighing more than what one's weight should be, taking height into consideration. It is classified by the WHO as shown on the table below on the basis of BMI. BMI is calculated by using the following formula:

BMI = your weight in kilogramme (kg)/your height in metre square (m^2)

Classification	BMI (kg/m2)
Obese	>30.0
Class I obesity	30.0-34.9
Class II obesity	35.0-39.9
Class III or morbid obesity	>40.0

Table 11. WHO classification of obesity

EFFECTS OF OBESITY ON PREGNANCY

Obesity affects over 300 million people worldwide. In the developed countries, for example the UK, the prevalence of obesity among pregnant women from 2003 to 2005 was between 16 and 19 out of 100, and in the same period, it was reported as a co-factor in 28 out of 100 deaths. In developing countries like Africa and Asia, there are no statistics on obesity.

Obesity in pregnancy is associated with increased risk of the following conditions:
- During pregnancy
  - miscarriage
  - abnormalities in babies
  - pre-eclampsia
  - gestational diabetes
  - clots formation (thromboembolism)
  - preterm labour
  - LFD baby
  - IOL
- In labour
  - slow progress of labour
  - shoulder getting stuck after delivery of baby's head
  - emergency Caesarean section
  - instrumental deliveries
  - bleeding after delivery
  - technical difficulties with intravenous access, epidural or spinal anaesthesia, and foetal surveillance in labour
- Wound infections.
- Anaesthetic complications
  - Epidural re-site rates are high. For these reasons, an early epidural may be advisable.
  - The risk of aspiration of gastric contents under general anaesthesia is significantly increased.
  - Difficulty in passing a tube into the throat (endotracheal intubation).
  - Post-operative collapse of part or (much less commonly) all of a lung.
  - Other complication of obesity namely high BP and heart disease.
- High risks of foetal death, neonatal death, and maternal death.
- Lower rate of breastfeeding.
- Infertility.
- Complications are more with excessive weight gain in pregnancy especially if you were obese before pregnancy. There may be retention of fat in the post-natal period.
- High chance of children being obese.

PREPREGNANCY CARE

The care is the same as discussed in chapter one of this book but with some modifications. Successful weight management in the preconception period reduces adverse outcomes.

- You should be given information and advice about the risks of obesity during pregnancy and childbirth and be supported to lose weight before conception if you are of childbearing age and your BMI is 30 or more. This will include dietary advice, exercise, drugs and information leaflets on them.

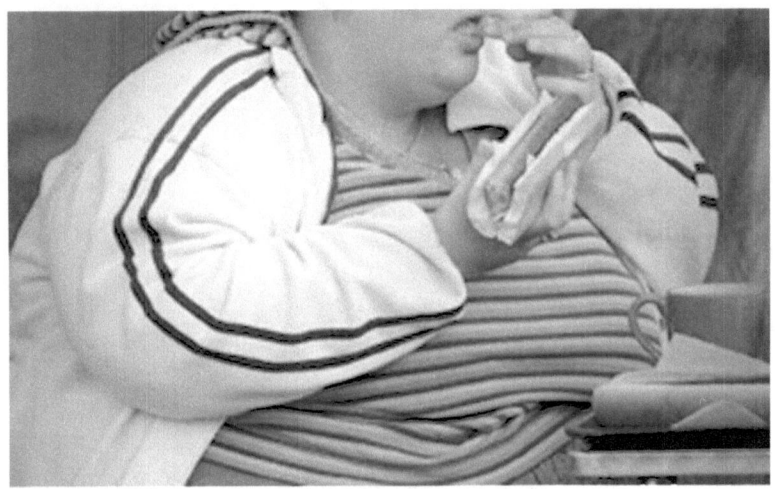

Figure 163. Obesity in pregnancy

- You should be taking folic acid 5 mg daily, starting from 1 month before conception and continue till the first trimester. This is because you are likely to have lower blood levels of folic acid when compared with somebody who is not obese.

ANTENATAL CARE

Your antenatal care will be as in non-obese patients but with some modifications.

- Your weight, height, and BMI will be taken at the booking clinic, preferably at 10 weeks of pregnancy; if it is 40 and more, the following will be done:
  - You should be referred to a dietician but it is important to note that weight loss is not advised in pregnancy. If your BMI is 35-39.9, referral will be considered.
  - You will be offered post-natal treatment to prevent blood clots formation in the veins of your legs or lungs regardless of your mode of delivery, and this will be continued for a minimum of 1 week after childbirth.

- An appropriate size of BP arm cuff will be used to measure your BP, and the size should be documented in your note.
- If your BMI is 35 and more, you have a significant risk of anaesthetic problems and an increased risk of PE. You should therefore have BP and urine check at each antenatal visit and anaesthetic assessment should be offered in the third trimester.
- If your BMI is 30 or more, you should be screened for gestational diabetes at 24-28 weeks of pregnancy.
- If the growth of baby is clinically difficult to assess, a growth scan at 28, 32, and 36 weeks will be organised.

PLANNING LABOUR AND DELIVERY

- If your BMI is 40 and above, in the third trimester of pregnancy, you will have a documented assessment of your specific needs for safe labour and delivery; these will include working loads of bed and theatre table, the provision of appropriate lateral transfer equipment, for example hoists, and appropriately sized stockings to prevent clots formation in your legs.
- If your BMI is 35 and more, you should give birth in a consultant-led obstetric unit with appropriate neonatal services. Home births and water births are discouraged due to the increased risk of problems (baby's shoulder getting stuck after delivery of the head and bleeding after childbirth) associated with obesity and the urgency of treatment that may be required.
- If you have had previous Caesarean section, decision about mode of delivery should be taken with your full involvement, taking into consideration the following facts:
    - Obesity is a risk factor for unsuccessful VBAC.
    - Morbid obesity carries a greater risk for uterine rupture during trial of labour and also injury to your newborn.
    - Emergency Caesarean section is associated with an increased risk of serious problem for you because anaesthetic and operative difficulties are more prevalent in the obese than in non-obese.

CARE IN LABOUR

- Obesity alone is not an indication for IOL in the absence of other obstetric or medical indications, so a normal vaginal birth will be encouraged.
- You will be encouraged to be mobile in labour, and adequate fluid will be given.
- TED stockings should be used in order to prevent blood clots formation in the legs.

- The midwife should ensure that the correct size of BP arm cuff is used for measuring your BP.
- You should have active management of the third stage of labour by giving you intravenous drug that contracts the womb.

If your BMI is 40 and above, the following will be applicable to you:

- There is an increased risk of pressure sores formation because of relative immobility, especially in labour. Therefore, potential pressure areas will be regularly inspected, and appropriate plans will be put in place with regard to body positions, repositioning schedules, skin care, and support surfaces.
- The duty anaesthetist covering labour ward will be informed immediately if delivery or operative intervention is anticipated. An early epidural may be advisable depending on the clinical scenario.
- You should have venous access established early in labour.

Care After Delivery for all Obese Women

You will be offered a routine post-natal care and also specific management and advice as enumerated below.

- Early mobilisation and adequate fluid intake is required.
- Prevention of blood clot formation if your BMI is more than 40; this is achieved by giving you a low-molecular-weight heparin (LMWH) (page xxx).
- The wound will be assessed and observed for signs of infection and breakdown if you have any operation.
- Breastfeeding will be encouraged.
- Advice will be offered on diet and regular exercise to promote weight loss and prevent further weight gain.
- Consideration will be given to referring you to a specialist that deals with obesity if you are morbidly obese.

Sources

- Confidential Enquiry into Maternal and Child Health (CEMACH). Saving Mothers Lives—2003-2005. London: RCOG Press; 2007.
- CMACE/RCOG joint guideline—Management of women with obesity in pregnancy, March 2010.
- Guelinckx I, et al. Maternal obesity: pregnancy complications, gestational weight gain and nutrition. Obes Rev. 2008;9:334-42.
- Heslehurst, N. et al. (2008) 'The impact of maternal BMI status on pregnancy outcomes with immediate short-term obstetric resource implications: a metaanalysis', *Obesity Reviews,* 9 (6), pp.635-683.

DIABETES IN PREGNANCY

Diabetes is a condition caused by too much glucose (sugar) in the blood. Normally, the amount of glucose in the blood is controlled by a hormone called insulin. It is classified into two types:
- Pre-existing diabetes—type I and type II
- Gestational diabetes

PRE-EXISTING DIABETES (TYPE I AND TYPE II)

TYPE I (IDDM)
- The body produces almost no insulin.
- It can run in a family and can be caused by virus.
- It presents in child or in young adults
- More in Europeans who are not overweight
- Clinical findings are mainly in untreated patients
- Treatment is with insulin

TYPE II (NON-INSULIN DEPENDENT DIABETES MELLITUS)
- This occurs when the body doesn't produce enough insulin or the cells that normally respond to insulin cease to do so (insulin resistance).
- It is treated by altering diet or with oral drugs that bring down the levels of blood glucose (oral hypoglycaemic agents); many are also treated with insulin.
- It occurs in all racial groups, adults, children, and adolescents.
- It is associated with decreased physical activity and obesity.
- It can present with a high glucose levels for a long time without clinical presentation; therefore, at the time of diagnosis, hidden complications will be looked for.
- Control of blood glucose level is helpful in preventing long-term complications.

CLINICAL PRESENTATION OF TYPE 1 AND TYPE 2 DIABETES
You should report to your doctor if you have any of the symptoms outlined below.
- Thirst
- Passing too much urine (polyuria)
- Blurred vision
- Weight loss

The presentation may be in the form of complications which are as follows:
- Thrush
- Skin infections

- Negative effect on larger blood vessels of the heart, brain, and peripheral blood vessels, causing stroke and heart attack (macrovascular arterial disease)
- Negative effect on smaller blood vessels (microvascular disease), causing problems in
  - the eyes, diabetic retinopathy
  - the kidneys, diabetic nephropathy
  - the nerves, diabetic neuropathy
- Reduced life expectancy due to the problem with blood vessels.

DIAGNOSIS OF DIABETES (TYPES 1 AND 2)

Criteria for diagnosis of diabetes are similar for children and adults, and they are as follows:

- Blood test for random blood glucose (RBG) should show its level to be more than or equals 11.1 mmol/L at any time of the day irrespective of the time since last meal in the presence of symptoms of diabetes.
- The oral glucose tolerance test (OGTT): Fasting blood glucose (no caloric intake for at least 8 hours before doing the blood test) should be more than or equals 7 mmol/L. You will then be given to drink 394 mL of lucozade, which is equivalent to 75 mg of glucose. Two hours after the glucose meal, blood will be taken for checking glucose level; it should be equals or more than 11.1 mmol/L.
- A pre-diabetic condition called impaired glucose tolerance is defined as OGTT showing 2-hour plasma glucose to be more than or equals 7.8 but less than 11.1 mmol/L.
- Another ingredient in the blood called glycosylated haemoglobin levels (HbA1c) can also help in the diagnosis of diabetes.
- High blood glucose levels may occur in acute infection, trauma, or other stress conditions but they normalise spontaneously after the cause is no more present. In that situation, your doctor will delay the confirmatory test for diabetes, but the cause will be dealt with anyway.

EFFECTS OF PREGNANCY ON DIABETES (TYPES I AND II)

- Normal pregnancy is associated with some degree of insulin resistance, so if you are on insulin, you will need increasing does of it as pregnancy progresses.
- Kidney function is likely to deteriorate if you already have diabetic kidney problem called nephropathy.
- Diabetic eye disease (retinopathy) is likely to get worse or develop newly in pregnancy. This is due to the increase in blood flow in the part of the eye called retina; it also occurs if there is rapid improvement in blood glucose control.

- Low blood glucose and unawareness of it is more common in pregnancy because of aggressive lowering of blood glucose.
- Feeling sick and vomiting in pregnancy can worsen diabetic control. Diabetic complication called ketoacidosis is rare in pregnancy but can occur in the presence of severe vomiting, infection, or steroid treatment in pregnancy.
- General anaesthesia can be associated with a higher rate of aspiration of stomach content due to higher resting stomach volume compared to women without diabetes.

EFFECTS OF PRE-EXISTING DIABETES (TYPES I AND II) ON PREGNANCY

EFFECTS ON MOTHERS
- Increased risk of miscarriage if diabetes is poorly controlled.
- Increased risk of preeclampsia.
- Increased Caesarean section rate to about 60% and also IOL.
- Preterm labour.
- Obstructed labour and shoulder getting stuck in labour.
- Diabetic kidney disease can cause severe swelling, especially of the legs, and anaemia that may only respond to treatment with a drug called recombinant erythropoietin.
- Increased risk of infection particularly of the womb, urinary and respiratory tracts after delivery and also wound infections.
- Thrush is very common.

EFFECTS OF PRE-EXISTING DIABETES (TYPES I AND II) ON THE FOETUS
- Increased risk of congenital abnormalities due to poor control of glucose levels at the time of conception, for example congenital heart defects, skeletal, neural tube, genital and urinary tracts defects.
- Increased risk of foetal death during pregnancy and child death during the first month of life.
- Polyhydramnios (increased amount of amniotic fluids around the baby).
- Preterm delivery.
- Foetal distress (low levels of oxygen in the baby).

EFFECTS OF PRE-EXISTING DIABETES (TYPES I AND II) ON THE NEWBORN DURING THE FIRST MONTH AFTER BIRTH (NEONATAL PERIOD)
- High glucose levels in your blood during pregnancy leads to a high glucose levels in foetal blood and therefore large for date baby (macrosomia)—birth weight more than 4.5 kg, which increases the risk

of traumatic birth. This in turn can lead to baby's shoulder getting stuck during delivery.

- Large organs, for example kidney, liver, and pancreas.
- Persistent foetal high blood glucose levels during pregnancy will change to low levels after birth because of the following reasons: the high levels supported by maternal blood are cut off, baby's organ called 'pancreas' continues to produce insulin, which gets rid of glucose from the blood.
- Low levels of minerals called calcium and magnesium in baby's blood.
- Respiratory distress syndrome meaning difficulties with breathing at birth, especially in IDDM.
- Specific heart problem called hypertrophic cardiomyopathy, which is characterised by enlargement of the muscle of the heart.
- Brain dysfunction (convulsion, etc.) caused by oxygen starvation in labour.
- A condition called polycythaemia, which is characterised by increased number of red blood cells in blood vessels, high levels of bilirubin, and neonatal jaundice(yellowness of the eyes.)
- Increased risk of the baby developing obesity and/or diabetes in later life.

DIABETIC CARE IN PREGNANCY

If you have pre-gestational diabetes, you should see your GP immediately at the very moment you feel pregnant because of the following reason:

- to optimise the control of your blood glucose levels and therefore reduce the risk of complications
- to confirm that you had prepregnancy care, and if not to offer it
- to confirm that you are pregnant
- to arrange a referral to obstetric team if pregnancy is confirmed

Early visit to a doctor is of particular importance, especially in developing countries, where diabetic women preparing for pregnancy rarely attend prepregnancy clinic. Antenatal care will be delivered by a multidisciplinary team consisting of your GP, obstetrician, a diabetic physician, a diabetic specialist nurse, a midwife and, a dietician.

Your antenatal schedules will be the same as for normal pregnancy (page 83) but with some modifications as outlined in the table below.

Appointment	Care for women with diabetes during pregnancy
First appointment (joint endocrine and antenatal clinic), before 7-9 weeks	• Diabetic complications will be looked for. • Your medications and its complications will be reviewed • Assessment of glycaemic control will be offered by checking your blood for a substance called HbA1c (first trimester only). • Advice and support in relation to optimising glycaemic control will be offered. • Eye and/or kidney assessment will be offered if they have not been undertaken in the past 12 months. • Plan will be put in place so that you have contact with the diabetic team every 1-2 weeks throughout pregnancy.
7-9 weeks	• You will have a scan to assess the viability of the pregnancy
Booking appointment (ideally by 11-13+6 weeks)	• Education and advice will be given about the effects of diabetes on you and your baby, labour and childbirth, and effects of pregnancy on the diabetes. • Routine 11-13+6 weeks assessment and advice (page xx) will be offered.
16-17 weeks	• Eye assessment will be offered if you showed signs of diabetic eye disease at the first antenatal appointment. • Routine care will be given as in non-diabetic patients.
22-23 weeks	• Anomaly scan will be performed. • Specialised foetal heart scan will be performed by a specialist.
28 weeks	• Ultrasound monitoring will be performed to check the foetal growth, liquor volume and blood flow in the baby. • Eye assessment will be offered if you have pre-existing diabetes and you showed no evidence of diabetic eye disease at your first antenatal clinic visit. • You will enter the care pathway if you have been diagnosed with GDM as a result of the antenatal screening.
32 weeks	• Ultrasound monitoring will be done to check the foetal growth, liquor volume and blood flow in the baby. • Routine care will be given as for non-diabetic women.

36 weeks	• Routine care will be given as for non-diabetic women.
	• Ultrasound monitoring will be done to check the foetal growth, liquor volume, and blood flow in the baby.
	• Intravenous insulin chart for labour will be completed at or before 36 weeks and placed in your obstetric notes.
	• Information and advice will be given about
	– timing, mode, and management of birth
	– pain relief in labour
	– changes to your diabetic drugs during and after birth
	– management of the baby after birth
	– initiation of breastfeeding and the effect of breastfeeding on blood glucose control
	– contraception and follow-up
38 weeks	IOL will be preferred or Caesarean section if indicated. Ultrasound monitoring will be done to check foetal growth, liquor volume, and blood flow in the baby if you are awaiting spontaneous labour.
39 weeks	Ultrasound monitoring will be done as above if not delivered yet.
40 weeks	Ultrasound monitoring will be done as above if not delivered yet.
41 weeks	Ultrasound monitoring will be done as above if not delivered yet.

Table 12. Timetable of antenatal appointments and care

Generally, from the twenty-eighth week, appointments are for every 2 weeks till 36 weeks unless otherwise needed and then weekly till delivery. Eye assessment will be performed at 4 weekly intervals if background eye problem is present or the level of HbA1c falls by more than 2%.

OTHER ASPECTS OF MANAGEMENT

- Complications: The diabetic team will manage different aspects of the condition during pregnancy including complications.
- Healthy eating and exercise.
- Treatment to lower blood glucose levels (hypoglycaemic treatment): In Type I diabetes, you will be on insulin, while in type II, you will either be on tablets alone or on both tablets and insulin.
- Assessment of blood glucose and control: Home blood glucose monitoring (HBGM) will be preferred.
    - You should check your fasting blood glucose levels (normal at 3.5-5.9 mmol/L) and also blood glucose levels 1 hour after every meal (normal at below 7.8 mmol/L).
    - You should test your blood glucose before going to bed if you are on insulin.

– If you have type 1 diabetes, you should be offered ketone-testing strips so that you can test for ketones in your urine or in your blood if your blood glucose becomes critically high (hyperglycaemia) or you become unwell.

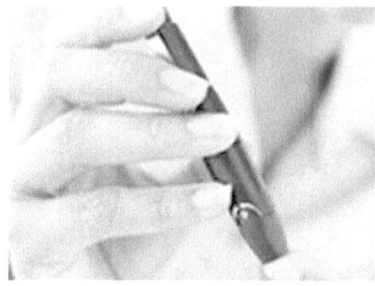 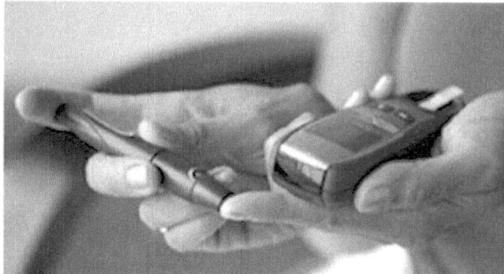

Figure 164a and b. Stabbing for blood glucose test

MANAGEMENT OF COMPLICATIONS

The complications are as follows:
* Low blood glucose (hypoglycaemia) and unawareness of it
* High BP (hypertension)
* Diabetic kidney disease (nephropathy)
* Diabetic ketoacidosis in pregnancy
* Diabetic eye disease
* Diabetic nerve disease
* Preterm labour

LOW BLOOD GLUCOSE (HYPOGLYCAEMIA) AND UNAWARENESS OF IT

Low blood glucose is defined as a blood glucose concentration below 50-55 mg/dL (2.7-3 mmol/L).

SYMPTOMS

Symptoms are divided into two categories:
* Those that are caused by the effect of low blood glucose on the nerves that control the activities of internal organs (neurogenic symptoms); they include the following:
  – anxiety
  – palpitations
  – sweating
  – shakiness
  – dry mouth
  – looking pale

- hunger
- unusual feeling on the skin (burning, pricking, etc.)
- Those that are caused by the effect of low blood sugar and an associated reduced oxygen levels on the brain (neuroglycopenic symptoms). These symptoms occur when glucose levels fall below 50-55 mg/dL (2.7 mmol/L). They are as follows:
  - feeling irritable
  - headache
  - difficult speaking
  - loss of balance
  - unusual feeling on the skin (burning, pricking, etc.)
  - abnormal thinking
  - seeing double
  - loss of strength in the hand and leg on one side of the body, for example left hand and left leg
  - loss of consciousness, seizure, coma, and even death if untreated

At the point that loss of strength in the legs and hands occur, you can still treat yourself by taking glucose, but after that, convulsion and coma can occur at level of glucose 1.5 mmol/L.

Lack of awareness of low blood glucose occurs in 25 out of 100 people with type 1 diabetes. The body fails to recognise low levels of glucose and therefore the initial neurogenic symptoms fail to occur. The presentations are therefore the neuroglycopenic symptoms.

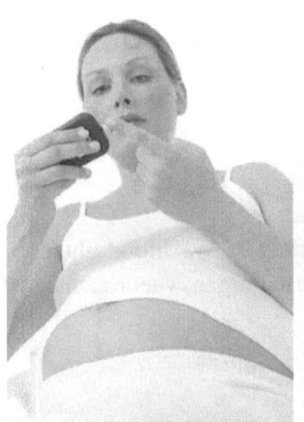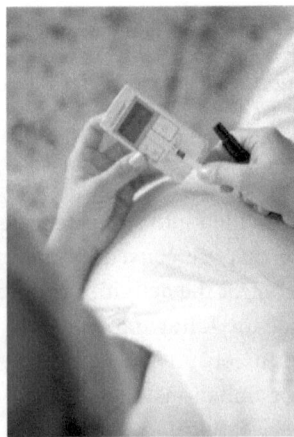

Figure 165a and b. Testing for glucose level

TREATMENT

About 15-20 g of glucose as glucose tablets are taken by mouth (3-5 g/10 kg body weight), or soft drinks containing pure glucose. A second administration dose of glucose may be required. The following are not used for the treatment:
- fruit juice, because it is absorbed more slowly than glucose
- honey, because it contains only 40-50% glucose and the same amount of fructose
- sucrose solution as granulated sugar in orange juice or milk, because it does not provide a quick rise in blood glucose levels

You should adhere to your original plan of treatment including HBGM, diet, insulin, and inter-meal snacks. In the case of loss of consciousness, the treatment is as follows:
- Intravenous injection of concentrated glucose solution.
- Glucagon injection 1 mg given under the skin. Effect peaks at 20 minutes to 1 hour. This can make you feel sick or vomit; therefore, careful monitoring of blood glucose levels will be continued until you are able to eat normally. Glucagon does not cross the placenta, so its use in pregnancy is safe.

You should carry something that identifies you as having diabetes so that you can be treated promptly if disabling low blood glucose occurs. The use of a type of insulin called the rapid-acting insulin analogues (aspart and lispro) when compared with regular human insulin has been associated with
- a fewer episodes of hypoglycaemia
- a reduction in high glucose levels after meal
- an improvement in overall blood glucose control

GESTATIONAL DIABETES MELLITUS

DEFINITION

Gestational diabetes occurs when the body cannot completely process the food nutrient called carbohydrate (sugars and starches) into a source of energy for the body, resulting in high levels of glucose of variable severity with first recognition during pregnancy. The diagnostic test for gestational diabetes is as in Type I and II diabetes but it is conducted at 26-28 weeks of pregnancy. About 50% of women with gestational diabetes go on to develop diabetes in later life. Rarely, diabetes presenting first in pregnancy is type 1 or 2 that is previously undiagnosed.

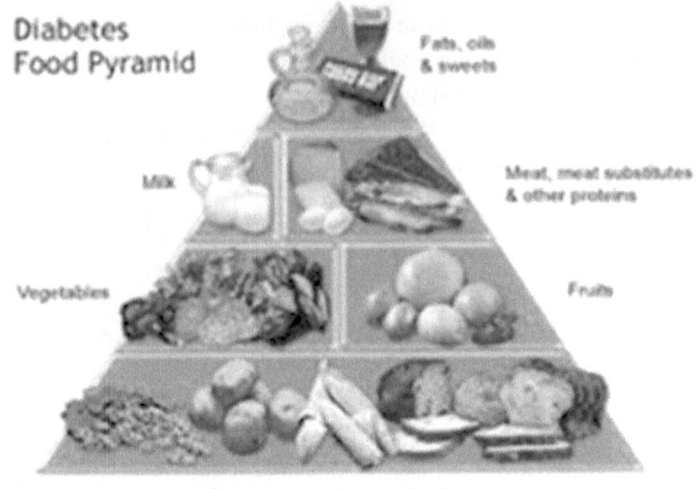

Figure 166. Healthy eating in diabetics

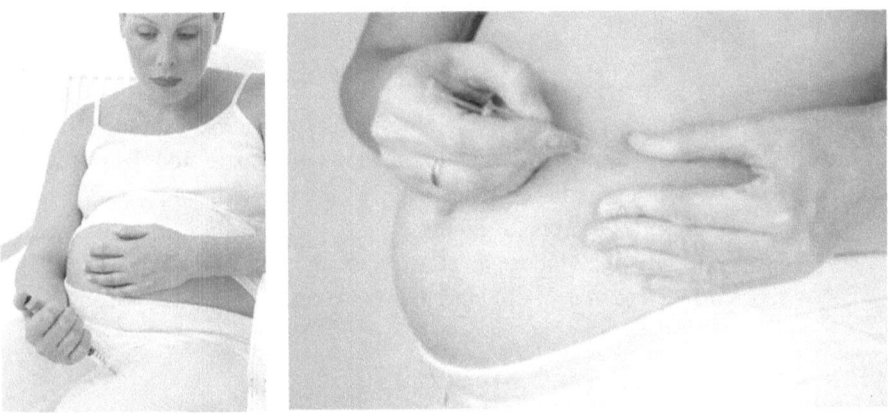

Figure 167a and b. Self injection of insulin

SCREENING FOR GESTATIONAL DIABETES

Screening for GDM is done differently in different hospitals and in different countries. In the UK, the NICE recommends screening using risk factors for GDM, which are to be looked for at the booking clinic. They are as follows:

- BMI more than 30 kg m^{-2}
- Diabetes in first-degree relative (your mother, father, brother, or sister)
- Previous big baby weighing 4.5 kg or more
- Family origin with a high prevalence of diabetes, including
  - South Asia (India, Pakistan, or Bangladesh)

– Black Afro-Caribbean
– Middle Eastern (Saudi Arabia, United Arab Emirates, Iraq, Jordan, Syria, Oman, Qatar, Kuwait, Lebanon, or Egypt).

Other risk factors that are not pointed out by the NICE guideline are as follows:
- Previous unexplained stillbirth
- Above 40 years old

The diagnostic test OGTT will be performed at 26-28 weeks of pregnancy if you have any of the above factors. It will also be performed at any stage during pregnancy if any of the following is applicable to you:
- Symptoms or signs suggestive of GDM, which are
  – glucose in your urine on two occasions when you are more than 20 weeks and once before 20 weeks of pregnancy
  – increased volume of amniotic fluids (polyhydramnios)
  – big baby during pregnancy
  – recurrent urinary tract infection or thrush (candidiasis)
- Blood glucose levels
  – RBG at booking (blood taken within 2 hours of eating) equals or is more than 7.0 mmol/L.
  – RBG (blood taken more than 2 hours after meal) is more than 5 mmol/L.
  – Fasting blood glucose is more than 5 mmol/L.
  – Blood taken one hour after glucose meal—50 g of glucose drink (263 mL of lucozade) at 26 weeks equals or is more than 8.0 mmol/L.

WOMEN WITH A PREVIOUS HISTORY OF GESTATIONAL DIABETES
Out of 100 women who had gestation diabetes in their previous pregnancy, 30-84 of them will develop it again in their next pregnancy; this figure rises to 75 out of 100 if you were treated with insulin during your previous pregnancy. The following will be done for you:
- You will be advised to attend a joint clinic at booking to see an obstetrician and an endocrinologist (a physician who deals with diabetes, thyroid problems, and other endocrine problems) for proactive monitoring and advice.
- You will be screened at booking for diabetes by doing a blood test called HbA1c, and appropriate action will be taken if elevated.
- You will be advised to start self-monitoring of blood glucose from the first trimester; diagnostic test OGTT will be performed at 16-18 weeks and repeated at 26-28 weeks if the results are normal.

- Diabetes controlled by diet alone or metformin for Caesarean section
- Delivery in diabetic eye disease

Your obstetrician and allied professionals will discuss all these situations with you.

INITIAL ASSESSMENT AND MANAGEMENT OF YOUR BABY AFTER DELIVERY.

In view of the complications that can occur in babies, the following management plan is advocated for the newborn:

- Your should give birth in a hospitals where professionals are well trained to recognise these complications and where advanced neonatal resuscitation skills are available 24 hours a day.
- Your baby will be given blood tests immediately after delivery to rule out the complications and his or her blood glucose level will be checked at 2-4 hours after birth.
- Specialised heart scan may also be performed to rule out heart problems
- Your baby should be with you unless there is a clinical complication or there are abnormal clinical signs that warrant admission for intensive or special care.
- Your baby may be admitted to a neonatal unit if he or she has complications or is borne before 34 weeks or between 34 and 36 weeks.
- Your baby can take about 72 hours to adapt to the new way of feeding after birth. Therefore, transfer to community care is not recommended before 24 hours of age and not before health care professionals are satisfied that he or she is maintaining blood glucose levels and has developed good feeding skills.
- Your baby should be fed as soon as possible after birth (within 30 minutes) and then at frequent intervals (every 2-3 hours) until feeding maintains pre-feed blood glucose levels at a minimum of 2.0 mmol/L.
- Your baby could be given additional measures such as tube feeding or intravenous dextrose if one of the following is applicable:
  - Blood glucose values are below 2.0 mmol/L on two consecutive readings despite maximal support for feeding.
  - There are clinical signs of low blood glucose.
  - Baby will not feed orally effectively.

MANAGEMENT OF MOTHERS AFTER DELIVERY

TYPE I AND II DIABETES

Insulin requirements and blood glucose levels fall in all women with diabetes following birth, and this is even more when breastfeeding. This means your blood glucose is likely to be low. The following are, therefore, recommended:

- The intravenous insulin infusion that you have been given during labour or Caesarean section will be halved.
- Blood glucose levels will be checked hourly during the infusion and for additional 4 hours after it has been stopped.
- The insulin infusion will be stopped when you start eating and your prepregnancy treatment, including insulin will be resumed immediately.
- For Type II diabetes the antidiabetic drugs that are normally used are metformin or glibenclamide. You may need to remain on insulin to maintain blood glucose levels.
- The following will be reviewed by the multidisciplinary team 6 weeks after your delivery:
  - Diabetic assessment
  - Discussion about future self-management of your diabetes
  - The implications of breastfeeding
  - Contraceptive advice

GESTATIONAL DIABETES AFTER CHILDBIRTH

In the post-natal period, the processing of glucose in your body (metabolism) can alter as follows:

- It may return to normal.
- There may be ongoing GDM.
- Frank diabetes (type 1 or type 2 diabetes that was unrecognised before pregnancy) may ensure.

Your care should, therefore, be modified as follows:

- Your insulin infusion will be stopped if you were on it.
- Your blood glucose will be checked 4 hours after childbirth.
- Your BP will then be checked 6 hourly for the first 24 hours; if it remains in the normal range, the monitoring will be stopped.
- You obstetrician will seek the opinion of the diabetic team, if your blood glucose measurements are elevated.
- You should be offered lifestyle advice, which are weight control, diet, and exercise; these measures should prevent progression of GDM to type 2 diabetes.

- Your fasting blood glucose level will be checked at 6 weeks after birth by your GP and then annually thereafter. In some hospitals, OGTT is offered at 12 weeks after birth.

PRECONCEPTION CARE IN PRE-EXISTING DIABETIC PATIENT

- General prepregnancy care, as outlined in chapter one is applicable with some modifications.
- Complication should be looked for and managed, especially high BP, eye and kidney problems and others.
- Optimisation of blood glucose level: Your blood will be taken for measuring the level of HbA1c; a value equals or less than 6.1% is acceptable (7.0% in the UK). It is repeated every 4 weeks until the best achievable control is attained. HBGM 4-7 times daily may be necessary. Acceptable values are as follows:
  - <6 mmol/L (fasting)
  - 7.8 mmol/L (1 hour post-meal)
  - 7 mmol/L (2 hours post-meal)

If you have Type I diabetes, you should be offered ketone-testing strips and advised to test for ketones in your urine or blood if your blood glucose levels goes up or you feel unwell.

- High dose of folic acid (5 mg/day) should be taken until 12 weeks of gestation.
- The development of the foetal organs occurs in the first 3 months of pregnancy, and so good control of glucose levels and avoidance of medications that could harm the developing foetus should be established before discontinuing contraception.
- All oral drugs that lower blood glucose level except metformin and glibenclamide will be discontinued before pregnancy, and insulin injection will be started. Metformin, glibenclamide, and insulin can be used at any stage in pregnancy.
- Insulin analogues are synthetic substances created by modifying the chemical structure of insulin to produce either faster-acting insulin, which is taken before meal, or longer-acting basal insulin, which is taken once a day. The rapid-acting analogues lispro and aspart are safe in pregnancy.
- Drugs used for the treatment of high BP called ACE inhibitors and angiotensin-II receptor antagonists will be discontinued while you are trying for a baby or as soon as pregnancy is confirmed because of the possible risk of birth defects associated with them. They will be replaced

with drugs that are safe in pregnancy, namely methyldopa, labetalol, and nifedipine.

- Anticholesterol drugs namely statins and fibrates should be discontinued before pregnancy or as soon as pregnancy is confirmed as cholesterol is important for foetal development.
- Aspirin can be continued in pregnancy if you are already on it.
- Investigation for infertility should be carried out if you fail to achieve pregnancy 6 months after achieving good diabetic control.

High Blood Pressure in Pregnancy

Classification
High BP in pregnancy is classified into the following categories based on the time of occurrence:
- Chronic high BP: It occurs before 20 weeks of pregnancy and also before pregnancy. It can be primary when no cause is found or secondary when a cause is found, for example kidney problem.
- Pregnancy-induced hypertension PIH is a high BP that occurs after 20 weeks.
- Preeclampsia PE is another high BP that occurs after 20 weeks of pregnancy, but on this occasion, it is associated with a significant amount of a substance called protein in the urine.

HIP is further classified on the basis of its severity into the following categories:
- Mild, BP equals 140-149/90-99
- Moderate, BP equals 150-159/100-109
- Severe, BP equals or more than 160/110

Pregnancy and Chronic High Blood Pressure

Prepregnancy Advice and Care
The general prepregnancy care, as outlined in chapter one is also applicable here with some modifications which are as following:
- Your medication should be reviewed before trying for a baby. Certain high BP drugs that can cause birth defects in baby will be stopped, and safer ones will be prescribed.

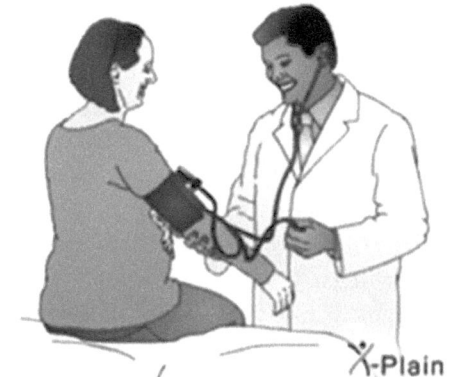

Figure 168. Taking blood pressure

- You should either keep your dietary sodium salt intake low or substitute it with some other salt; sodium salt worsens high BP.

MANAGEMENT DURING PREGNANCY

- If you do not have any complication, your BP will be maintained at less than 150/100. If you have complications, for example kidney disease, the aim of the treatment will be to keep your BP lower than 140/90 mmHg.
- If your hypertension is secondary to other problem, for example heart or kidney problem, you will be referred to a specialist physician.
- Based on your needs and those of your baby, additional antenatal appointments will be arranged.
- If your BP has been controlled, timing of birth will not be before 37 weeks.
- If your BP is persistently above 160/110 and not responding to treatment, you will be offered delivery; if you are less than 36 weeks pregnant, you should be offered steroid for maturation of baby's lungs before delivery.

MANAGEMENT AFTER BIRTH

- The aim will be to keep your BP below 140/90; it will be monitored
  - daily for the first 2 days after birth.
  - at least once between day 3 and day 5 after birth.
  - as clinically indicated if treatment is changed after birth.
- The antenatal BP treatment will be continued.
- Methyldopa should be stopped within 2 days of birth if you have been on it during pregnancy, and the BP treatment that you were taking before pregnancy should be restarted.
- Long-term BP treatment will be reviewed 2 weeks and then 6-8 weeks after birth by your GP.

PREGNANCY AND PREGNANCY-INDUCED HYPERTENSION

- It is normally diagnosed in the antenatal clinic or in the community by midwives or incidentally when women present with some other problems to the maternity day unit or labour ward. You should immediately be referred to an obstetrician.
- You will be asked specific questions to find out if you have any sign of PE.
- Your doctor will decide whether to place you on a medication(methyldopa, nifedipine, labetalol) or not(Table 13).
- Your BP measurement and urine test for protein will be carried out twice weekly and blood tests weekly if you are receiving outpatient care after being treated in the hospital for severe PIH.
- You will not be offered delivery before 37 weeks if BP has been lower than 160/110 with or without BP treatment. Your senior obstetrician should discuss the timing with you.
- You will be offered delivery if your BP is persistently above 160/110 and not responding to treatment; steroid will be given if you are less than 36 weeks.

MANAGEMENT AFTER BIRTH

- Your BP will be measured
  - daily for the first 2 days after birth.
  - at least once between day 3 and day 5 after birth.
  - as clinically indicated if antihypertensive treatment is changed after birth.
- You will continue taking the anti BP drugs that you were on during the antenatal period; the dose may be reduced if your BP falls below 140/90 mmHg.
- You should be given another BP tablet within 2 days of birth if you were on methyldopa during pregnancy.
- You should be started on BP drug if you were not on medication during pregnancy and your BP becomes higher than 149/99 after delivery.
- Your GP should see you for a medical review at 2 and 6-8 weeks after birth. If you remain on BP tablets during these visits, a medical review will be arranged for you.

Pregnancy-induced hypertension			
Degree of hypertension	Mild (from 140/90 to 149/99)	Moderate (from 150/100 to 159/109)	Severe (160/110 mmHg)
Admission to hospital	No	No	Yes, until BP is 159/109 or lower
Treatment	No	Labetalol as first-line treatment to keep BP at less than 150/100	
Measurement of BP	Not more than once a week. Twice weekly if you develop PIH before 32 weeks of pregnancy or you are at high risk of developing PE(Page 342).	At least twice a week	At least 4 times a day
Testing for protein in the urine	At each visit to the antenatal clinic. Twice weekly if you develop PIH before 32 week or you are at high risk of developing PE (Page 342).		Daily
Blood tests	No	Blood tests to rule out PE at presentation. No further blood tests if no protein in the urine at subsequent visits	Blood tests to rule out PE at presentation and then weekly

Table 13. Some aspects of management of PIH
(British National Institute for Clinical Excellence, NICE, 2011)

PRE-ECLAMPSIA

PE is classified on the basis of the period in pregnancy when it starts, into the following categories:

- Early PE, before 34 weeks
- Intermediate PE, 34-37 weeks
- Late PE, after 37 weeks

The presentations are as follows:
- High BP
- Protein in the urine
- Placenta is affected and can therefore give rise to
  - small-for-age baby
  - decreased amniotic fluid volume AFV
  - baby can become distressed
  - foetal death can occur
- PE can also present with its complications which are as follows:
  - eclampsia, which is a life-threatening condition and occurs in the form of fits or convulsion
  - kidney failure
  - liver failure
  - lung failure
  - HELLP syndrome, which is characterised by breakdown of red blood cells, abnormal results of liver function test LFT, and low platelets levels
- Symptoms of severe PE, indicating high risk of fitting, are as follows:
  - severe headache
  - blurring vision or flashing before the eyes
  - severe pain in the upper part of the abdomen
  - vomiting
  - sudden swelling of the face, hands, or feet
  - Brisk reflexes (knee or elbow jacks) and clonus (resistance on trying to move the foot upward)

SCREENING FOR PE

At your booking clinic, assessment will categorise you into 'moderate' or 'high risk' for preeclmpsia.

HIGH RISK FACTORS
- Previous history of PE
- Chronic hypertension
- Chronic kidney disease
- Diabetes
- Certain substances in the blood that can predispose to blood clot formation—aPLs
- Others

MODERATE RISK FACTORS
- First pregnancy
- Age 40 years or older

- Pregnancy interval of more than 10 years
- BMI of 35 or more
- Family history of PE (mother or sister)
- Multiple pregnancy
- First pregnancy with a new partner
- Pregnancy from egg donation
- Booking clinic
  - your lower BP equals or more than 80 mmHg
  - significant amount of protein in your urine

Unfortunately, these risk factors (high and moderate) can predict only 330 out of 1,000 women who will develop early onset PE, 278 out of 1,000 for intermediate, and 245 out of 1,000 for late PE. The above screening tool, therefore, has been improved by adding the following, which are assessed in the first and second trimesters:
- Blood flow in the artery that supplies blood to the womb (page xx)
- Your mean BP
- Biochemical tests

This combined model of screening will predict 91 out of 100 women who will develop early onset PE, 794 out of 1000 for intermediate, and 609 out of 1,000 for late PE.

PREVENTION OF PE
- If you have any of the features under the high-risk group or more than one under the moderate-risk group, you should be given aspirin 75 mg from 12 weeks of pregnancy until the birth of your baby.
- During pregnancy, you will have frequent BP measurements and urine tests for protein if you have any of the risk features as enumerated above.

MANAGEMENT OF PE
- You should seek immediate advice from a health care professional if you experience any of the symptoms of severe PE, which are outlined above. Unfortunately, these early warning signs and symptoms do not always occur.
- You should be given medication(labetalol, methyldopa and nifedipine) if you need it.
- Some aspects of the management are as outlined in table 13.

TIMING OF BIRTH AND FURTHER MANAGEMENT
- No delivery before 34 weeks if you and your baby are fine.
- Delivery is offered for mild or moderate hypertension after 37^{+0} weeks. Delivery for this severity of the disease at 34^{+0} to 36^{+6} weeks depends on your condition and that of your baby, other risk factors, and availability of neonatal intensive care.

- Indications for delivery at any GA are as follows:
  - eclampsia
  - severe PE not responding to treatment
  - mild or moderate hypertension and abnormal blood results

If any of the three conditions is applicable to you and decision has been taken to deliver your baby, then you will be placed on a special protocol that includes the following:
- Treatment for prevention of convulsion.
- Treatment of high BP.
- Fluid restriction.
- Steroid for maturation of baby's lungs if you are between 24 and 34 weeks; it may be given if you are between 35 and 36 weeks.

The protocol is meant to prevent the development of fits and stabilise you before labour; if you have developed it, it aims at preventing further fits. The protocol will be continued during labour and for 24 hours after delivery or after the last fit (whichever is the longer).

Mode of delivery in severe hypertension and severe PE or eclampsia will depend on the existing clinical circumstances and your preference. For mild and moderate PE, vaginal birth is indicated.

Management After Birth

- If you had severe PE or eclampsia, your management will continue in the high dependent unit of the labour ward or in the intensive care unit of the hospital depending on your condition.
- If you have not been on high BP medication,
  - your BP will be taken
    - ➢ at least 4 times a day while you are still in the hospital.
    - ➢ at least once between day 3 and day 5 after birth or on alternate days if BP was abnormal.
  - you will be started on treatment if your BP becomes 150/100 or higher.
- You will be assessed for the signs and symptoms of severe PE each time your BP is measured.
- If you have been on high BP treatment,
  - your BP will be taken
    - ➢ at least 4 times a day while you are still in the hospital.
    - ➢ every 1-2 days for up to 2 weeks after discharge or until you are off treatment and have no hypertension.
  - you will continue on your treatment.
  - your drug may be reduced if your BP falls below 140/90 mmHg.

- – your drug must be reduced if your BP falls below 130/80 mmHg.
- If you were on methyldopa during pregnancy, it will be stopped within 2 days of birth.
- If the following conditions are met, you will be discharged home:
  - – no symptoms of PE
  - – BP, with or without treatment, is 149/99 or lower
  - – blood test results are stable or improving
- If you have high BP, you should be offered appointment to see your GP for a medical review at 2 and 6-8 weeks after birth. If you remain on BP tablets during these visits, a medical review will be arranged for you.

BLOOD RESULTS AFTER CHILDBIRTH

- Blood test will be performed 48-72 hours after birth or step-down from critical care. It will not be repeated if results are normal but if results are improving but still within the abnormal range, the test will be repeated as clinically indicated and also at the 6-8 weeks post-natal review.
- Urine dipstick for protein will be performed at the post-natal review (6-8 weeks after birth); if you still have proteinuria (1+ or more), a further review at 3 months after birth will be offered to assess kidney function and consideration will be given to referring you for a specialist kidney assessment.

FURTHER INFORMATION ON HIP
AFTER DISCHARGE FROM THE HOSPITAL

- For PIH or PE, there is an increased risk of
  - – developing high BP and its complications in later life.
  - – developing PIH and PE in future pregnancy.
- For PE,
  - – The relative risk of developing kidney disease is increased.
  - – There is no risk of recurrence of PE in future pregnancy if inter-pregnancy interval is up to 10 years.
- Before next pregnancy, it is necessary to achieve and keep BMI within the healthy range of 18.5-24.9.

SOURCES

- Guideline for Practice. Harris Birthright Research Centre for Fetal Medicine, King's College Hospital, London, 2011.
- RCOG information leaflet. PE: what you need to know. Published November 2007.
- Hypertension in pregnancy: the management of hypertensive disorders during pregnancy, NICE Guideline. August 2010, revised January 2011.

OBSTETRIC CHOLESTASIS

Obstetric cholestasis (OC) is a disease of the liver that occurs in pregnancy and is characterised by the following signs and symptoms:

EFFECTS ON YOU
- Intense itching (especially involving the palms and soles of the feet with no rash) and therefore sleep deprivation.
- Abnormal results of LFTs and/or raised bile acids in the blood.
- Pale stool, dark urine, and yellow eyes (jaundice).
- Vaginal bleeding after childbirth.

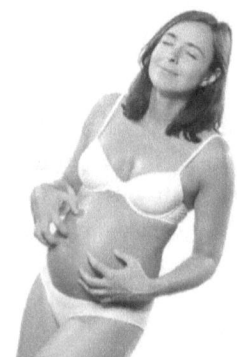

Figure 169. Itching in cholestasis

EFFECTS ON YOUR BABY
- Increased chance of baby dying during pregnancy and within 1 month after delivery; in developed countries, this is in the order of 57 in 10,000 pregnant women.
- Preterm birth.
- Increased likelihood of baby doing a poo (meconium) in the womb; baby can aspirate meconium during labour and delivery, and this can adversely affect him or her.

RISK FACTORS
If any of the following is applicable to you, you are at high risk of developing OC during pregnancy:
- Personal or family history of OC
- Multiple pregnancy
- Hepatitis C
- Gallstones

PREVALENCE

Its prevalence is influenced by genetic and environmental factors and varies between populations worldwide. In developed countries, for example England, OC affects 7 out of 1,000 pregnant women, but in developing countries of India or Pakistan, it occurs in 12-15 out of 1,000 women. We do not have the figures for people living on the African continent, but it is likely to be high.

DIAGNOSIS

It is based on the occurrence of the following:

- The maternal and foetal effects as described above.
- The diagnosis is made after excluding other causes of itching and of liver dysfunction by doing a series of blood tests and ultrasound scan of the liver.
- The tests will be repeated every 1-2 weeks to rule out OC if you have persistent itching and normal LFT results.

MANAGEMENT AND MONITORING

In most cases, you will not be admitted to the hospital after the diagnosis has been confirmed. The management is as follows:

- Weekly assessment of LFTs and review by your obstetrician until delivery.
- Weekly BP measurement and urine tests to rule out associated PE.
- A clotting screen will be performed when the diagnosis is made; it may be abnormal.
- Twice weekly trace of baby's heart.
- Foetal death cannot currently be predicted by biochemical tests, ultrasound, or by trace of baby's heart. There is no evidence of placental involvement in OC, so SGA and decreased liquor volume are not features of the disease.

TREATMENT

- Topical treatment aimed at relieving itching include calamine lotion and similar substances. They may provide slight temporary relief of itching.
- Systemic treatments aimed at relieving itching include
  - Colestyramine: It may also worsen vitamin K deficiency in the baby and has been associated with bleeding into baby's brain.
  - Piriton: It may make you feel sleepy.
- Tablets of ursodeoxycholic acid improve itching and liver function.
- Water-soluble vitamin K, 5-10 mg, is taken by mouth daily; higher dose of 10 mg is indicated when blood clotting test is abnormal.
- It is not advisable to take vitamin K in late pregnancy and labour because of a possible risk to the baby—anaemia in newborn caused by breaking down of red blood cells and neonatal jaundice. So it will be taken till you are 36 weeks pregnant.

DELIVERY

- IOL should be offered after 37^{+0} weeks of pregnancy, especially if your LFT is significantly abnormal due to the inability to predict stillbirth.
- Management of labour will be as in any other high-risk pregnancy.
- Continuous foetal monitoring will be offered in labour.

FOLLOW-UP AT 6 WEEKS AFTER DELIVERY

The purpose of the follow-up appointment is as follows:

- To ensure that the LFTs have returned to normal. LFT results may get worse in the first 10 days after delivery; therefore, its routine measurement will be deferred beyond this time.
- To ensure that itching has resolved.
- To ensure that all investigations carried out during the pregnancy have been reviewed and you fully understood the implications of OC.
- To give further advice on OC, which includes
  - no long-term effect on you or your baby
  - a high recurrence rate of 45-90%
  - increased incidence of OC in your family members
  - avoidance of oestrogen-containing contraceptives that can give rise to the same presentations as OC

SOURCES

- RCOG Green-top Guideline No. 43. Obstetric cholestasis, April 2011.
- RCOG information for patient. Obstetrics Cholestasis. Information for you. Published May 2012.
- Kenyon AP, Tribe RM, Nelson-Piercy C, Girling JC, Williamson C, Seed PT, et al. Pruritus in pregnancy: a study of anatomical distribution and prevalence in relation to the development of obstetric cholestasis. Obstet Med 2010;3:25-9.

BLOOD CLOTS FORMATION IN PREGNANCY AND AFTER BIRTH

DEFINITIONS AND PREVALENCE

Blood clots, also called thromboses or emboli, can form in either vein or artery; when it occurs in the vein, it is called VTE or thrombosis. Veins have valves as shown below; they are blood vessels that take blood towards the heart and lungs, while arteries carry blood away from them. When blood clots form in the deep veins of the calf muscles or in the veins of the pelvic area, it is called DVT. If the clots move to the lung and block the veins there, it is called pulmonary thromboembolism (PTE).

Blood Clot Diagram

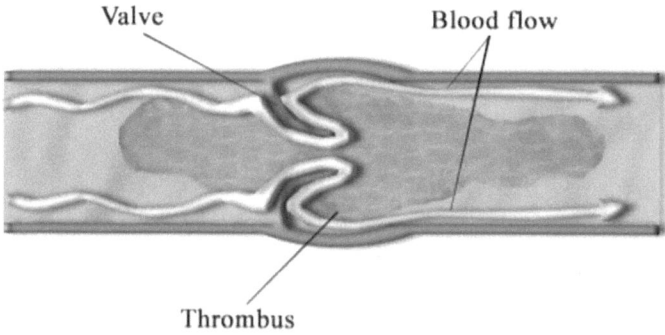

Figure 170. Blood clot in the vein

PTE remains one of the leading direct causes of maternal death in developed countries, especially in the UK. It is rarely diagnosed in many developing countries because of lack of diagnostic tools, especially in Africa. The risk of VTE in pregnancy is increased four to six-fold when compared with non-pregnant women. The absolute risk of VTE is low, with an overall incidence in pregnancy and post-delivery of 1-2 out of 1,000.

CLINICAL PRESENTATION OF BLOOD CLOTS IN PREGNANCY

Blood clots in the veins can occur at any stage of pregnancy, but during the six weeks after birth, the risk is at its peak. The signs and symptoms of VTE include the following:

DVT
- a red and hot swollen leg (usually in one leg)

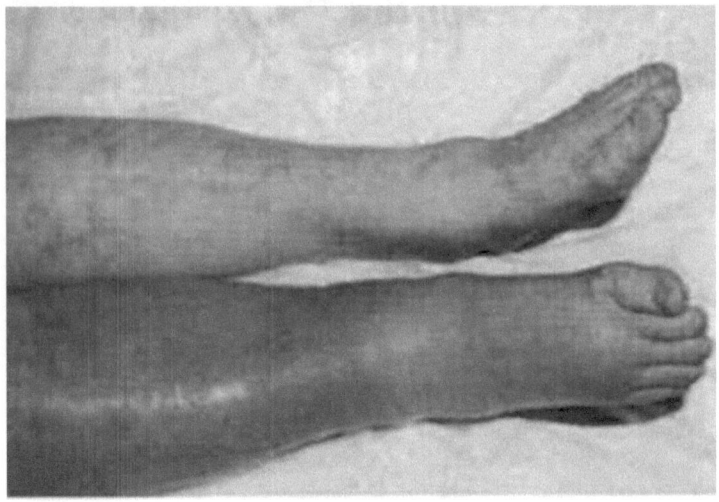

Figure 171. Deep vein thrombosis

- pain and/or tenderness in the leg—you may only experience this when standing or walking, or it may just feel heavy
- lower abdominal pain
- back pain
- low-grade temperature

DVT can travel from the legs or pelvis to the lungs and cause PTE; this occurs more in the above-knee DVT.

PTE
- Sudden unexplained difficulty in breathing
- Tightness in the chest or chest pain
- Coughing up blood
- Feeling very unwell, collapsing, or shock—presentations of massive PTE, when the blood clot is very big
- Death

If you develop any of the symptoms for DVT and PTM, you should call your maternity unit or doctor immediately.

DIAGNOSIS AND INITIAL TREATMENT OF DVT
If you have signs and/or symptoms suggestive of VTE, the following will be done:
- Ultrasound scan of the lower limbs to confirm the diagnosis of DVT.

- When pelvic vein thrombosis is suspected (back pain and swelling of the entire limb), a test called venography (examination of veins) may be considered.
- Treatment with a drug called LMWH will be started immediately and continued until the diagnosis is excluded unless treatment is strongly contraindicated. The LMWH does the following:
  - prevents the blood clot getting any bigger so your body can gradually dissolve it.
  - reduces the risk of the DVT progressing to PTE.
  - reduces the risk of another venous thrombosis developing
- You should wear graduated elastic compression stockings.

Further management will depend on the findings of the ultrasound scan. If the scan does not confirm the diagnosis, the treatment will be stopped but if it confirms it or there is a strong clinical suspision, the following will be done:
- The LMWH will be continued, the affected leg elevated when lying down and an elastic compression stocking will be applied to reduce swelling.
- You should be encouraged to mobilise while wearing the stocking; mobilisation improves pain and swelling that is normally associated with DVT and prevents the development of further complications.
- Further management of DVT for those cases that are resistant to treatment, severe complications like venous gangrene (death of part of the lower limb), and the use of venous filters are not discussed in this book.

Diagnosis and Initial Treatment of Acute Presentation of Blood Clots in the Lungs (PTE)

Once PTE is suspected, the following will be done:
- Treatment with LMWH will be started immediately until PTE is ruled out.
- You should wear graduated elastic compression stockings.
- Chest X-ray to rule out other illnesses, for example infection of the lungs, will be performed. The radiation dose to the foetus from a chest X-ray performed at any stage of pregnancy is negligible.
- Ultrasound of both lower legs may be carried out to rule out associated DVT. A diagnosis of DVT may indirectly confirm a diagnosis of PTE and further investigation may not be necessary.
- Specialised imaging procedures called ventilation/perfusion (V/Q) lung scan and/or scan of the lungs called computed tomography pulmonary angiogram (CTPA) may be performed to confirm the diagnosis. The

ventilation component of the V/Q scan can often be omitted during pregnancy, thereby minimising the radiation dose for the foetus.

- Alternative or repeat testing may be carried out where V/Q scan or CTPA and Doppler ultrasound are normal, but the clinical suspicion of PTE is high.

Risks	V/Q scan	CTPA
Childhood cancer in the baby	1/2,800,000	1/1,000,000
Maternal breast cancer	Background risk, that is risk for every woman of 1 in 200 is not increased	Lifetime background risk increased by 13.6%
Altered foetal or neonatal thyroid function	Not applicable	Can be caused by the iodinated contrast used with CTPA
Radiation to you and your baby	Small and not associated with a substantial increased complication	More than with V/Q scan but still negligible

Table 14. Risks associated with V/Q scan and CTPA

Despite the potential advantages of CTPA of accurately diagnosing blood clots, many hospitals continue to recommend V/Q scanning as first-line investigation in pregnancy because if the test shows that there is no blood clot, that is very likely to be correct and also because of its substantially lower radiation dose to pregnant breast tissues.

BASELINE BLOOD INVESTIGATIONS
(APPLICABLE TO VTE AND PTE)

Before anticoagulant therapy is commenced, blood will be taken for the following investigations:

- Full blood count to measure the number of different cells in your blood.
- Blood clotting test to assess the clotting status of your blood.
- Blood test to assess kidney and liver function. This test is necessary because the drug that is used for the treatment of blood clots, LMWH, passes through the liver and the kidney; confirmation of normal function of these organs is therefore important.
- Blood test to check whether you have a sticky blood condition (thrombophilia) or not. The thrombophilia is a group of disorder that can cause blood clots in your blood vessels.

MAINTENANCE TREATMENT OF VTE

- You will be taught Self-injection of the LMWH and managed as an outpatient until delivery.
- You will continue to inject the treatment dose of LMWH during the remainder of the pregnancy because there is a significant risk of the VTE happening again.
- Warfarin is not used for antenatal VTE treatment because of its adverse effects on the baby.

ANTICOAGULATION TREATMENT IN SPECIAL CIRCUMSTANCES

MANAGEMENT OF MASSIVE LIFE-THREATENING PTE IN PREGNANCY

This subject is not discussed further in this book.

ANTICOAGULANT THERAPY DURING LABOUR AND DELIVERY

- If spontaneous labour occurs and you are receiving treatment doses of unfractionated heparin injected under the skin (subcutaneous), careful monitoring for its adequacy with blood test is required. If the blood test shows that you are receiving too much heparin, an antidote of heparin called protamine sulphate will be given to you to counteract its action; this will reduce the risk of bleeding.
- If you are given unfractionated heparin under the skin, it is normally stopped 12 hours before IOL or regional anaesthesia (epidural or spinal); if you receive it through the vein, then the duration is 6 hours.
- For delivery by elective Caesarean section, the treatment doses of LMWH will be omitted for 24 hours before surgery. A dose of LMWH that prevents blood clots formation (not treatment dose) will be given 3 hours after operation (but more than 4 hours after removal of the epidural catheter). The treatment dose will be recommenced in the evening if the Caesarean section was done in the morning hours.
- If either unfractionated heparin or LMWH is used, there is a 2 out of 100 risk of blood clots forming in the operation wound following Caesarean section.
- If you are on therapeutic doses of LMWH, wound drains will be considered at Caesarean section and the skin incision will be closed with staples or interrupted sutures to allow drainage of any blood clots (haematoma).

ANTICOAGULANT TREATMENT FOR THOSE AT HIGH RISK OF HAEMORRHAGE

Any woman who is considered to be at high risk of bleeding and in whom continued heparin treatment is considered essential will be managed with intravenous, unfractionated heparin until the risk factors for bleeding have resolved. Risk factors include the following:

- You have had major APH
- changes in blood clotting, which predisposes to more bleeding
- medical illness that causes bleeding such as von Willebrand disease, haemophilia
- progressive wound blood clot
- suspected bleeding in the abdomen
- You have had post-partum haemorrhage
- risk of major bleeding, for example if your afterbirth is low-lying
- Low platelet count, less than
- acute stroke in the last 4 weeks
- severe kidney disease
- severe liver disease
- uncontrolled high BP (when it is greater than 200/120)

POST-NATAL ANTICOAGULATION

- Treatment dose of anticoagulant therapy will be continued for the duration of the pregnancy and for at least 6 weeks after birth; in total at least 3 months of treatment will be given.
- Either LMWH or oral anticoagulant warfarin will be used.
- Treatment with warfarin after delivery will be avoided until at least the third day after childbirth if you have increased risk of bleeding. Daily blood tests (called international normalised ratio INR) will be undertaken from day 2 of treatment with warfarin for at least 10 days to monitor the treatment during the changeover from LMWH to warfarin. Heparin treatment will be continued until the INR is greater than 2. The normal values are 2-3.
- Heparin (unfractionated or LMWH) or warfarin can be taken when breastfeeding.
- The continuing risk of thrombosis will be assessed, including a review of personal and family history of VTE, before discontinuing treatment.
- Arrangements will be made to repeat the tests for sticky blood conditions (thrombophilia tests) after anticoagulation treatment has been stopped.

GENERAL INFORMATION ON HEPARIN, WARFARIN AND GRADUATED ELASTIC COMPRESSION STOCKINGS.

The following are used in the treatment and prevention of blood clots formation:

- Fractionated heparin called LMWH, for example Clexane, dalteparin (Fragmin), and tinzaparin
- Unfractionated heparin
- Warfarin
- Graduated elastic compression stockings

LOW-MOLECULAR-WEIGHT HEPARIN

- It is the agent of choice.
- It is at least as effective as and safer than unfractionated heparin.
- It is less associated with low platelets levels in your blood and brittle bone disease in prolonged use than the conventional unfractionated heparin.
- The dose of LMWH is based on your weight before pregnancy or at booking clinic. Routine monitoring of the dose of LMWH by doing a special blood test called 'peak anti-Xa activity' is recommended in the following situations:
  - extremes of body weight (less than 50 kg or 90 kg or more)
  - kidney impairment
  - recurrent VTE
- Caution should be taken if you have any risk factor for bleeding, as outlined above; if you do, the decision to give the drug will be based on careful consideration of the balance between the risk of bleeding and clots formation. Unfractionated heparin may be preferable.

UNFRACTIONATED HEPARIN

It has a shorter half-life than LMWH, and its effect can be completely reversed by a drug called protamine sulphate. Occasionally, it may be used around the time of delivery in women at very high risk of thrombosis in the following situations:

- LMWH cannot be used because regional anaesthetic techniques may be required.
- You are at increased risk of haemorrhage, for example in labour.

A typical situation is when you have been on the blood clots prevention dose of LMWH and you are in labour. In this situation, if the LMWH has not been given for 24 hours, a prophylactic dose of 5,000 IU of unfractionated heparin can be given and repeated every 12 hours until LMWH can be resumed after delivery. The required interval between a prophylactic dose of unfractionated heparin and regional anaesthesia is less (4 hours) when compared with LMWH (12 hours), and there is less concern regarding formation of blood clots in the epidural or spinal space with unfractionated heparin.

Unfractionated heparin decreases platelets count; therefore, the count will be monitored every 2-3 days from day 4 of treatment until heparin is stopped.

If you develop heparin-induced low platelets, it means you have heparin allergy, and therefore, you will be treated with other anticoagulant drugs, namely the heparinoid, danaparoid sodium, or fondaparinux under specialist advice.

WARFARIN

Warfarin use in pregnancy is restricted to a few situations where heparin is considered unsuitable, for example some women with mechanical heart valves. Its restriction is due to the following reasons:

- It crosses from your blood through the placenta to your baby's blood. It can therefore lead to an increased risk of birth defects in approximately 5 out of 100 foetuses that are exposed to it between 6 and 12 weeks of pregnancy. This figure is higher if greater than 5 mg per day is used.
- It increases the risk of spontaneous miscarriage, stillbirth, and Neurological problems in the baby.
- You and your baby in the womb are at an increased risk of bleeding.

GRADUATED ELASTIC COMPRESSION STOCKINGS OR THROMBOEMBOLIC DETERRENT STOCKINGS TED

The use of properly applied graduated compression stockings of appropriate strength is recommended in pregnancy and after childbirth in the following situations:

- If you are hospitalised for post-Caesarean section and considered to be at particularly high risk of VTE (combined with LMWH).
- If you had previous VTE or a thrombophilia, you should wear it throughout pregnancy and for 6-12 weeks after delivery (usually combined with LMWH).
- If you travel long distance for more than 4 hours.

PREVENTION OF BLOOD CLOTS FORMATION IN PREGNANCY AND AFTER CHILDBIRTH

Firstly, you will be assessed with a view of identifying the predisposing factors to blood clots formation. The assessment is carried out in the prepregnancy clinic, at the booking clinic, whenever you are admitted to the hospital, after delivery and whenever there is an acute episode of blood clots formation both during pregnancy and after delivery.

Categories	Risk factors		
	High Risk	**Intermediate risk**	**Low risk**
Personal Medical History	Recurrent VTE	A known sticky blood condition	Gross varicose veins
	Previous Single VTE + sticky blood condition	Single previous VTE, provoked by a transient major risk factor that is no longer present. No family history of VTE nor sticky blood	Current systemic infection (requiring antibiotics or admission to hospital) e.g. pneumonia, pyelonephritis, postpartum wound infection,
	Single VTE + Your first degree family member has a sticky blood condition	Medical conditions, e.g. heart or lung diseases, cancer, inflammatory bowel disease, sickle cell disease, connective tissue disorders, etc.	
	Previous unprovoked or estrogen/ pregnancy-related VTE		
	Severe thrombophilia [x]		
Family History			VTE
Demographic features			Age > 35 years
			Number of children = 3 and more
		BMI more than 40 (based on booking weight)	Obesity (BMI > 30 kg/ m2) either prepregnancy or in early pregnancy i.e at booking.
Social History		Intravenous drug user	Smoker
Obstetric History			Pre-eclampsia
			Dehydration/Severe vomiting in early pregnancy hyperemesis/ Ovarian hyperstimulation syndrome
			Multiple pregnancy
			Assisted reproduction technique

Labour, childbirth and post delivery		Emergency caesarean section in labour	Elective caesarean section
		Surgical procedure in pregnancy or at less than 6 weeks after birth	Forceps delivery (midcavity or rotational)
			Prolonged labour – more than 24 hours
			Blood loss after delivery of more than 1 litre
Transient risk factor			Current systemic infection
			Immobility for 3 or more days
			long-distance travel – 4 hours and more.
Combined risks	After delivery, 2 persistent factors from the intermediate category or more than 3 factors from the low risk category	3 or more risk factors from the "low risk category" during pregnancy.	2 and less risk factors from the low risk category during pregnancy
		2 or more risk factors from the low risk category after delivery.	
		2 or more risk factors from the "low risk category" if admitted to the hospital during pregnancy	

*   **– Antithrombin deficiency**

– More than one thrombophilic defects

– Homozygous factor V Leiden

– Homozygous prothrombin G20210A

– Thrombophilia and additional risk factors

Table 15. Risk factors for VTE in pregnancy and after childbirth.

MANAGEMENT

HIGH RISK

- You should be given a daily injection of LMWH throughout the pregnancy and for 6 weeks after childbirth.
- You will be required to wear a pair of TED stockings.
- You will also be referred to a specialist in blood problems.

EFFECTS OF GDM ON MOTHER AND BABY

The effects are the same as in pre-existing diabetes in pregnancy except that in GDM, there are no miscarriages and congenital abnormalities and less or no involvement of vital organs namely kidney, eyes, and peripheral nerve.

MANAGEMENT

- You will enter the 'care pathway for women with diabetes during pregnancy' (as in Table 12 above) at 26-28 weeks.
- Full clinical assessment will be carried out.
- Educational package on GDM in general including the complications and possible outcomes of pregnancy should be given to you.
- You will be taught the HBGM—fasting and 1-hour after meals.
- Diet and exercise: About 82-93 out of 100 women with gestational diabetes will achieve blood glucose control on diet and exercise alone. Indications for other treatment are as follows:
    - Diet and exercise fail to maintain blood glucose targets during a period of 1-2 weeks. This happens in 10-20 out of 100 women.
    - Ultrasound suggests that your baby is big.
- Oral agents (metformin and glibenclamide) and/or insulin (regular human insulin or rapid-acting insulin analogues) will be used to control the blood glucose levels where diet and exerscise fail.

LABOUR AND DELIVERY IN TYPE I, II, AND GESTATIONAL DIABETES

TIMING AND MODE OF BIRTH

Routine IOL at 38-39 weeks of pregnancy reduces the risk of stillbirth and the chance of the shoulder getting stuck in labour without increasing the risk of Caesarean section. Diabetes is not a contraindication to attempting vaginal birth after caesarean section VBAC.

BLOOD GLUCOSE CONTROL DURING LABOUR AND BIRTH

It is mandatory that in labour, your glucose levels are monitored hourly and maintained at normal 4-7 mmol/L. This is because labour is stressful and stress can give rise to high blood glucose levels, which can be associated with

- foetal distress and
- low blood glucose level in the baby after birth

OTHER ASPECTS OF DIABETIC LABOUR THAT REQUIRE SPECIFIC MANAGEMENT ARE AS FOLLOWS:

- Pain relief in labour
- Diabetics on insulin undergoing elective Caesarean section
- Diabetes controlled by diet alone or metformin in labour

INTERMEDIATE RISK
- You may be given LMWH during pregnancy, but after delivery, daily injection of the drug will definitely be given for 7 days.
- You will be required to wear TED stockings.
- You will be referred to a specialist in blood problems.
- You will be advised to continue the drug LMWH if the risk factor is persistent after delivery, until the risk factor is no longer present.

Generally, in all situations where the blood-thinning drug is required, it will be given as early in pregnancy as practical, preferably in the first trimester. For previous recurrent VTE before pregnancy, if you are not on warfarin, you should be started on LMWH as soon as you have a positive pregnancy test. If you were on warfarin before pregnancy, you should stop taking it and change to LMWH as soon as pregnancy is confirmed, ideally within 2 weeks of the missed period but at worst, before the sixth week.

LOW RISK
- You will be encouraged to mobilize early after childbirth and to avoid dehydration by drinking more fluid.

PREVENTION OF BLOOD CLOTS FORMATION DURING LABOUR AND DELIVERY, INCLUDING THE USE OF REGIONAL ANAESTHESIA AND ANALGESIA
- If you are on LMWH during the antenatal period and you have any vaginal bleeding or labour begins, you should not inject any further LMWH. You should go to the maternity ward immediately. Your obstetrician should assess you and ask for the opinion of a specialist in blood problems (haematologist) before restarting you on blood thinning drug.
- Since pregnancy-associated predisposition to formation of blood clots is maximal immediately following delivery, it is desirable to continue LMWH during labour or delivery if you are receiving antenatal thromboprophylaxis with LMWH. However, if a regional anaesthetic (epidural for labour or spinal for Caesarean section) is to be used, you are advised to discontinue LMWH at the onset of labour or prior to planned delivery.
- If you are receiving high doses of LMWH to prevent blood clot formation, the dosage should be reduced from the high to the normal prophylactic level on the day before IOL and, if appropriate, continued in this level during labour.
- To minimise or avoid the risk of blood clot formation in the epidural space, regional anaesthesia will not be used until at least

- 12 hours after the prophylactic dose of LMWH.
- 24 hours after the treatment dose of LMWH.
- LMWH can be given 4 hours after operation or 4 hours after removal of the epidural catheter; the catheter will not be removed within 10-12 hours of the most recent LMWH injection.

- If you are on prophylactic dose of LMWH and you are to have elective Caesarean section, you should receive the LMWH on the day before delivery. On the day of the delivery, any morning dose will be omitted and the operation should be performed that morning.
- If you are at high risk of bleeding and prevention of blood clots formation is needed, you may be more conveniently managed with unfractionated heparin and/or graduated compression stockings instead of LMWH.
- If you have VTE, excess blood loss and blood transfusion are risk factors for it, so prophylaxis should be begun or reinstituted as soon as the immediate risk of bleeding is reduced.

SOURCES

- Thromboembolic disease in pregnancy and the puerperium: acute management. The Royal College of Obstetricians and Gynaecologists (RCOG), February 2007.
- Venous thrombosis in pregnancy and after birth, Information for you. The Royal College of Obstetricians and Gynaecologists (RCOG), September 2008.
- RCOG Green-top Guideline No. 37a. Reducing the risk of thrombosis and embolism during pregnancy and the puerperium, November 2009.

Glossary

- **Abdomen:** It is also called belly or tummy. It is the part of the body between the chest and the pelvis. The region enclosed by the abdomen is termed the abdominal cavity.
- **Abdominal circumference:** The distance around foetal abdomen at the level of the navel.
- **Acid and base:** Acid is a substance which in water solutions tastes sour, turns litmus paper red, and reacts with certain metals, such as zinc, to yield hydrogen gas. Bases is a substance which in water solutions taste bitter, turn litmus paper blue, and feel slippery. When a water solution of acid is mixed with a water solution of base, water and a salt are formed.
- **Albumin:** A protein that can appear in your urine when you are pregnant. It can be a sign of an infection or PE. Your midwife will test your urine for albumin at your antenatal check-ups.
- **Amniocentesis:** A test in which a thin needle is inserted into the uterus through the abdominal wall to take a sample of the fluid surrounding the baby.
- **AFV:** Amniotic fluid volume.
- **Amniotic sac:** The bag of fluid that surrounds and cushions your baby in the womb.
- **Amniotomy:** It is the procedure of using a plastic hook inserted through a woman's vagina to release the waters (called amniotic fluid) around the baby.
- **Anaesthetics:** Medicines that reduce or take away pain.
- **Androgen:** This is the male sex hormone. The primary and most well-known androgen is testosterone.
- **Antenatal:** This means 'before birth' and refers to the whole of pregnancy, from conception to birth.
- **Antenatal care:** This is the care that is offered by the health care professionals during your pregnancy. They will check you and your baby to confirm that both of you are well.
- **Antibiotics:** These are medicines that can be used to treat infections caused by micro-organisms, usually bacteria or fungi.
- **Antibodies:** These are your body's natural defence against any foreign substance that enters your blood. It is a protein that is produced by the body to neutralise or destroy disease-carrying organisms and toxins.
- **Anti-embolism stockings:** These are tight stockings (also known as 'compression stockings') specially designed to reduce the risk of developing a blood clot in your legs. The stockings squeeze your feet, lower legs, and thighs, helping your blood to circulate around your legs more quickly.
- **Antiphospholipid antibodies:** These are antibodies directed against phosphorus-fat components of your cell membranes called

phospholipids; certain blood proteins bind with phospholipids and form the complexes. They are associated with different obstetric problems like RM, FGR, PE, and so on, and clots formation in blood vessels.

- **Aromatherapy:** is a form of alternative medicine that uses plant materials and aromatic plant oils, including essential oils, and other aromatic compounds for the purpose of altering one's mood, cognitive, psychological or physical wellbeing.

- **Baby blues:** Feeling sad or mildly depressed a few days after your baby is born. The baby blues are very common—8 out of 10 new mothers feel like this. They can be caused by hormone changes, tiredness, or discomfort and usually only last a week. More severe depression or anxiety that lasts longer than a week could be post-natal depression.

- **Balanced diet:** A diet that provides a good balance of nutrients.

- **Birth plan:** A written record of what you would like to happen during pregnancy, labour, and childbirth.

- **Body mass index:** Your weight in kilograms (kg) divided by the square of your height in metres (m^2).

- **Breech birth:** When a baby is born bottom rather than head first.

- **Caesarean section:** An operation to deliver a baby by cutting through the mother's abdomen and then into her uterus. If you have a Caesarean, you will be given an epidural or general anaesthetic.

- **Cardiovascular diseases:** Conditions that affect the heart and blood vessels, for example high blood pressure.

- **Catheter:** A thin, flexible, hollow plastic tube that can be used to perform various diagnostic and/or therapeutic procedures. Catheters may be used for the injection of fluids or medications into an area of the body or for drainage, such as from a surgical site. They are also frequently used to allow physicians to access the body with surgical instruments.

- **Centile charts:** They show the position of a measured parameter within a statistical distribution. They do not show if that parameter is normal or abnormal. They merely show how it compares with that measurement in other individuals. If a parameter such as height is on the 3rd centile, this means that for every 100 children of that age, 3% would be expected to be shorter and 97 taller.

- **Cerebrovascular diseases:** Conditions that affect the supply of blood to the brain, for example stroke.

- **Cervix:** The neck of the uterus. It is normally almost closed, with just a small opening through which blood passes during monthly periods. During labour, your cervix will dilate (open up) to let your baby move from your uterus into your vagina.

- **Cervical length:** Length of the neck of the uterus (womb).

- **Chemotherapy:** It is a treatment of an illness or disease with a chemical substance, for example in the treatment of cancer.
- **Chorion:** The future placenta that delivers life-sustaining oxygen and nutrients to your baby and carries away waste products.
- **Chorionic villus sampling:** A test to detect genetic disorders, particularly chromosomal disorders such as Down's syndrome. It is usually carried out at around 11 weeks.
- **Chromosomes:** These are tiny thread-like structures found in all the cells of the body, and they carry the genes. They are 23 pairs in number. Genes determine the characteristics that we inherit from our parents, for example hair and eye colour, nose, blood group, height, and build.
- **Chronic:** It usually means a condition that continues for a long time or keeps coming back.
- **Colostrum:** The milk that your breasts produce during the first few days after your baby is born. It is very concentrated and full of antibodies to protect your baby against infections. It is sometimes quite yellow in colour.
- **Conception:** The start of a pregnancy when an egg (ovum) is fertilised and then moves down the fallopian tube to the uterus, where it attaches itself to the uterus lining.
- **Conception:** This is a process that begins with the egg and sperm cell meeting in the fallopian tube (fertilisation of an egg), then transformation and migration of the fertilised egg to the uterus, and ends with the attachment or implantation of the transformed fertilised egg into a woman's uterus.
- **Contagious:** A disease or infection is said to be contagious when it can be easily passed from one person to another.
- **Contraception (also known as birth control):** It prevents or reduces your chances of getting pregnant.
- **Cot death (sudden infant death syndrome):** The sudden and unexpected death of an apparently healthy infant during his or her sleep.
- **Crohn's disease:** A digestive condition that causes abdominal pain and diarrhoea.
- **Diseases:** This is an illness or condition that interferes with normal body functions.
- **Down's syndrome:** A lifelong condition caused by an abnormal number of chromosomes. People with Down's syndrome have learning disability and an increased risk of some health problems. It also affects their physical growth and facial appearance.
- **DNA:** DNA stands for deoxyribonucleic acid. It is the genetic material of a cell. The chromosomes inside the nucleus (control centre) of the cell are made up of DNA, lots and lots of DNA. It is very fine and tightly coiled, but there may be as much as a metre in a single cell. DNA is really a code. It is divided up into sections. These sections are genes,

which carry all the instructions for making up our body. So there is a gene that tells the body to have brown hair, and so on. Each gene is a code for a particular protein. Our bodies are made up of proteins. So the genes dictate how we are made and what our bodies look like. You inherit half your DNA from your mother and half from your father.

- **Ectopic pregnancy:** An ectopic pregnancy occurs when a fertilised egg implants and grows not in the usual place the womb but in other places namely the fallopian tube, cervix, ovaries, or abdomen. The fertilised egg cannot develop properly and has to be removed.
- **Ejaculation:** It is the ejection of semen (usually carrying sperm) from the male reproductive tract and is usually accompanied by orgasm. It is usually the final stage and natural objective of male sexual stimulation and an essential component of natural conception.
- **Ejaculatory ducts:** The tube through which sperm passes out of the penis.
- **Embryo:** The term used for the developing baby in the very early weeks up until 8 weeks of pregnancy.
- **Entonox (gas and air):** A form of pain relief offered during labour. It is a mixture of oxygen and another gas called nitrous oxide, which is breathed in through a mask or mouthpiece.
- **Epidural:** An anaesthetic that numbs the lower half of the body. It can be very helpful for women who are having a long or particularly painful labour or who are becoming very distressed. A thin catheter is passed between the backbones and secured so that medicine can be delivered to the nerves in the spinal cord.
- **Episiotomy:** A surgical incision made in the area between the vagina and the anus (perineum). This is done during the last stages of labour and delivery to expand the opening of the vagina to prevent tearing during the birth of the baby.
- **Fallopian tubes:** Branch-like tubes that lead from the ovaries to the uterus. Eggs are released from the ovaries into the fallopian tubes each month. Fertilisation takes place in one of the fallopian tubes.
- **Fertilisation:** It takes place if a sperm joins with an egg and fertilises it in the fallopian tube.
- **Foetus:** The term used for the developing baby from week 8 of pregnancy.
- **Foetus:** A foetus is an unborn baby, from the eighth week of pregnancy until birth.
- **Folic acid:** One of the B group of vitamins, which is found naturally in foods, including green leafy vegetables, fortified breakfast cereals and brown rice. Folic acid is important for pregnancy as it can help prevent birth defects known as neural tube defects. If you are pregnant or trying to get pregnant, you should take a 400-μg folic acid tablet every day until you are 12 weeks pregnant.

- **Follicle:** This is a female reproductive unit and is made up of a group of cells including the egg inside it. The development starts from the last few days of female menstruation and continues throughout the menstrual cycle.
- **Fontanelle:** A diamond-shaped patch on the front and top of a baby's head where the skull bones have not yet fused together. During birth, the fontanelle allows the bony plates of the skull to flex so that the baby's head can pass through the birth canal. The bones usually fuse together and close over by a child's second birthday.
- **Formula milk:** It is the cows' milk that has been processed and treated so that the babies can digest it. It comes in powder or liquid form.
- **Fundus:** The top of the uterus.
- **General anaesthetic:** An anaesthetic that puts you to sleep.
- **Genetic counselling:** This is the process by which patients or relatives, at risk of an inherited disorder, are advised of the consequences and nature of the disorder, the probability of developing or transmitting it, and the options open to them in management and family planning.
- **Genitals:** These are the sex or reproductive organs that are visible on the outside of the body. In females, this is the vulva, labia, and clitoris. In males, this is the penis, scrotum, and testicles.
- **Haemoglobin (Hb):** It is found in red blood cells and carries oxygen from the lungs to all parts of the body. Pregnant women need to produce more haemoglobin because they produce more blood. If you don't produce enough, you can become anaemic, which will make you feel very tired. Your haemoglobin levels are tested during antenatal check-ups. Health as per WHO—health is 'a state of physical and mental well-being, not merely an absence of disease or infirmity'.
- **Head circumference:** The distance around foetal skull at the level of the most outmost part of the skull called parietal eminence.
- **Heart attack:** A heart attack happens when there is a blockage in one of the arteries in the heart.
- **Hepatitis:** Inflammation of the liver and characterised by the presence of inflammatory cells in the tissue of the organ.
- **Home birth:** Giving birth at home, with care provided by a midwife. This is usually planned!
- **Homeopathy:** is a complementary or alternative medicine (CAM). This means that homeopathy is different in important ways from treatments that are part of conventional Western medicine.
- **Hormones:** Both men and women have hormones, which are chemicals that circulate in the bloodstream. They carry messages to different parts of the body and result in certain changes taking place. Female hormones, which include oestrogen and progesterone, control many of the events of

a woman's monthly cycle, such as the release of eggs from her ovaries and the thickening of her uterus lining.

- **Hydrotherapy:** Water treatment.
- **Hyperandrogenaemia:** High level of the male hormone androgen in the blood.
- **Hyperinsulinaemia:** This means high level of insulin in the blood.
- **Immune system:** The immune system is the body's defence system, which helps to protect it from disease, bacteria, and viruses.
- **Inflammation**: Inflammation is the body's response to infection, irritation, or injury, which causes redness, swelling, pain, and sometimes a feeling of heat in the affected area.
- **Implantation:** This is the process in which the developing fertilised egg attaches itself to the lining of the womb.
- **Induction of labour:** A method of artificially or prematurely stimulating labour. A baby can be induced if they are getting too big, if the pregnancy has gone past the 42-week mark, or if there are health risks to either the baby or the mother if the pregnancy continues.
- **Insulin resistance:** Insulin resistance is not a disease as such but rather a state in which a person's body tissues have a lowered level of response to insulin, a hormone secreted by the pancreas that helps to regulate the level of glucose (sugar) in the body. As a result, the person's body produces larger quantities of insulin to maintain normal levels of glucose in the blood. It is associated with or contributing to a range of serious health problems, including type 2 diabetes, the metabolic syndrome, obesity, and polycystic ovary syndrome.
- **Intravenous treatment:** The drugs administered directly into the vein.
- **Jaundice:** The development of a yellow colour on a baby's skin and a yellowness in the whites of their eyes. It is caused by an excess of the pigment called bilirubin in the blood. Jaundice is common in newborn babies and usually occurs approximately 3 days after birth. It can last for up to 2 weeks after birth or up to 3 weeks in premature babies. Severe jaundice can be treated by phototherapy, where a baby is placed under a very bright light. Babies who are jaundiced for longer than 2 weeks should be seen by a doctor as they may need urgent treatment. See page 149 for more information.
- **Lanugo:** Very fine, soft hair that covers your baby at approximately 22 weeks. The lanugo disappears before birth.
- **Low-residue foods:** Foods that are easy to digest and are low in fibre and other substances that the body finds it hard to digest.
- **Lungs:** They are a pair of organs in the chest that control breathing. They remove carbon dioxide from the blood and replace it with oxygen.
- **Lymph glands:** Small organs found throughout the body such as in the neck, groin, or armpit, may be swollen.

- **Macrosomia:** Large-for-date babies.
- **Mastitis:** Inflammation or infection in the breasts caused by blocked milk ducts. Symptoms include hot and tender breasts and flu-like symptoms.
- **Meconium aspiration:** Baby aspirating his or her own poo that is passed in the womb.
- **Menarche:** The first menstrual discharge; it occurs normally between the ages of 9 and 17. Factors such as hereditary, diet, and overall health can accelerate or delay the onset of menarche.
- **Maternity team care:** A team of midwives, obstetricians, anaesthetists, neonatologists, and other specialists who provide care to women who have complex pregnancies.
- **Meconium:** The first stools that your baby passes; this can happen while in the womb or after birth. It is made up of mucus and other materials that your baby has ingested during his or her time in the womb. It is sticky like tar and has no odour.
- **Midwifery care:** Care for pregnant women whereby the midwife is the lead professional. It is suitable for women who have an uncomplicated pregnancy.
- **Midwifery-led unit:** A unit close to a labour ward or a separate unit that provides care led by midwives, with a minimum of medical interventions and in a home-like environment. Different phrases may be used to describe this type of unit. If you are not sure, ask your doctor or midwife.
- **Mittelschmerz:** Pain over the lower abdomen at the time of ovulation; it is a German word for ovulation pain.
- **Mobility:** This means movement
- Molar pregnancy: This is an unsuccessful pregnancy where the placenta and foetus do not form properly and a baby does not develop. Molar pregnancies are caused by an imbalance in genetic material (chromosomes) in the pregnancy. Most often, this occurs when an egg that contains no genetic information is fertilised by a sperm, or when a normal egg is fertilised by two sperm.
- **Morbidly adherent placenta:** A rare condition in which the placenta attaches abnormally to the wall of the womb. It can cause severe bleeding.
- **Neck of the womb (cervix):** This is the part of the womb that partly lies under the bladder and protrudes into the vaginal space. It is normally closed, with just a small opening through which blood passes out during monthly menstrual periods. During labour, your cervix will dilate (open up) to let your baby move from the uterus into your vagina.
- **Neonatal care:** The care given to sick or premature babies. It takes place in a neonatal unit, which is specially designed and equipped to care for them.
- **Neonatal death:** Baby dying within 1 week after birth.
- **Nuchal translucency scan:** An ultrasound scan to help identify whether you are at risk of having a baby with Down's syndrome. The scan is

carried out at 11-13 weeks of pregnancy and measures the thickness of the fluid behind the neck of the baby. Babies at risk of Down's syndrome tend to have a bigger thickness. At the same time, the age of the pregnancy will be confirmed with scan and major abnormalities in the baby will be looked for.

- **Obstetrician:** A doctor who has received specialised training and experience in the care of women during pregnancy and childbirth.
- **Obstetric cholestasis:** A potentially dangerous liver disorder. Symptoms include severe generalised itching without a rash, particularly in the last 4 months of pregnancy.
- **Oedema:** Another word for swelling, most often of the feet and hands. It is usually nothing to worry about, but if it gets worse suddenly, it can be a sign of PE.
- **Osteoporosis:** A medical condition in which the bones become weak and brittle.
- **Ovulation:** Ovulation occurs when an egg (ovum) is released from a woman's ovaries during her monthly menstrual cycle. If the egg is fertilised during this time, she will get pregnant. This is the time of the month when you are most likely to conceive.
- **Oxytocin:** A hormone naturally produced by the body that causes the womb to contract. A synthetic copy of this hormone is sometimes used during childbirth to increase or start contractions of the womb.
- **Paediatrician:** A doctor who is a specialist in children illness.
- **Perinatal:** The time shortly before and after the birth of a baby.
- **Perinatal mental health:** Mental health problems that develop during pregnancy and that can last for up to 1 year after childbirth.
- **Placenta:** The organ attached to the lining of the uterus, which separates your baby's circulation from your circulation. Oxygen and food from your bloodstream are passed to your baby's bloodstream through the placenta and along the umbilical cord. Waste is also removed this way.
- **Placenta praevia:** A condition in which the placenta is low-lying in the womb and covers all or part of the entrance to the womb, so interfering with normal delivery.
- **Post-natal:** The period beginning immediately after the birth of a baby until they are about 6 weeks old.
- **Post-natal care:** The professional care provided to you and your baby from the birth until your baby is about 6-8 weeks old. It usually involves home visits by midwives to check that both the mother and the baby are well. Classes may also be available.
- **Post-natal depression:** Feelings of depression and hopelessness after the birth of a baby. These feelings are more severe than the 'baby blues'

(see page 178). Post-natal depression affects 1 in 10 women and can be serious if left untreated. See page 82 for more information.

- **Pre-eclampsia:** A condition that happens in the second half of pregnancy and that can cause serious problems for you and your baby if it is not detected and managed. Signs of pre-eclampsia are high blood pressure, protein in the urine, and/or swelling of the hands, feet, ankles, and sometimes the face.
- **Pre-eclampsia:** A condition that only occurs during pregnancy. Symptoms include high blood pressure, protein in urine, bad headaches, vision problems, and the sudden swelling of the face, hands, and feet. It usually develops after the twentieth week of pregnancy but can occur earlier. Although most cases are mild and cause no trouble, it can be serious for both the mother and the baby.
- **Premature birth:** The birth of a baby from 24 weeks of pregnancy to before the standard period of pregnancy, which is 37 completed weeks.
- **Premature labour:** When labour starts from 24 weeks of pregnancy and before the standard period of pregnancy, which is 37 completed weeks.
- **Puberty:** The period of development in which the reproductive organs become functional and the secondary sex characteristics are expressed.
- **Rectum:** The storage area at the end of the colon that holds the stools until they are passed out of the anus.
- **Regional anaesthetic:** A type of anaesthetic that numbs the lower part of your body. Spinal and epidural anaesthetics are types of regional anaesthetics. The anaesthetic drugs are either given through an injection into the spine before the start of the operation or run into your spine through a small tube (catheter). The catheter may have been put in place as part of the epidural used for pain relief during labour or at the time of the operation.
- **Reproduction:** Process by which an organism produces or reproduces its species.
- **Respiratory diseases:** Conditions that affect breathing.
- **Retina:** Light-sensitive layer of the eye.
- **Rhesus disease:** A woman who is rhesus negative can carry a baby who is rhesus positive if the baby's father is rhesus positive. This can cause problems in second or later pregnancies. If she gets pregnant with another rhesus positive baby, the immune response will be quicker and much greater. The antibodies produced by the mother can cross the placenta and attach to the D antigen on her baby's red blood cells. This can be harmful to the baby as it may result in a condition called haemolytic disease of the newborn, which can lead to anaemia and jaundice.
- **Rhesus negative:** People who do not have a substance known as D antigen on the surface of their red blood cells are known as rhesus negative. This can cause problems in second or later pregnancies (see above).

369

- **Rhesus positive:** People who have a substance known as D antigen on the surface of their red blood cells are known as rhesus positive.
- **Rubella (German measles):** A virus that can seriously affect unborn babies if the mother gets it during the early weeks of pregnancy. Most women have been immunised against rubella so they are not at risk.
- **Sex chromosomes:** They are paired chromosomes that determine the sex, XX in a woman and XY in a man. At fertilisation, the future baby (zygote) acquires one chromosome from each parent. If the egg which always contains the X chromosome is fertilised by a sperm containing an X chromosome, the baby will be a girl (XX). If the sperm contains a Y chromosome, the baby will be a boy (XY).
- **Speculum:** A plastic or metal instrument used to separate the walls of the vagina and also used for vagina swab test.
- **Spermatogenesis:** Production of sperm.
- **Sporadic:** Occurring at irregular intervals; having no pattern or order in time.
- **Stillbirth:** Delivering a dead baby.
- **Ultrasound scans:** An imaging technique that uses high-frequency sound waves to create an image of the baby in the uterus. It shows the baby's body and organs as well as the surrounding tissues.
- **Umbilical cord:** The cord that attaches the baby to the placenta, linking the baby and the mother. Blood circulates through the cord, carrying oxygen and food to the baby and carrying waste away again.
- **Ureters:** The urinary pipe that takes urine from the kidneys to the bladder.
- **Urethra:** The urinary pipe through which urine passes from the bladder to outside.
- **Vernix:** This is a sticky white coating that covers a baby when it is in the uterus. It mostly disappears before birth, but there may be some left on your baby when they are born.
- **Vertebrae:** The spine is made up of 33 irregularly shaped bones called vertebrae. Each vertebra has a hole in the middle through which the spinal cord runs.
- **Zygote:** The product of binding of a sperm to an egg is called zygote, and the process of binding is called fertilisation. A zygote is a single cell, with a complete set of chromosomes (46), that normally develops into an embryo, foetus, and then baby.

Index

www.ingramcontent.com/pod-product-compliance
Lightning Source LLC
Chambersburg PA
CBHW020724180526
45163CB00001B/92